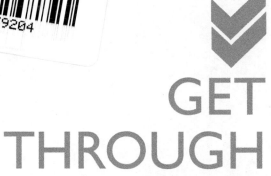

GET THROUGH

MRCPsych
Paper B: Mock
Examination Papers

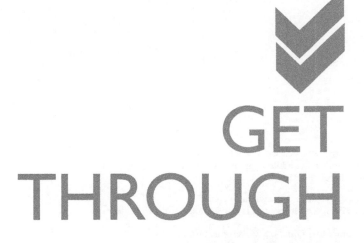

GET THROUGH

MRCPsych
Paper B: Mock
Examination Papers

Melvyn WB Zhang MBBS, DCP, MRCPsych
National HealthCare Group, Singapore

Cyrus SH Ho MBBS, DCP, MRCPsych
National University of Singapore

Roger Ho MBBS, DPM, DCP, Gdip Psychotherapy,
MMed (Psych), MRCPsych, FRCPC
National University of Singapore

Ian H Treasaden MB, BS, LRCP, MRCS, FRCPsych, LLM
West London Mental Health NHS Trust,
Imperial College Healthcare NHS Trust, and
Bucks New University, UK

Basant K Puri MA, PhD, MB, BChir, BSc (Hons) MathSci,
DipStat, PG Dip Maths, MMath, FRCPsych, FSB
Hammersmith Hospital and Imperial College London, UK

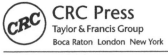

CRC Press
Taylor & Francis Group
Boca Raton London New York

CRC Press is an imprint of the
Taylor & Francis Group, an **informa** business

CRC Press
Taylor & Francis Group
6000 Broken Sound Parkway NW, Suite 300
Boca Raton, FL 33487-2742

© 2016 by Taylor & Francis Group, LLC
CRC Press is an imprint of Taylor & Francis Group, an Informa business

No claim to original U.S. Government works

Printed and bound by Ashford Colour Press Ltd.
Version Date: 20160426

International Standard Book Number-13: 978-1-4822-4744-2 (Paperback)

Visit the Taylor & Francis Web site at
http://www.taylorandfrancis.com

and the CRC Press Web site at
http://www.crcpress.com

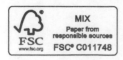

CONTENTS

INTRODUCTION

This book consists of over 1000 questions and answers, which are set out as five individual revision mock examination papers. They correspond to the new format of Paper B of the Royal College of Psychiatrists' examinations, which has been revised recently. The questions (a mixture of both multiple-choice questions and extended matching items) have been set so as to reflect the type and the standard of the questions of the MRCPsych examination, at the time of writing.

Some of the questions featured in this book have been modeled against the core themes that have been tested in the recent MRCPsych examination. A large proportion of the questions have been set based on recent advances in research, as published in the *British Journal of Psychiatry* and *Advances in Psychiatric Treatment*. Unlike other books, the critical appraisal and research methodology and statistics question have been set based on data extracted from papers that the authors have published in high-impact journals. The authors have provided explanation for each of the questions included in the mock examination paper. Readers are provided with references to which they could refer to, if they are in doubt with regard to any of the theoretical concepts. Readers who are preparing for the MRCPsych examination are, however, still encouraged to keep themselves up to date with the latest regulations and guidance issued by the Royal College of Psychiatrists.

We welcome any feedback from those of you who are using this book. Please also let us know further type of questions you would like to see in the next edition of this book.

We wish to thank again all the authors who have contributed to this revision guidebook.

Melvyn WB Zhang
Cyrus SH Ho
Roger CM Ho
Basant K Puri
Ian H Treasaden

AUTHORS

Dr Melvyn Zhang, MBBS, DCP, MRCPsych, is a specialist registrar/senior resident at the National Healthcare Group, Singapore. He graduated from the National University of Singapore and received his postgraduate training with the Royal College of Psychiatrists (UK). He is currently working with the Institute of Mental Health, Singapore. He has a special interest in the application of web-based and smartphone technologies for education and research and has been published extensively in this field. He is a member of the Public Education and Engagement Board (PEEB), Royal College of Psychiatrists (UK), as well as a member of the editorial board of the *Journal of Internet Medical Research (Mental Health)*. He has published extensively in the *British Medical Journal (BMJ), Lancet Psychiatry* and *BJPsych Advances.*

Dr Cyrus SH Ho, MBBS, DCP, MRCPsych, is an associate consultant psychiatrist and clinical lecturer from the National University Hospital, Singapore. He graduated from the National University of Singapore, Yong Loo Lin School of Medicine and subsequently obtained the Diploma of Clinical Psychiatry from Ireland and Membership of the Royal College of Psychiatrists from the United Kingdom. As a certified acupuncturist with the Graduate Diploma in Acupuncture conferred by the Singapore College of Traditional Chinese Medicine, he hopes to integrate both Western and Chinese medicine for holistic psychiatric care. He is actively involved in education and research work. His clinical and research interests include mood disorders, neuropsychiatry, pain studies and medical acupuncture.

Dr Roger Ho, MBBS, DPM, DCP, Gdip Psychotherapy, MMed (Psych), MRCPsych, FRCPC, is an assistant professor and consultant psychiatrist at the Department of Psychological Medicine, National University of Singapore. He graduated from the University of Hong Kong and received his training in psychiatry from the National University of Singapore. He is a general adult psychiatrist and in charge of the Mood Disorder Clinic, National University Hospital, Singapore. He is a member of the editorial board of *Advances of Psychiatric Treatment*, an academic journal published by the Royal College of Psychiatrists. His research focuses on mood disorders, psychoneuroimmunology and liaison psychiatry.

Dr Ian H Treasaden, MB, BS, LRCP, MRCS, FRCPsych, LLM, is currently an honorary consultant forensic psychiatrist at West London Mental Health NHS Trust and Imperial College Healthcare NHS Trust, as well as a visiting senior lecturer at Bucks New University.

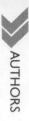

Until 2014, he was a consultant forensic psychiatrist at Three Bridges Medium Secure Unit, West London Mental Health NHS Trust, where he was also the clinical director, College and Coordinating Clinical Tutor for the Charing Cross Rotational Training Scheme in Psychiatry, and tutor in law and ethics and honorary senior clinical lecturer at Imperial College London.

He has authored papers on forensic and general psychiatry, and he is co-author of the books *Textbook of Psychiatry* (3 editions), *Mental Health Law: A Practical Guide* (2 editions), *Emergencies in Psychiatry, Psychiatry: An Evidence-Based Text* and *Revision MCQs and EMIs for the MRCPsych* and the forthcoming *Forensic Psychiatry: Fundamentals and Clinical Practice*.

He qualified in medicine from the London Hospital Medical College, University of London, in 1975 where he was awarded the James Anderson Prize in Clinical Medicine. He undertook training in forensic psychiatry at the Maudsley & Bethlem Royal Hospitals in London and Broadmoor Special Hospital, Berkshire, England between 1982 and 1984.

Basant K Puri, MA, PhD, MB, BChir, BSc (Hons) MathSci, DipStat, PG Dip Maths, MMath, FRCPsych, FSB, is based at Hammersmith Hospital and Imperial College London, United Kingdom. He read medicine at St John's College, University of Cambridge. He also trained in molecular genetics at the MRC MNU, Laboratory of Molecular Biology, Cambridge. He has authored or co-authored more than 40 books, including the second edition of *Drugs in Psychiatry* (Oxford University Press, 2013), third edition of *Textbook of Psychiatry* with Dr Ian Treasaden (Churchill Livingston, 2011) and, with the publisher of the present volume, the third edition of *Textbook of Clinical Neuropsychiatry and Neuroscience Fundamentals* with Professor David Moore (2012).

GET THROUGH MRCPSYCH PAPER B MOCK EXAMINATION

Total number of questions: 191 (116 MCQs, 75 EMIs)
Total time provided: 180 minutes

Question 1
A 58-year-old man drinks eight units of alcohol after work each night. He becomes violent when drinking and is hospitalized after an alcohol-related brawl. He tells the psychiatrist that he has been drinking for many years and is not willing to cut down on his alcohol intake. He also rejects a hotline number to an additional treatment facility nearby. According to the stages of change, which stage is he in?
 a. Action
 b. Contemplation
 c. Maintenance
 d. Precontemplation
 e. Preparation

Question 2
A 20-year-old pregnant woman is heroin dependent. She insists on undergoing heroin withdrawal and asks you for advice. In this case, in which period would withdrawal cause least harm to the baby?
 a. After delivery
 b. All three trimesters
 c. First trimester
 d. Second trimester
 e. Third trimester

Question 3
Which of the following statements regarding the correlation coefficient is false?
 a. A correlation coefficient can be strong but statistically non-significant because of the sample size.
 b. Correlation describes the strength of the linear relationship between variables, which is denoted by the correlation coefficient (r).

c. Spearman's and Kendall's rank coefficients are the non-parametric alternatives to Pearson's correlation coefficient.
d. The value of the correlation coefficient can range from –2 to +2.
e. A value of 0.2–0.5 signifies moderate correlation.

Question 4
Which of the following statements regarding standard deviation (SD) is true?
a. For a sample size of 20, a good estimate of population SD can be obtained by using 20 in the denominator of the equation.
b. SD can have negative values.
c. SD has the same units as the original observation.
d. SD is more difficult to calculate than quartile distribution.
e. Variance is the square root of the SD.

Question 5
A 52-year-old man drinks eight bottles of beer every other night. He reports feeling jittery if he does not drink, and he uses shots of alcohol to get him through the day. He is seeing a psychologist, who uses a technique that is described using the acronym FRAMES. Which of the following is not part of the acronym FRAMES?
a. Advice
b. Feedback
c. Menu
d. Resistance
e. Self-efficacy

Question 6
A 37-year-old woman lies in bed all day. She cries herself to sleep every night and has lost 18 kg over the past 2 years. She has attempted suicide several times and is currently hospitalized for her most recent attempt. Which of the following treatment options is contraindicated in the initial stage of her condition?
a. Brief psychodynamic therapy
b. Cognitive behavioural therapy (CBT)
c. Electroconvulsive therapy
d. Inpatient treatment
e. Pharmacotherapy

Question 7
Based on the latest evidence on the treatment for mild cognitive impairment, which of the following demonstrates the strongest evidence?
a. Cholinesterase inhibitors do not reduce the frequency of incident dementia.
b. Donepezil improves cognition over 48 months.
c. Huannao Yicong improves cognition and social functioning.
d. Nicotine improves attention over 6 months.
e. Pribedil improves cognition over 6 months.

Question 8
Which of the following is the least common feature of Cushing's syndrome of endogenous origin?
a. Cognitive impairment
b. Delusion of guilt
c. Depression
d. Mania
e. Second-person auditory hallucination

Question 9
The percentage of patients with delirium who have abnormal tracing detected on their EEG is
a. 10%
b. 20%
c. 50%
d. 75%
e. 90%

Question 10
Which of the following statements about the neurobiology of ageing is incorrect?
a. In normal ageing, there is a slow reduction in the weight and the volume of the human brain with an increase in the size of the ventricles after the age of 50 years.
b. All neuroanatomical areas in the brain show significant loss of neurons with normal ageing.
c. The absolute rate of nerve cells loss is around 1% per year after the age of 60 years.
d. Lipofuscin accumulates in the cytoplasm of the nerve cells from childhood.
e. Tau protein is involved in the linking of neurofilaments and microtubules and accumulates in a small proportion of ageing nerve cells.

Question 11
What is the approximately incidence of delirium amongst old people who are hospitalized?
a. 1%
b. 10%
c. 30%
d. 50%
e. 70%

Question 12
Based on the 10th Revision of *International Classification of Disease* (ICD-10) criteria, which of the following statements regarding moderate mental retardation is false?
a. Independent living is rarely achieved.
b. The intelligence quotient (IQ) score range is usually below that of 49.
c. It is often associated with epilepsy and neurological and other disabilities.

d. Simple practical work is possible.
e. At least 20% of neurofibromatosis type I (NF-1) sufferers present with moderate-to-severe learning disability (LD).

Question 13
Which of the following is not a characteristic of children with Prader–Willi syndrome?
a. Inverted V-shaped upper lip
b. Hyperphagia
c. Hypogonadism
d. Obesity
e. Spasticity

Question 14
Which of the following syndromes does not present with microcephaly?
a. Angelman syndrome
b. Cornelia de Lange syndrome
c. Cri du chat syndrome
d. DiGeorge syndrome
e. Neurofibromatosis

Question 15
Which of the following conditions is most frequently seen with autism?
a. Enuresis
b. Gilles de la Tourette's syndrome
c. Hyperkinetic disorder
d. Pica
e. Measles, mumps and rubella vaccination

Question 16
An 18-year-old lady complains of low mood, irritability and insomnia prior to her menses. Which of the following medications would you recommend?
a. Sertraline
b. Sex hormone such as progesterone
c. St John's wort
d. Low-dose sulpiride
e. Sleeping pills

Question 17
Which of the following with regard to depression in multiple sclerosis (MS) is true or false?
a. Major depressive disorder (MDD) occurs more when MS involves the cerebellum rather than the spinal cord.
b. MDD occurs in up to 50% of patients during their lifetime.
c. Selective serotonin reuptake inhibitor (SSRI) should be used with caution, as it may increase spasticity.

d. Rates of depression in first-degree relatives of depressed patients with MS are higher than the rates of depression in first-degree relatives of people who do not have MS.
   e. MS-induced cognitive impairment is not a risk factor for suicide.

Question 18
Which of the following statements about the treatment of depression in patients with Parkinson disorder is incorrect?
   a. Remeron should not be considered, as it may worsen sleep quality.
   b. It is important to optimize treatment of motor symptoms.
   c. SSRI has been considered to be the first-line treatment for depression.
   d. Bupropion is contraindicated due to its side effect profile.
   e. Tricyclic antidepressant should be avoided.

Question 19
Which of the following is most likely to be associated with juvenile delinquency?
   a. Oppositional defiant disorder in parents when they were younger
   b. Family history of depression
   c. High intelligence
   d. Parental criminality
   e. Small family size

Question 20
Which of the following is the best predictor of future violent behaviour?
   a. Availability of weapons
   b. History of past violence
   c. History of substance abuse
   d. Presence of first-rank symptoms
   e. Morbid jealousy

Question 21
The most common precipitating factor leading to deliberate self-poisoning and self-injury in children and adolescents under 16 years of age is related to which of the following?
   a. Relationship difficulties with friends
   b. Relationship difficulties with parents
   c. School-related problems
   d. Social isolation
   e. Presence of underlying psychiatric disorder

Question 22
A recent study has found that a single-nucleotide polymorphism (SNP) of the dopamine receptor-3 (DRD3) gene (rs167771) is associated with autism. Which of the following neuroanatomical areas is associated with the alleles of the rs167771 SNP and explains symptoms of autism?
   a. Amygdala
   b. Corpus callosum

c. Frontal lobe
d. Hippocampus
e. Striatum

Question 23
Which of the following modalities of treatment has been shown to be most effective for children with conduct disorder?
a. Cognitive therapy
b. Behavioural therapy
c. Interpersonal therapy
d. Multimodal therapy
e. Solution-focused therapy

Question 24
Which of the following statements about obsessive-compulsive disorder (OCD) is incorrect?
a. OCD affects an approximate 3% of adults and children.
b. Relief of anxiety reduction is an important maintaining factor of the obsessive-compulsive symptoms.
c. The association between OCD and suicidality is weak.
d. Most patients respond to serotonin reuptake inhibitors, irrespective of their symptoms' severity.
e. Some patients continue with a chronic or a chronic relapsing course.

Question 25
With regard to suicide and violence in schizophrenia, which of the following is incorrect?
a. Approximately 10% of patients with schizophrenia do commit suicide.
b. The prevalence of violence amongst outpatients with schizophrenia has been estimated to be 5%.
c. Suicide in schizophrenia usually occurs late into the illness.
d. Paranoid schizophrenics are more likely to commit suicide compared with other subtypes of schizophrenics.
e. Verbal aggression is the most common type of violence seen amongst schizophrenics.

Question 26
A 35-year-old male with a history of schizophrenia presents to the outpatient clinic with prominent cognitive impairments. Which of the following would you recommend as an adjunct medication?
a. Cholinergic agent
b. Dopaminergic agent
c. Gamma-aminobutyric acid (GABA) agonist
d. Glutamatergic agent
e. Noradrenergic agent

Question 27
First-degree relatives of individuals with hyperkinetic disorder are particularly prone towards the development of which of the following?
a. Major depressive disorder
b. Cyclothymia
c. Dissociative disorder
d. Specific phobia
e. Bipolar disorder

Question 28
The mother of a 14-year-old boy with attention deficit hyperactivity disorder (ADHD) wants to ask you about the side effects of methylphenidate medication. Which of the following statements is incorrect?
a. Methylphenidate almost always delays physical growth.
b. A drug holiday is required to facilitate growth.
c. Methylphenidate suppresses appetite.
d. Methylphenidate combined with clonidine is better than placebo in controlling tics and ADHD symptoms.
e. Dependence is common in patients who continue methylphenidate long-term.

Question 29
A 35-year-old woman suffering from schizophrenia has been well treated, and her last admission was 1 year ago. For the last month, she has been having symptoms of poor appetite, insomnia and feelings of hopelessness. The most likely diagnosis is
a. Complicated schizophrenia
b. Post-schizophrenia depression
c. Reactive depression
d. Schizoaffective disorder
e. Schizophrenia with negative symptoms

Question 30
With regard to the aetiology of depression in patients suffering from Parkinson disease, which of the following is least likely to be a predisposing factor?
a. Having a family history of depression
b. History of right-sided brain injuries
c. Low dopamine levels in the mesolimbic system
d. Presence of cognitive impairment
e. Loss of functional independence

Question 31
A 13-year-old obese boy with learning disability has been referred to the learning disability clinic. His mother claimed that he has been having irresistible hunger drive associated with incessant skin picking. In addition, he also tends to talk to himself. Which other psychiatric comorbidity is highly prevalent in his condition?
a. Generalized anxiety disorder
b. Obsessive-compulsive disorder

c. Panic disorder
d. Depressive disorder
e. Psychotic disorder

Question 32
What is the estimated prevalence of schizophrenia in people with mental retardation?
  a. 1%–2%
  b. 3%–5%
  c. 9%–8%
  d. 9%–11%
  e. 12%–14%

Question 33
Hypermethylation of which of the following genes is most likely to be associated with antisocial personality disorder?
  a. Dysbindin gene
  b. Enolase gene
  c. Monoamine oxidase A promoter gene
  d. Nicotinamide adenine dinucleotide phosphate-oxidase gene
  e. Serotonin transporter (5HTT) gene

Question 34
Approximately what percentage of elderly individuals suffer from major depressive disorder?
  a. 1%
  b. 2%
  c. 3%
  d. 4%
  e. 10%

Question 35
Which of the following is a technique used in Moreno's psychodrama?
  a. Cognitive restructuring
  b. Free association
  c. Representational role reversal
  d. Psychoeducation
  e. Systematic desensitization

Question 36
A 29-year-old woman tells her psychotherapist that everything has been going well for her and that she is making good progress in her treatment. She leaves the therapy session and engages in self-harm. Which of the following best describes the above phenomenon?
  a. Acting in
  b. Acting out

c. Resistance

d. Regression

e. Transference

Question 37

Which one of the following statements regarding the standard error of the mean (SEM) is false?

a. As sample size increases, SEM decreases.

b. As the SD increases, SEM increases.

c. It is used in constructing confidence intervals for a mean or proportion.

d. It measures the variability of the sample statistic (mean or proportion) in relation to the true but unknown population characteristic.

e. It is a measure of the variability of the observations.

Question 38

Which of the following regarding student's *t*-test is false?

a. Calculated *t*-value is an observed difference in means/standard error of the difference in means.

b. Calculated *t*-value is compared with a critical *t*-value from tables at a predetermined significance level and appropriate degrees of freedom. The larger the value of *t* (±), the smaller the value of *p* and the stronger the evidence that the null hypothesis is untrue.

c. Independent sample *t*-test is used to compare the effects of two drugs on a particular patient at different points in time.

d. Paired *t*-tests compare the means of two small paired observations, either on the same individual or on the matched individual.

e. The SDs must be approximately the same in the two groups.

Question 39

In a study to investigate the general public's perspective on traditional Chinese medicine, participants are first identified based on certain characteristics and are then required to provide the names of other potential participants. What type of sampling method is this?

a. Cluster sampling

b. Convenience sampling

c. Quota sampling

d. Snowball sampling

e. Systematic sampling

Question 40

A 36-year-old man is diagnosed with heroin dependence. Which of the following symptoms would he not develop tolerance to?

a. Constipation

b. Hallucinations

c. Insomnia

d. Myoclonus

e. Sedation

Question 41

A 21-year-old man was at a social event, and his friend offered him a recreational drug. He took the drug knowing that it would not cause physical withdrawal symptoms if he were to abruptly stop taking it subsequently. Which of the following is the most likely drug?

a. Barbiturates
b. Amphetamine
c. Cocaine
d. Ecstasy
e. Lysergic acid diethylamide (LSD)

Question 42

Which of the following antidepressants is the most appropriate if a patient has pre-existing sexual dysfunction and has been referred to the National Health Service (NHS) mental health service for depression?

a. Agomelatine
b. Amineptine
c. Moclobemide
d. Dothiepin
e. Bupropion

Question 43

A 35-year-old woman has been taking first-generation antipsychotic for her schizophrenia condition throughout her pregnancy. Which of the following would her infant be most susceptible to?

a. Premature delivery
b. Post-term delivery
c. Low birth weight
d. Small for gestational age
e. Large for gestational age

Question 44

Which of the following genes has been found to be implicated in hyperkinetic disorder and has been linked to an enhanced response to psycho-stimulants?

a. Dopamine D4 receptor gene
b. Dopamine transporter (DAT1) gene
c. Alpha 2A gene
d. Catechol-O-methyltransferase (COMT) gene
e. Norepinephrine transporter gene

Question 45

A 35-year-old woman has been having difficulties with sleep. Over the past couple of months, she has been frequently having the urge to move her legs as a result of unpleasant sensations while she is resting. At times, even with movement, there is no relief of her symptoms. She has decided to seek help from her general

practitioner (GP). You would advise the GP to consider commencement of the following medications, with the exception of
a. Clonazepam
b. Gabapentin
c. Levodopa
d. Fluoxetine
e. Iron tablets

Question 46
With regard to paraphrenia, which of the following personality types is a predisposing factor?
a. Schizoid personality disorder
b. Schizotypal personality disorder
c. Borderline personality disorder
d. Paranoid personality disorder
e. Obsessive-compulsive personality disorder

Question 47
A 28-year-old university student presents to the emergency department with the following features: auditory hallucinations, visual hallucinations, paranoid delusions, thought disorders and passivity experiences. His room-mate informs you that the patient has been abusing drugs such as amphetamine lately. Which of the following clinical signs and symptoms would make you suspect that this is more likely to be substance-induced psychotic disorder versus that of an underlying schizophrenia?
a. Auditory hallucinations
b. Visual hallucinations
c. Thought disorder
d. Paranoid delusions
e. Passivity experiences

Question 48
Based on the Randomized Injectable Opioid Treatment Trial (RIOTT), which of the following statements is correct?
a. Oral methadone treatment showed clear benefits over supervised injectable heroin in health and social outcomes.
b. Supervised injectable heroin treatment showed clear benefits over oral methadone in health and social outcomes.
c. Supervised injectable methadone treatment showed clear benefits over oral methadone in health and social outcomes.
d. Both supervised injectable heroin treatment and supervised injectable methadone treatment showed clear benefits over optimized oral methadone in health and social outcomes.
e. Neither supervised injectable heroin treatment nor supervised injectable methadone treatment showed benefits over optimized oral methadone in health and social outcomes.

Question 49

Which of the following definitions is incorrect?

a. Absolute risk reduction is the difference in risk of a given event between two groups.
b. Confidence interval is the range of values within which one can be 95% certain that the true reference population value lies.
c. Number needed to treat is the number needed to treat to get one bad outcome.
d. Relative risk is the ratio of the risk of a given event in one group of subjects compared with another group.
e. Relative risk reduction is the proportion of the initial or baseline risk that was eliminated by a given treatment or by avoidance of exposure to a risk factor.

Question 50

Which of the following statements is false for case–control studies?

a. They are not ideal for rare diseases/outcomes.
b. They are poor for rare exposures.
c. Temporal relationships may be difficult to establish.
d. There may be selection bias.
e. There may be recall bias.

Question 51

Which of the following definitions best describes face validity?

a. How well a category appears to describe an illness.
b. How internally consistent a measure is.
c. How well a category predicts a pertinent aspect of care.
d. How often the same diagnosis is assigned by different assessors.
e. Whether a category has meaning in terms of what it is designed to describe.

Question 52

Which of the following statements best describes Cronbach's alpha?

a. It determines whether a test measures what it purports to measure.
b. It indicates the internal consistency of the test.
c. It examines the extent of agreement between a present measurement and one in the future.
d. It describes the level of agreement between assessments of the same material made by two or more assessors at roughly the same time.
e. It is a measure of agreement in which allowance is made for chance agreement.

Question 53

A 40-year-old woman suffering from schizophrenia has been taken haloperidol for the past 10 years. Her QTc is 500 ms. She wants to find out the potential medical complications if she continues to take haloperidol. Which of the following complications is least likely?

a. Atrial fibrillation
b. Palpitations
c. Sudden cardiac death

d. Torsade de pointes
e. Ventricular fibrillation

Question 54
Which of the following symptoms is least likely to be different between young and old people suffering from depressive disorder?
a. Behavioural disturbances
b. Complaints of loneliness
c. Poor concentration and memory
d. Paranoid and delusional ideation
e. Sleep disturbances

Question 55
For management of depression in old people, which of the following statements is incorrect?
a. Newer antidepressants such as SSRI and serotonin and norepinephrine reuptake inhibitors (SNRIs) are better tolerated as they have lesser side effects.
b. Tricyclic antidepressants are absolutely contraindicated in old people.
c. Depressed elderly presenting with delusion may require the addition of an antipsychotic.
d. Electroconvulsive therapy (ECT) is the most effective treatment for life-threatening depressive disorder.
e. Depressed elderly who show resistance to first-line treatment tend to do well with lithium augmentation.

Question 56
Which of the following is considered to be a good prognostic factor for elderly depression?
a. Female gender
b. Male gender
c. Active medical illness or poor physical health
d. Atypical features of depression
e. History of dysthymia

Question 57
Which of the following is the most common cause of mental retardation?
a. Head injury
b. Down syndrome
c. Foetal alcohol syndrome
d. Fragile X syndrome
e. Lesch–Nyhan syndrome

Question 58
What is the approximate proportion of people with Down syndrome at age 60–69 years who will develop Alzheimer's disease?
a. 10%
b. 20%

c. 40%
d. 60%
e. 80%

Question 59

A 22-year-old male has been admitted to the gastroenterology unit for hepatic dysfunction. He has been diagnosed with liver disease since he was a teenager. The core trainee has evaluated him and found that apart from him having depressed mood, he also has some elements of cognitive impairment. The medical team is particularly concerned currently about the neurological complications arising from his condition. Based on your knowledge, which of the following is the most likely modality of inheritance for the disease that this 22-year-old male has?

a. Autosomal dominant
b. Autosomal recessive
c. Mitochronical inheritance
d. Spontaneous mutation
e. Polygenetic inheritance

Question 60

Stress and depression often increase the risk of coronary artery disease (CAD). Which of the following biological markers is least likely to be involved?

a. Fibrinogen
b. Interleukin-6
c. Natural killer cells
d. Interleukin-10
e. von Willebrand factor

Question 61

Which of the following statements regarding criminal behaviour in patients with schizophrenia is false?

a. It increases with comorbid substance use.
b. Patients with schizophrenia have higher rates of offending compared with the general population.
c. Patients with schizophrenia usually assault a known person rather than a stranger.
d. Violence is a common precipitant prior to the first admission to psychiatric ward.
e. Violence in patients with schizophrenia is not always a result of psychosis.

Question 62

Which of the following statements regarding offending in patients with epilepsy is false?

a. Low intelligence is associated with violence in patients with epilepsies.
b. Offending in epileptics is usually during the ictal phase of the illness.
c. There is an approximately twofold increase in the prevalence of epilepsy in prisoners compared with the general population.
d. The rate and type of offending by those with epilepsy are similar to the general population.
e. There is no excess of violent crimes in epileptic prisoners.

Question 63
What percentage of children with autism is also diagnosed with severe or profound mental retardation?
a. 10%
b. 30%
c. 40%
d. 50%
e. 75%

Question 64
Previous research into the genetics associated with conduct disorder has demonstrated that conduct disorder is associated with the inheritance of antisocial traits from parents who demonstrate criminal behaviours. All of the following are biological factors that have been implicated in the aetiology of conduct disorder except
a. Excess testosterone
b. History of head injury
c. Low plasma serotonin level
d. Low plasma dopamine level
e. Low testosterone

Question 65
A 35-year-old female has recently given birth to her son. After delivery, her husband noted that there has been a change in her personality and behaviour. She has been evaluated by the mental health team and has been admitted to the ward, as she is believed to be suffering from post-partum psychosis. The medical student attached to the team is curious: Which of the following is not a common clinical feature of post-partum psychosis?
a. Presence of auditory hallucinations
b. Presence of catatonic-like symptoms
c. Being either excessively withdrawn or elated and labile in mood
d. Presence of mood-incongruent delusions of reference and persecution
e. Presence of first-rank symptoms

Question 66
Which of the following forensic offences is most highly associated with individuals diagnosed with Asperger syndrome?
a. Shoplifting
b. Road traffic–related offences
c. Fire setting
d. Substance misuse
e. Theft

Question 67
Based on the findings of the Multimodal Treatment of Attention Deficit Hyperactivity Disorder (MTA) Study, which of the following is true with regard to the incidence of substance abuse in children with ADHD?
a. No increment
b. Two times increment

c. Three times increment
d. Four times increment
e. Eight times increment

Question 68

A 55-year-old female has been diagnosed with breast cancer recently, has undergone surgery and is currently now on tamoxifen. If her mood is low, which antidepressant could she be started on, with minimal interactions with tamoxifen?
a. Fluoxetine
b. Paroxetine
c. Sertraline
d. Doxepin
e. Venlafaxine

Question 69

A 30-year-old man has been brought into the emergency department. He is noted to have increased heart rate, associated with euphoria and hyperactivity. His friends, who have accompanied him, informed that he has been abusing khat for the past year. Which of the following is not a complication associated with chronic usage?
a. Psychosis
b. Depression
c. Diminished sexual drive
d. Reduction in suicidal ideations
e. Myocardial infarction

Question 70

Which of the following is false?
a. Routine investigations include U & Es, liver function tests, serum calcium and phosphate.
b. In patients with suspected hypoparathyroidism, 25(OH)D3 is a reliable indicator of total body stores of vitamin D.
c. Chronic hypocalcaemia causes alopecia, cataracts and papilloedema.
d. Treatment of hypoparathyroidism involves a combination of alfacalcidol and calcitriol.
e. The multiple endocrine neoplasia type I (MEN 1) syndrome involves parathyroid tumour, pituitary adenoma and phaeochromocytoma.

Question 71

Which of the following statements best describes criterion validity?
a. It refers to predictive and concurrent validity together.
b. It refers to face and content validity together.
c. It refers to convergent and divergent validity together.

d. It refers to construct validity and predictive validity together.
e. It refers to the level of agreement between assessments by one rater of the same material at two or more different times.

Question 72
Which of the following represents a technique of randomization such that contamination between intervention and control group is being minimized?
a. Simple randomization
b. Block randomization
c. Stratified randomization
d. Covariate randomization
e. Cluster randomization

Question 73
Which of the following studies produces Figure 1.1?
a. Cochrane review
b. Data mining
c. Qualitative study
d. Meta-analysis
e. Systemic review

Question 74
Based on Figure 1.1, which of the following studies has the largest sample size?
a. Ko et al. (2008).
b. Ko et al. (2009).
c. There is no difference in sample size between studies.
d. Yoo et al. (2004).
e. Yen et al. (2009).

Study name	Statistics for each study					Odds ratio and 95% CI
	Odds ratio	Lower limit	Upper limit	Z-Value	p-Value	
Ko et al. (2009)	2.162	1.521	3.074	4.295	0.000	
Yen et al. (2009)	2.875	2.125	3.888	6.850	0.000	
Ko et al. (2008)	5.091	2.371	10.932	4.174	0.000	
Yoo et al. (2004)	3.280	1.759	6.117	3.736	0.000	
	2.847	2.147	3.774	7.274	0.000	

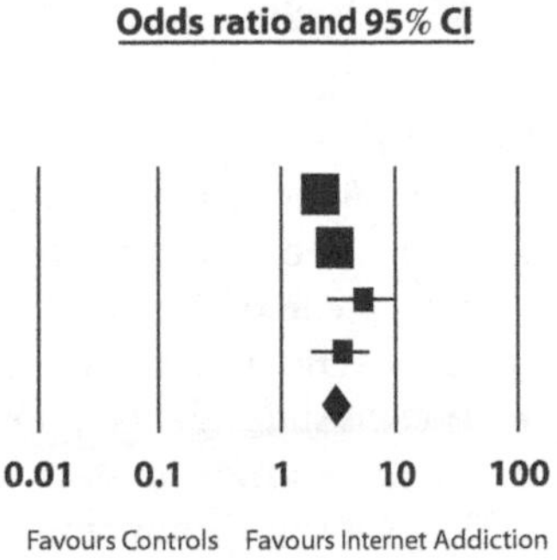

0.01   0.1   1   10   100

Favours Controls   Favours Internet Addiction

Figure 1.1 Forest plot comparing the odds ratios of having co-morbid ADHD amongst patients suffering from Internet addiction (IA) versus controls without IA. (From Ho RC, Zhang MW, Tsang TY, Toh AH, Pan F, Lu Y, Cheng C, Yip PS, Lam LT, Lai CM, Watanabe H, Mak KK (2014 Jun 20). The association between Internet addiction and psychiatric co-morbidity: A meta-analysis. *BMC Psychiatry*, 14: 183.)

Question 75

In Figure 1.1, the odds ratio is indicated for each study. Which of the following is the correct formula for odds ratio?
   a. (The number of controls without ADHD times the number of controls with ADHD)/(The number of IA [Internet addiction] participants with ADHD times the number of IA without ADHD)
   b. (The number of controls with ADHD times the number of IA without ADHD)/(The number of IA participants with ADHD times the number of controls without ADHD)
   c. (The number of IA participants with ADHD times the number of controls with ADHD)/(The number of controls without ADHD times the number of IA without ADHD)
   d. (The number of IA participants with ADHD times the number of controls without ADHD)/(The number of controls with ADHD times the number of IA without ADHD)
   e. (The number of IA participants with ADHD times the number of IA without ADHD)/(The number of controls without ADHD times the number of controls with ADHD)

Question 76

Referring to the study conducted by Yoo et al. (2009) in Figure 1.1, there is a horizontal line drawing across the box. What is represented by the horizontal line?
   a. Interquartile range of the odds ratio in the study conducted by Yoo et al. (2009)
   b. Interquartile range of the standardized mean differences in severity of ADHD between IA and controls
   c. 95% confidence interval of the odds ratio
   d. 95% confidence interval of the standardized mean differences in severity of ADHD between IA and controls
   e. 99% confidence interval of the standardized mean differences in severity of ADHD between IA and controls

Question 77

Based on Figure 1.1, what is the estimated heterogeneity between different studies?
   a. There is not enough information provided to determine where there is heterogeneity or not.
   b. There is no heterogeneity.
   c. There is significant but low level of heterogeneity.
   d. There is significant but moderate level of heterogeneity.
   e. There is significant but high level of heterogeneity.

Question 78

Which of the following is the correct conclusion drawn from Figure 1.1?
   a. People suffering from ADHD are less likely to develop IA compared with controls.
   b. People suffering from ADHD are more likely to develop IA compared with controls.

c. People suffering from IA are less likely to develop ADHD compared with controls.
d. People suffering from IA are more likely to develop ADHD compared with controls.
e. There is no difference between patients suffering from IA and controls in the risk of the developing ADHD.

Question 79
Which of the following is not a sign of resistance in psychoanalysis?
a. Asking irrelevant questions
b. Blurting things out without censoring them
c. Fidgeting
d. Intellectualizing events
e. Late for appointments

Question 80
Which of the following is a mature defence mechanism?
a. Anticipation
b. Idealization
c. Intellectualization
d. Introjection
e. Repression

Question 81
The following are features of pseudo-dementia, with the exception of
a. Usually acute in onset
b. Presence of lack of motivation and does not attempt to answer the questions
c. Memory deficits are often reported by others
d. Intact arithmetic skills
e. Intact paired associate learning

Question 82
All of the following are common clinical symptoms found in the elderly with mania, except
a. Rapid flight of ideas
b. More circumstantial speech
c. More paranoid ideations
d. Less hyperactivity
e. More cognitive impairment

Question 83
Down syndrome is a condition that is caused usually by trisomy 21. Investigators have made use of techniques that induce X-chromosome inactivation to silence the activity of the extra gene. Which of the following is the correct terminology for such a process/technique?
a. Translation
b. Transcription

c. Silencing
d. Mutation
e. Lyonization

Question 84
Which of the following is not a feature of Rett syndrome?
a. Choreoathetoid movements
b. Hypertrophic feet
c. Seizures
d. Spasticity
e. Truncal ataxia and apraxia

Question 85
You are a doctor working in the British Army and encounter soldiers who develop post-concussion symptoms after head injury. Which of the following factors are most significant predisposing factors for post-concussion symptoms amongst soldiers?
a. Depression and injury occur during military operation
b. Depression and severity of body injury
c. Depression and post-traumatic stress
d. Injury occurs during military operation and severity of body injury
e. Post-traumatic stress and severity of body injury

Question 86
Approximately what percentage of patients eventually kill themselves in 1 year following deliberate self-harm (DSH)?
a. 1%
b. 2%
c. 3%
d. 4%
e. 5%

Question 87
Which of the following is not used to treat sexual offenders?
a. Cognitive behavioural therapy
b. Cyproterone
c. Fluoxetine
d. Medroxyprogesterone
e. Testosterone

Question 88
During a forensic assessment of an accused who has recently committed rape, he tells the forensic psychiatrist that he did it on impulse. When he was asked about whether he considered the potential consequences, he denied doing so. He also has had a history of poor work record and has used heroin in the past. Based on the classification of rapists by Trick et al. (1981), he will be classified as
a. Situational stress rapist
b. Sociopathic rapist

c. Sexually inadequate rapist
d. Sadistic rapist
e. Psychotic rapist

Question 89
Based on the Isle of Wight study, the age of onset of oppositional defiant disorder is before
a. 3 years
b. 4 years
c. 8 years
d. 12 years
e. 16 years

Question 90
Which of the following medications is most effective in treating aggression in conduct disorder based on recent research?
a. Haloperidol
b. Lithium
c. Quetipaine
d. Risperidone
e. Thioridazine

Question 91
A 13-year-old boy has dropped out from secondary school. He is odd and is not accepted by his classmates. Your consultant recommends ruling out Asperger's syndrome. Which of the following features would not support such a diagnosis?
a. Restricted and repetitive behaviours
b. Marked clumsiness
c. Socially withdrawn
d. Worries about the welfare of his classmates
e. Language delay

Question 92
With regard to the treatment of OCD, poor prognostic factors include all of the following, with the exception of
a. Symptoms involving the need for symmetry and exactness
b. Predominance of phobic ruminative ideas, with the absence of compulsions
c. Presence of hopelessness and hallucinations
d. Family history of OCD
e. Continuous, episodic course

Question 93
All of the following are known to be risk factors for suicide, except
a. Low social class
b. Middle social class
c. High social class
d. Divorced individuals
e. Poor social support

Question 94
A 22-year-old man presents to the clinic with white patches and gingival fibromata. He attends a special school because of learning difficulties and receives medical outpatient follow-up for epilepsy. A whole body scan shows tumours in the spleen, kidney and lungs. Which of the following conditions does he have?
  a. Neurofibromatosis
  b. Phenylketonuria
  c. Sanfilippo syndrome
  d. Tay–Sachs disease
  e. Tuberous sclerosis

Question 95
What has been the estimated prevalence of mania in elderly?
  a. 1%
  b. 5%
  c. 10%
  d. 15%
  e. 20%

Question 96
A patient with anxiety disorder is keen to go for hypnotherapy to relieve her symptoms. Which of the following statements about hypnotherapy is correct?
  a. Evidence shows that hypnosis can help recall in psychotherapy, leading to better outcomes.
  b. It is superior to relaxation exercises.
  c. It is recommended in the National Institute for Health and Care Excellence (NICE) guidelines for treatment of anxiety disorders.
  d. Sudden removal of symptoms by suggestion under hypnosis can lead to rebound depression and anxiety.
  e. Suggestion with hypnosis is found to be superior to suggestion without hypnosis.

Question 97
A medical student wants to look at the number of outpatients who experience postural hypotension with chlorpromazine treatment versus those who are not on treatment. Which of the following statistical tests is most appropriate in comparing the two groups?
  a. Chi-square test
  b. One-way analysis of variance (ANOVA)
  c. Paired t-test
  d. Student's t-test
  e. Z-test

Question 98
A core trainee is seeing a 27-year-old woman in the specialist clinic. He gathers from her that she has an ideal weight she is aiming for and that she purges to lose

weight. Which of the following would be more indicative and characteristic for diagnosing her with bulimia instead of anorexia?
   a. Restriction of energy and food intake leading to a significantly low body weight
   b. Intense fear of weight gain
   c. Persistent behaviour that interferes with weight gain
   d. Body image disturbances
   e. Poor impulse control with persistent preoccupation with eating and an irresistible craving for food

Question 99
A researcher wants to compare the effectiveness of asenepine treatment versus CBT in treatment of borderline personality disorder. Subjects are randomized into two groups. The first group will be administered asenapine for 12 weeks, after which they will be administered CBT for 12 weeks. The second group will undergo the reverse. Subjects will be given questionnaires to complete at the first and second 12th week. What type of study design is this?
   a. Case–control study
   b. Cohort study
   c. Crossover study
   d. Cross-sectional study
   e. Randomized control trial

Question 100
Based on the current literature, which of the following is not one of the recommended non-stimulant medications that are indicated for ADHD?
   a. Imipramine
   b. Bupropion
   c. Clonidine
   d. Atomoxetine
   e. Duloxetine

Question 101
Approximately what percentage of young people with conduct disorder eventually develops dissocial personality disorder?
   a. 5%
   b. 10%
   c. 20%
   d. 40%
   e. 60%

Question 102
Which of the following is the most common psychiatric condition associated with Cushing syndrome?
   a. Bipolar disorder
   b. Depression
   c. Amnesia

d. Attentional deficit disorder

e. Psychosis

Question 103

Which of the following is not a feature of Cornelia De Lange syndrome?

a. Feeding difficulties

b. Microcephaly

c. Mild-to-moderate learning disability

d. Stereotypic movements

e. Short stature

Question 104

Which of the following tools is not used for predicting sex offence recidivism?

a. Rapid Risk Assessment for Sex Offence Recidivism (RRASOR)

b. Sex Offender Risk Appraisal Guide (SORAG)

c. Sexual Violence Risk-20 (SVR-20)

d. Structured Anchored Clinical Judgement (SACJ)

e. Violence Risk Appraisal Guide (VRAG)

Question 105

If lithium is started in an elderly with mania, what is the maximum recommended total daily dose based on the current treatment guidelines?

a. 200 mg/day

b. 300 mg/day

c. 400 mg/day

d. 500 mg/day

e. 600 mg/day

Question 106

Your patient is a 15-year-old girl who has a history of repeated DSH and a poor relationship with her parents. You are keen to start her on family therapy. However, her parents are busy with their work, and they prefer family therapy that focuses on presenting communication difficulties with less frequent sessions. Which one of the following types of family therapy would you recommend?

a. Eclectic family therapy

b. Family communication focused therapy

c. Structural family therapy

d. Strategic family therapy

e. Systemic family therapy

Question 107

A 40-year-old alcoholic has been referred by his local GP to the addiction service. He has been drinking at least eight bottles of beer on a daily basis for the past 8 years. He has tried to stop drinking previously but relapsed due to the strong cravings that he had. Which of the following medications would help him deal with his strong cravings?

a. Acamprosate

b. Naltrexone

c. Naxolone
d. Disulfiram
e. Lorazepam

Question 108
A 34-year-old woman arrives at the emergency department with euphoria, visual hallucinations, arrhythmias, nausea and diaphoresis. Which of the following substances is she likely to be intoxicated with?
a. Barbiturates
b. Cannabis
c. Cocaine
d. Heroin
e. LSD

Question 109
Which of the following defence mechanisms is associated with phobias?
a. Denial
b. Reaction formation
c. Repression
d. Splitting
e. Undoing

Question 110
Which of the following medications does not need to be held off at the time of ECT to ensure successful treatment?
a. Bupropion
b. Clozapine
c. Fluoxetine
d. Lithium
e. Zopiclone

Question 111
Which of the following disorders is not associated with 5HTT gene polymorphisms?
a. Autism
b. Attention deficit hyperactivity disorder (ADHD)
c. Increased fear and anxiety-related behaviours
d. Obsessive-compulsive disorder (OCD)
e. Suicidal behaviour in depressed patients

Question 112
Which part of brain dysfunction has been suggested to be implicated in OCD?
a. Amygdala
b. Basal ganglia
c. Nucleus accumbens
d. Hippocampus
e. Substantia nigra

Question 113

A medical student wants to study whether cannabis is a risk factor for the development of schizophrenia. He plans to survey 100 patients with schizophrenia and 100 aged-matched controls with regard to their cannabis usage history. What type of study is this?

a. Case–control study
b. Cohort study
c. Crossover study
d. Cross-sectional study
e. Randomized control trial

Question 114

An elderly woman suffers from somatoform pain disorder, and her son wants to find out from you whether this condition is common in the community. What is the 1-year prevalence of this condition?

a. 8%
b. 18%
c. 28%
d. 38%
e. 48%

Question 115

A 35-year-old woman presents with a major depressive episode with a background of borderline personality disorder. You are keen to start her on treatment. Which of the following is true?

a. Cognitive behavioural therapy is more effective than medication.
b. Cognitive behavioural therapy is more effective than interpersonal psychotherapy.
c. Interpersonal psychotherapy is more effective than cognitive behavioural therapy.
d. Neither cognitive behavioural therapy nor interpersonal psychotherapy is effective.
e. Only medication is required, and there is no need for psychological treatment.

Question 116

Which of the following is the most common neuropsychiatric condition that usually arises from Addison disease?

a. Memory impairment
b. Bipolar disorder
c. Anxiety
d. Paranoia
e. Psychosis

Extended-Matching Items

Theme: Adult Psychiatry – Personality Disorders

Options:

a. Anankastic personality disorder
b. Anxious–avoidant personality disorder

c. Dependent personality disorder
d. Dissocial personality disorder
e. Emotionally unstable personality disorder, borderline type
f. Histrionic personality disorder
g. Narcissistic personality disorder
h. Paranoid personality disorder
i. Schizoid personality disorder

Lead in: Choose one possible diagnosis for each of the following clinical scenarios. Each option may be used once, more than once or not at all.

Question 117
A 49-year-old man refuses to see the registrar at the clinic and insists on seeing the consultant psychiatrist. He declares that he is an important person and has no time for young doctors. He insists on seeing the psychiatrist immediately. He tells the psychiatrist he will soon be one of the top in his profession and will have hundreds of employees' fates in his hands. (Choose one option.)

Question 118
A 27-year-old woman enjoys being the centre of attention and dresses seductively to draw the attention she wants. She has had multiple relationships, each lasting from a few days to a few months and none lasting more than 6 months. She bursts out crying when describing her past relationships and laughs as she reminisces about the happier times. (Choose one option.)

Question 119
A 37-year-old woman has had several suicide attempts, each prompted by quarrels with her boyfriend. She uses suicidal threats whenever her boyfriend suggests breaking up with her. She has changed psychiatrists three times over the past year as she thinks they are not concerned enough about her. (Choose one option.)

Theme: Psychotherapy
Options:
a. Bion
b. Catharsis
c. Denial
d. Dependency
e. Internalizing factors
f. Foulkes
g. Lewin
h. Pratt
i. Social norms
j. Yalom

Lead in: Select the ONE most appropriate answer for each of the following questions. Each option may be used once, more than once or not at all.

Question 120
List one of Yalom's therapeutic factors in group therapy. (Choose one option.)

Question 121
The founder of group analysis who propounded the idea of a social matrix. (Choose one option.)

Question 122
List one of Bion's three basic assumptions. (Choose one option.)

Theme: Research Methodology
Options:
  a. Continuous scale
  b. Interval scale
  c. Norminal scale
  d. Ordinal scale
  e. Ratio scale

Lead in: Match the ONE appropriate scale with the description below. Each option may be used once, more than once or not at all.

Question 123
The body mass index (BMI) of patients with schizophrenia in the outpatient psychosis clinic. (Choose one option.)

Question 124
The temperature of the psychiatric ward in Fahrenheit. (Choose one option.)

Question 125
The ethnicity of patients in a suicide research study. (Choose one option.)

Question 126
The temperature of the psychiatric ward in Kelvin. (Choose one option.)

Question 127
Hamilton Rating Scale for Depression (HAM-D) score <11 = mild depression = '1'. (Choose one option.)

Theme: Research Methodology
Options:
  a. Ascertainment bias
  b. Berkson bias
  c. Misclassification bias
  d. Neyman bias
  e. Recall bias

f. Selection bias

g. Volunteer bias

Lead in: Match the one correct bias to the following scenarios. Each option may be used once, more than once or not at all.

Question 128
A researcher wishes to perform a study to assess the effect of exercise on stress levels and mental health. He places his advertisements for subject participation outside a gym. He subsequently receives many interested participants, who happen to be members of that gym. (Choose one option.)

Question 129
A psychiatrist is conducting a randomized controlled trial studying the effects of placebo and antidepressants. He is concerned about his depressed patients and decides to place those with higher depression scores in the group receiving antidepressants. (Choose one option.)

Question 130
A researcher conducts a retrospective study to compare patients with schizophrenia and normal controls to identify risk factors for schizophrenia. He finds that these patients smoked a lot before the onset of their symptoms. He then concludes that smoking leads to schizophrenia. (Choose one option.)

Theme: Substance Abuse
Options:
  a. 6 hours
  b. 24 hours
  c. 48 hours
  d. 3 days
  e. 8 days

Lead in: Match one correct length of time that the following illicit drugs can be detected in a urine drug screen. Each option may be used once, more than once or not at all.

Question 131
Phencyclidine. (Choose one option.)

Question 132
Ecstasy. (Choose one option.)

Question 133
Amphetamine. (Choose one option.)

Question 134
Lysergic acid diethylamide (LSD). (Choose one option.)

Theme: Old-Age Psychiatry

Options:
a. Computed tomography (CT) brain scan
b. Magnetic resonance imaging (MRI) brain scan
c. Dopamine transporter (DAT) single photon emission computerized tomography
d. Perfusion hexamethylpropyleneamine oxime (HMPAO) single photon emission computed tomography (SPECT)

Lead in: Match one imaging technique that should be used in each of the following scenarios. Each of the options may be used once, more than once or not at all.

Question 135
A 75-year-old man presents with cognitive impairment, fluctuating consciousness and visual hallucinations. On physical examination, he has hypertonia and hypersalivation. The Mini Mental State Examination (MMSE) score is 18/20. His symptoms worsen after he is started on a low dose of risperidone. (Choose one option.)

Question 136
An 82-year-old woman presents with fluctuating, progressive memory loss and emotional incontinence. She has a history of falls and multiple medical problems, including old strokes, hypertension and diabetes. Her family says her personality is preserved. (Choose one option.)

Question 137
A 25-year-old woman complained of vomiting, vertigo and bilateral numbness of the hands 2 years ago. These symptoms lasted for 1 month before she recovered, albeit gradually. Her numbness subsequently relapsed a few months later and spread to weakness of all four limbs to the extent that she is unable to balance herself. She is also suffering from increasing muscle spasms affecting mainly the lower limbs. There is urgency of micturition and diplopia. (Choose one option.)

Theme: Learning Disability

Options:
a. Cat-like cry
b. Cleft palate with cardiac problems
c. Down-turned fishlike mouth with Greek warrior helmet face
d. Excessive weight gain and skin pricking
e. Elfin-like features with social disinhibition
f. Flapping hand movements
g. Hamartomatous tumours
h. Overlapping of fingers over thumb
i. Rocker bottom feet
j. Self-hugging and a hoarse voice
k. Self-mutilation, dystonia and writhing movements
l. Simian crease with almond-shaped eyes

m. Short stature, webbed neck
n. Tall with small testicles

Lead in: Match one clinical feature with each of the following genetic conditions. Each option may be used once or more than once or not at all.

Question 138
Angelman syndrome. (Choose one option.)

Question 139
Down syndrome. (Choose one option.)

Question 140
Cri du chat. (Choose one option.)

Question 141
Smith–Magenis syndrome. (Choose one option.)

Question 142
Patau syndrome. (Choose one option.)

Question 143
Williams syndrome. (Choose one option.)

Question 144
Turner syndrome. (Choose one option.)

Question 145
Tuberous sclerosis. (Choose one option.)

Question 146
Di George syndrome. (Choose one option.)

Question 147
Edwards syndrome. (Choose one option.)

Question 148
Lesch–Nyhan syndrome. (Choose one option.)

Question 149
Klinefelter syndrome. (Choose one option.)

Question 150
Prader–Willi syndrome. (Choose one option.)

Question 151
Wolf–Hirschhorn syndrome. (Choose one option.)

Theme: Learning Disability

Options:
- a. 2
- b. 3
- c. 5
- d. 10
- e. 15
- f. 20
- g. 30
- h. 35
- i. 45
- j. 50
- k. 85
- l. 90

Lead in: Match one number to each of the following disabilities. Each option may be used once, more than once or not at all.

Based on the ICD-10 criteria, what is the lower IQ limit for the following:

Question 152
Mild learning disability. (Choose one option.)

Question 153
Moderate learning disability. (Choose one option.)

Question 154
Severe learning disability. (Choose one option.)

Theme: Genetic Risk of Schizophrenia

Options:
- a. 0%–4%
- b. 5%–9%
- c. 10%–14%
- d. 15%–19%
- e. 20%–24%
- f. 25%–29%
- g. 30%–34%
- h. 35%–50%
- i. 60%–65%
- j. 70%–75%
- k. 80%–85%

Lead in: A 30-year-old man has been receiving treatment for schizophrenia over the past 3 years. He is currently stable and plans to get married and start a family. He is concerned about the genetic risks of schizophrenia in his offspring.

Match one percentage above with each of the following questions. Each option may be used once, more than once or not at all.

Question 155
The risk of schizophrenia in his child if his wife does not have schizophrenia. (Choose one option.)

Question 156
The risk of schizophrenia in his child if his wife has schizophrenia. (Choose one option.)

Question 157
The risk of schizophrenia if he adopts a child with velocardiofacial syndrome. (Choose one option.)

Question 158
The risk of schizophrenia in his half-sibling. (Choose one option.)

Question 159
The risk of schizophrenia in his younger cousin. (Choose one option.)

Question 160
The risk of schizophrenia in his nephews or nieces. (Choose one option.)

Question 161
The risk of schizophrenia in his biological uncles or aunts. (Choose one option.)

Question 162
The percentage of people with schizophrenia who smoke. (Choose one option.)

Question 163
The percentage of people with schizophrenia who do not continue with antipsychotic medication after 1 year. (Choose one option.)

Theme: Obsessive-Compulsive Disorder

Options:
   a. Fear of contamination
   b. Doubting
   c. Fear of illness, germs or bodily fear
   d. Symmetry
   e. Sexual or aggressive thoughts
   f. Checking
   g. Washing
   h. Counting

Lead in: Match one compulsion/obsession with each of the following questions. Each option may be used once, more than once or not at all.

Question 164
Which one is the most common and prevalent obsession? (Choose one option.)

Question 165
Which one is the most common and prevalent compulsion? (Choose one option.)

Question 166
Which one is the least prevalent obsession? (Choose one option.)

Question 167
Which one is the least prevalent obsession? (Choose one option.)

Theme: Congenital Abnormalities and Medications
Options:
a. Pulmonary hypertension
b. Agitation and irritability
c. Foetal heart defects
d. Reduction in gestational age
e. Reduction in birth weight
f. Spontaneous abortion
g. Neural tube defect
h. Oral clefts

Lead in: Match the congenital abnormalities with each of the following questions. Each option may be used once, more than once or not at all.

Question 168
The usage of SSRIs for the treatment of depressive disorders in pregnancy could lead to which of the above abnormalities? (Choose four options.)

Question 169
Paroxetine is contraindicated for usage in pregnancy due to the potential for it inducing which one of the above abnormalities? (Choose one option.)

Question 170
The usage of paroxetine and venlafaxine in pregnancy for the treatment of depressive disorder has been linked to the development of which one of the above abnormalities? (Choose one option.)

Question 171
The usage of lithium in pregnancy has been linked to the development of which one of the above abnormalities? (Choose one option.)

Question 172
The usage of valproate in pregnancy might lead to the development of which one of the above abnormalities? (Choose one option.)

Question 173
Lamotrigine is a medication that requires further evaluation as it is not routinely used in pregnancy. It might result in the development of which one of the above abnormalities? (Choose one option.)

Theme: Child Psychiatry

Options:
  a. Multisystemic therapy
  b. Duty to inform the police if not reported yet
  c. Obtain informed consent from the child and his or her parents
  d. Parent management training
  e. Family therapy
  f. Methylphenidate
  g. Risperidone

Lead in: Please match the above options with each of the respective clinical scenarios.

Question 174
A 12-year-old male has just been involved in a fight with his classmates. He has been quite defiant towards his parents, and they are struggling to cope with his behaviours. He does not have any psychiatric history.

Question 175
A 16-year-old boy's parents have taken a court order against him as he has been physically aggressive towards them and others. He was offered a course of psychotherapy, but his parents did not find the psychological intervention helpful. Which pharmacotherapy treatment is likely to be helpful for his condition?

Question 176
A core trainee consults the consultant as he has received a request from a GP with regard to the forensic evaluation of a 15-year-old male who has been involved in a criminal activity.

Question 177
A core trainee has been tasked to assess a 15-year-old boy. He has been recently arrested by the police for setting fire to a school. He has been previously arrested for shoplifting as well as fights.

Question 178
A 7-year-old boy has been having frequent loss of temper. This has lead to arguments with parents, and he is irritable only at home and not at school. Which of the following is recommended?

Theme: Old-Age Psychiatry and Neuroimaging

Options:
  a. CT brain scan
  b. MRI brain scan
  c. Dopaminergic iodine-123-radiolabelled 2β carbomethoxy-3β (4-iodophenyl)-N-(3-fluoropropyl) nortropane (FP-CIT) SPECT or DaTSCAN
  d. Perfusion HMPAO SPECT

Lead in: Match the above imaging techniques to the following scenarios. Select one most appropriate imaging technique.

Question 179

A 75-year-old man presents with cognitive impairment, fluctuating levels of consciousness, particularly confusion and bizarre behaviour in the evenings. His daughter claims that he has been seeing ghosts and not able to turn in his bed. On physical examination, he is found to have hypertonia and hypersalivation. The score on MMSE is 15/30. These above symptoms worsen following the commencement of antipsychotic medication.

Question 180

An 80-year-old man presents with fluctuating, progressive memory loss and emotional incontinence. He has history of falls and is being treated for hypertension by his GP. His relatives say that his personality is preserved.

Question 181

A 22-year-old woman complained of vertigo, vomiting and numbness of both hands 3 years ago. These symptoms lasted a month and she recovered fully, albeit gradually. She remained well until 8 months later when she had numbness of both hands and the left leg. These conditions improved spontaneously after 2 weeks. Twelve months after the initial symptoms, she again had numbness of both hands, but this time also with weakness of all four limbs so that she became chair-bound because she could not balance herself. She also suffered from increasing muscle spasm affecting mainly the lower limbs. There was also urgency of micturition and diplopia.

Theme: Psychotherapy

Options:
- a. Aversive conditioning
- b. Chaining
- c. Flooding
- d. Habituation
- e. Insight learning
- f. Latent learning
- g. Penalty
- h. Premack's principle
- i. Reciprocal inhibition
- j. Shaping
- k. Systematic desensitization
- l. Token economy

Lead in: From the above list of behavioural techniques, select the option that best matches each of the following examples. Each option might be used once, more than once or not at all.

Question 182

A 6-year-old boy is put in a maze to look for the toy box. After a few trials, he learns the cognitive map of the maze and needs a shorter time to find the toy box. (Choose one option.)

Question 183
A 2-year-old child is undergoing toilet training. The complex behaviour is broken down into simpler steps. She is rewarded with a sticker if she informs her mother when she has the urge to urinate. The positive reinforcement continues until she can inform her mother reliably without failures. Then the contingencies are altered, and she needs to go to the toilet on her own before the sticker is given. (Choose one option.)

Question 184
A patient with moderate learning disability has an aggressive tendency and tends to assault other residents in the hostel. The staff have devised a plan in response to his aggressive behaviour. His main pleasurable activity is watching television. He will be removed from the TV room and put in a single room for a 2-hour time-out period if he assaults any resident. (Choose one option.)

Theme: General Adult Psychiatry: Prevention and Treatment
Options:
  a. Attendance records
  b. Changing the settings
  c. Dropout rates
  d. Follow-up studies
  e. Prevalence rate
  f. Services load data
  g. Skill training
  h. Stress management

Lead in: Identify which of the above items best describe(s) the following prevention strategies established by the Department of Health. Each option may be used once, more than once or not at all.

Question 185
Gathering evidence that long-term prevention goals are met. (Choose one option.)

Question 186
Identifying prevention targets by gathering evidence for the suspected vulnerability of a specific target group. (Choose one option.)

Question 187
Prevention strategies aiming at increasing the coping capacity of a population. (Choose two options.)

Question 188
Prevention strategies aiming at reducing the environmental risks associated with a disease. (Choose one option.)

Theme: Substance Abuse and Addictions

Options:
- a. Advertising controls
- b. Community responses
- c. Controls on prescribed drugs
- d. Crop-control measures
- e. Educational efforts
- f. Interception and interdiction measures
- g. Redesign the chemical structure of a psychoactive drug
- h. Safe drinking limit
- i. Taxation and legislative controls on tobacco and alcohol

Lead in: Identify which of the above prevention strategies best describe the following classification. Each option may be used once, more than once or not at all.

Question 189
Demand reduction (Choose two options.)

Question 190
Harm reduction (Choose one option.)

Question 191
Supply or availability reduction (Choose four options.)

GET THROUGH MRCPSYCH PAPER B MOCK EXAMINATION

Question 1 Answer: d, Precontemplation

Explanation: In this example, the man's level of motivation is consistent with the precontemplation stage, as he has little or no motivation to change his behaviour. Prochaska and DiClemente's stages of change applied to alcohol abuse or dependence describe an individual's level of motivation for recovery. The model consists of five stages of change:

1. Precontemplation, where there is no interest in change in the foreseeable future (next 6 months).
2. Contemplation, where the individual considers change in the next 1–6 months but not immediately.
3. Preparation, which involves planning on change in the next month.
4. Action, where meaningful changes were made in the recent past (6 months).
5. Maintenance, which refers to maintaining change for 6 months or more.

Reference: DiClemente CC, Schlundt D, Gemmell L (2004). Readiness and stages of change in addiction treatment. *Am J Addict*, 13: 103–119.

Question 2 Answer: d, Second trimester

Explanation: If a pregnant woman decides to withdraw from heroin, it should be done during the second trimester, as it then poses the least harm to the baby and has the lowest association with miscarriage. Withdrawal during the first trimester may cause spontaneous abortion and during the third trimester poses a risk of delivering premature babies, which have a poorer chance of survival and greater incidence of permanent disability. The patient should be put on methadone maintenance treatment after withdrawal. Methadone maintenance improves birth weight but may depress respiration in the newborn and may lead to a more severe and prolonged withdrawal syndrome, with higher frequencies of seizures. Newborn infants should be kept in hospital for at least 2 weeks. Respiratory depression may be treated with naloxone and seizures and withdrawal by sedatives such as diazepam.

Reference: Puri BK, Treasaden I (eds) (2010). *Psychiatry: An Evidence-Based Text*. London: Hodder Arnold, pp. 717, 809, 1034–1035.

Question 3 Answer: d, The value of the correlation coefficient can range from –2 to +2.

Explanation: The correlation coefficient is an index that quantifies the linear relationship between a pair of variables. Various correlation coefficients are available, all taking values between –1 and 1, with the extreme values indicating a perfect linear relationship and the sign indicating the direction of the relationship. A value of 0 indicates that there is no linear relationship between the two variables, although there may be a more esoteric nonlinear relationship. The most common of such coefficient is Pearson's product moment correlation coefficient, which acts as an estimator of the population correlation in a bivariate normal distribution. The degree of correlation is represented by the *r*-value. *r*-value (degree of correlation): 0–0.2 (negligible), 0.2–0.5 (weak), 0.5–0.8 (moderate) and 0.8–1.0 (strong).

References: Lewis GH, Sheringham J, Kalim K, Crayford TJ (2008). *Mastering Public Health*. London: Royal Society of Medicine Press, p. 99; Everitt BS (2006). *Medical Statistics from A to Z* (2nd edition). Cambridge, UK: Cambridge University Press, pp. 60–61.

Question 4 Answer: c, Standard deviation (SD) has the same units as the original observation.

Explanation: SD is the most commonly used measure of the spread of a set of observations. It is equal to the square root of the variance. A low SD indicates that the data points tend to be very close to the mean (also called expected value); a high SD indicates that the data points are spread out over a large range of values. A useful property of SD is that, unlike the variance, it is expressed in the same units as the data. For a sample size of 20, the denominator should be 19, degree of freedom = $n - 1$. SD is always positive.

Reference: Lewis GH, Sheringham J, Kalim K, Crayford TJ (2008). *Mastering Public Health*. London: Royal Society of Medicine Press, p. 79.

Question 5 Answer: d, Resistance

Explanation: The acronym 'FRAMES' stands for

- Personalized *feedback* or assessment results detailing the target behaviour and associated effects and consequences on the individual
- Emphasizing the individual's *responsibility* for change
- Giving *advice* on how to change
- Providing a *menu* of options for change
- Expressing *empathy* through behaviours conveying caring, understanding and warmth
- Emphasizing *self-efficacy* for change and instilling hope that change is not only possible but also within reach

Reference: Puri BK, Treasaden I (eds) (2010). *Psychiatry: An Evidence-Based Text*. London: Hodder Arnold, p. 1038.

Question 6 Answer: a, Brief psychodynamic therapy

Explanation: Specific contraindications for brief psychodynamic therapy are severe depression, acute psychosis and borderline personality disorder. General contraindications are when the therapist is unable to make effective contact with the patient and when there is evidence of a need for extended work with the patient. According to a review of empirical data, there is evidence for the efficacy of brief psychodynamic therapy for the following disorders: depressive disorders, anxiety disorders, post-traumatic stress disorder, somatoform disorder, bulimia nervosa, anorexia nervosa, borderline personality disorder, cluster C personality disorder and substance-related disorders. Brief psychodynamic therapy is also contraindicated when the patient has high tendency for serious self-harm.

Reference and Further Reading: Leichsenring F (2005). Are psychodynamic and psychoanalytic therapies effective? A review of empirical data. *Int J Psychoanal*, 86: 841–868; Puri BK, Treasaden I (eds) (2010). *Psychiatry: An Evidence-Based Text*. London: Hodder Arnold, p. 936.

Question 7 Answer: a, Cholinesterase inhibitors do not reduce the frequency of incident dementia.
Explanation: Based on a systematic review recently published, 41 studies were looked into. The review has highlighted that cholinesterase inhibitors did not appear to reduce the frequency of mild cognitive impairment leading towards dementia. Single trials have highlighted that cognition did improve for a psychological intervention over 6 months, usage of a dopamine agonist over 3 months and donepezil over 48 weeks.

Reference: Claudia C et al. (2013). Treatment for mild cognitive impairment: Systematic review. *Br J Psychiatry*, 203: 255–264.

Question 8 Answer: d, Mania
Explanation: Mania is less common than depression in Cushing's syndrome of endogenous origin, but the converse holds true in exogenous cases, in which mania is common.

Further Reading: Puri BK, Treasaden I (eds) (2010). *Psychiatry: An Evidence-Based Text*. London: Hodder Arnold, p. 574.

Question 9 Answer: e, 90%
Explanation: Amongst patients suffering from delirium, approximately 90% of them have abnormal electroencephalographic (EEG) traces. Delta activities, asymmetry in the waves and localized spike and sharp wave complexes, occur more frequently in those with intracranial pathology. Alpha activities correlate with cognitive functioning, and delta activities correlate with the duration of illness.

Recently, in a study conducted amongst a group of non-sedated patients who had undergone cardiothoracic surgery, it was observed that two electrodes in a frontal-parietal derivation could easily distinguish amongst patients who had delirium versus those who did not have.

References: Puri BK, Hall AD, Ho RC (2014). *Revision Notes in Psychiatry*. Boca Raton, FL: CRC Press, p. 691; Van der Kool AW, Zaal IJ, Klijin FA, Koek HL, Meijer RC, Leigten FS, Slooter AL (2015). Delirium detection using EEG: What and how to measure. *Chest*, 147(1): 94–101.

Question 10 Answer: b, All neuroanatomical areas in the brain show significant loss of neurons with normal aging.
Explanation: The brain is overprovided with neurons; hence, a loss of neurons does not necessarily result in a loss of function. Some neuroanatomical areas of the brain show no loss in the number of neurons with normal aging (e.g. the dentate nucleus of the cerebellum). Great losses in neurons and neuronal connection are largely found in the frontal cortex, hippocampus, locus coeruleus and substantia nigra.

Reference: Puri BK, Hall AD, Ho RC (2014). *Revision Notes in Psychiatry*. Boca Raton, FL: CRC Press, p. 681.

Question 11 Answer: b, 10%
Explanation: Statistics have shown that the incidence of delirium amongst old people who are hospitalized is between 5% and 10%. The prevalence increases in cardiac surgery patients, hip fracture patients, intensive care patients and patients with advanced cancer to 30%, 50%, 70% and 80%, respectively.

Procedures such as total joint replacement do cause elderly to be predisposed towards delirium. In a recent meta-analysis, it was found that 17% of patients who underwent total joint replacement (TJR) developed delirium during hospital admission. Hence, it is important for health professionals to recognize delirium early and to institute appropriate treatment.

References: Puri BK, Hall AD, Ho RC (2014). *Revision Notes in Psychiatry*. Boca Raton, FL: CRC Press, p. 682; Scott JE, Mathias JL, Kneebone AC (2015). Incidence of delirium following total joint replacement in older adults: A meta-analysis. *Gen Hosp Psychiatry*, 37: 223–229.

Question 12 Answer: e, At least 50% of neurofibromatosis type I (NF-1) sufferers presents with moderate-to-severe learning disability (LD).
Explanation: International Classification of Diseases (ICD) defines mental retardation as being a condition of being arrested or incomplete development of the mind, especially characterized by impairment of skills manifested during the developmental period, which contribute to the overall level of intelligence including cognitive, language, motor and social abilities. The intelligence quotient (IQ) range for moderate mental retardation is 35–49, for mild retardation is 50–69, for severe mental retardation is 20–34 and for profound mental retardation is <20. Those with moderate mental retardation have varying profiles of abilities; language use and development are also variable (may be absent). There is a delay in achievement of self-care. Simple practical work is possible, but independent living is rarely achieved.

Option (e) is incorrect, as previous research found that learning disabilities affect at least 50% of children with NF-1 diagnosis. In particular, they have had problems with academic achievements.

References: Puri BK, Hall AD, Ho RC (2014). *Revision Notes in Psychiatry*. Boca Raton, FL: CRC Press, p. 663; Hyman SL et al. (2006). Learning disabilities in children with Neurofibromatosis type 1: Subtype, cognitive profile, and attentive-deficit-hyperactivity disorder. *Dev Med Child Neurol*, 48(12): 973–937.

Question 13 Answer: e, Spasticity

Explanation: Prader–Willi syndrome is an autosomal dominant disorder with deletion of chromosome 15q11-13, of paternal origin. Patients present with hypotonia rather than spasticity, which leads to feeding difficulties and failure to thrive during infancy. During childhood, orthopaedic problems such as congenital dislocation of hip and scoliosis are common. In adolescence, behavioural disorders such as overeating and obesity, self-injurious behaviour, compulsive behaviour, aggression, excessive daytime sleepiness, skin picking, hoarding and anxiety may be present. Insatiable appetite is diagnostic.

In addition, psychiatric disorders such as psychosis are quite prevalent in adults with this syndrome. For children, oppositional defiant disorder (ODD) was the most common diagnosis and is present in approximately 20% of children with this syndrome. Age, gender and genetic subtype do not mediate the association.

References: Puri BK, Hall AD, Ho RC (2014). *Revision Notes in Psychiatry*. Boca Raton, FL: CRC Press, pp. 673–674; Lo ST, Collin PJ, Hokken-Koelega AC (2015). Psychiatric disorders in children with Prader-Willi syndrome—Results of a 2 year longitudinal study. *Am J Med Genet A*, 167A(5): 983–91.

Question 14 Answer: e, Neurofibromatosis

Explanation: NF presents with macrocephaly rather than microcephaly. Other syndromes that cause microcephaly include Wolf–Hirschhorn syndrome and Rubinstein syndrome. NF is autosomal dominant with 50% of cases caused by sporadic mutations. There is abnormal production of neurofibromin. Clinical features include short stature, macrocephaly, optic nerve glioma, hypertension, tumours arising from the connective tissue of nerve sheaths, café au lait spots, cutaneous neurofibromas, freckling of groin or armpit, skeletal deformities and lisch nodules.

Reference: Puri BK, Hall AD, Ho RC (2014). *Revision Notes in Psychiatry*. Boca Raton, FL: CRC Press, p. 673.

Question 15 Answer: c, Hyperkinetic disorder

Explanation: 70% of children with autism would have associated mental retardation, mild-to-moderate mental retardation (30%) and severe-to-profound mental retardation (50%). There might be associated academic learning problems in literacy or numeracy. In addition, in around 50% of children, they have associated attention-deficit hyperactivity disorder (ADHD) as well.

Reference: Puri BK, Hall AD, Ho RC (2014). *Revision Notes in Psychiatry*. Boca Raton, FL: CRC Press, p. 627.

Question 16 Answer: a, Sertraline

Explanation: Selective serotonin re-uptake inhibitors (SSRIs) are efficacious in treating both physical and psychological symptoms of premenstrual syndrome.

Reference: Henshaw CA (2007). Premenstrual syndrome: Diagnosis, aetiology, assessment and management. *Adv Psychiatr Treat*, 13: 139–146.

Question 17 Answer: d, Rates of depression in first-degree relatives of depressed patients with multiple sclerosis (MS) are higher than the rates of depression in first-degree relatives of people who do not have MS.

Explanation: MS is a relapsing and remitting autoimmune disorder with diverse neurological signs as a result of plaques of demyelination and degeneration axonal loss throughout the white matter, with the exception of the peripheral nerves. The common psychiatric manifestations include fatigue (80%), depression (14%–27%), anxiety (14%–25%), mania (2%) and pathological laughter and crying (10%).

Option (d) is incorrect. Compared with depressive illness, genetic linkage for MS is much reduced. The rate of depression in first-degree relatives of depressed patients with MS is much lower than the rate of depression in first-degree relatives of depressed individuals who do not have MS.

Recent research has demonstrated that cortisol has a role in the fatigue experienced in those diagnosed with relapsing-remitting MS. Cortisol in itself is a key regulator of the immune system, energy metabolism and stress.

References: Kaufman DM, Milstein MJ (2013). *Kaufman's Clinical Neurology of Psychiatrist* (7th edition). Philadelphia, PA: Saunders, p. 340; Puri BK, Hall AD, Ho RC (2014). *Revision Notes in Psychiatry*. Boca Raton, FL: CRC Press, p. 502.

Question 18 Answer: d, Bupropion is contraindicated due to its side effect profile.

Explanation: The prevalence of depressive disorder has been estimated to be around 20%. Depressive symptoms usually precede motor symptoms in 30% of cases. Psychiatrists should focus on low mood, irritability, pessimism and suicidal thoughts when assessing depression in patients with Parkinson disease depression. With regard to treatment, it is always essential to exclude underlying organic causes such as hypothyroidism. It is essential to optimize treatment of motor symptoms. SSRI has been considered to be the first-line treatment for depression in Parkinson's disease. Tricyclic antidepressants should be avoided as they cause confusion and cognitive impairment. In the event that SSRI and bupropion fail, psychiatrists should consider electroconvulsive therapy (ECT). ECT can also cause transient improvement in motor symptoms.

Current research studies have suggested that the choice of an antidepressant should be based mainly on the comorbidities and the unique characteristics of each patient. Antidepressants of choice include citalopram, sertraline, bupropion and venlafaxine. As a result, bupropion is not contraindicated in treating depression for patients suffering from Parkinson's disease.

References: Puri BK, Hall AD, Ho RC (2014). *Revision Notes in Psychiatry*. Boca Raton, FL: CRC Press, p. 489; Costa FH, Rosso Al, Maultasch H, Nicaretta DH, Vincent MB (2012). Depression in Parkinson's disease: Diagnosis and treatment. *Arq Neuropsiquiatr*, 70(8): 617–620; Raskin S, Durst R (2010). Bupropion as the treatment of choice in depression associated with Parkinson's disease and it's various treatment. *Med Hypotheses*, 75(6): 544–546.

Question 19 Answer: d, Parental criminality

Explanation: Juvenile delinquency is defined as law-breaking behaviour by 10- to 20-year-old people. The aetiology is multifactorial and is not associated with an established psychiatric disorder. Factors associated with the development of delinquency include unsatisfactory child rearing, low IQ, conduct disorder in childhood, parental criminality and large family size. Factors that may improve the prognosis with respect to adult criminality include establishing good relationship with a parent or counsellor, improvement in the home environment, good experience in school, good peers, successful employment and good marital relationship between parents. Approximately 50% will have stopped their delinquent behaviour by the age of 19.

Reference: Puri BK, Hall AD, Ho RC (2014). *Revision Notes in Psychiatry*. Boca Raton, FL: CRC Press, p. 723.

Question 20 Answer: b, History of past violence

Explanation: A history of past violence is the best predictor of future violence. Other predictors of violence include history of misuse of substances or alcohol; previous expression of intent to harm others; previous use of weapons; previous dangerous impulsive acts; denial of previous established dangerous acts; antisocial, explosive or impulsive personality traits or disorders and active symptoms of schizophrenia or mania, in particular, delusions or hallucinations focused on particular person, command hallucination, preoccupation with violent ideas, delusion of control (particularly with violent theme), agitation, overt hostility and suspiciousness.

Reference: Puri BK, Hall AD, Ho RC (2014). *Revision Notes in Psychiatry*. Boca Raton, FL: CRC Press, p. 725.

Question 21 Answer: a, Relationship difficulties with parents

Explanation: Previous analysis of the data collated of attempted suicide between the years of 1976 and 1993 has demonstrated that the most frequent problems for 16-year-olds are mainly due to relationship difficulties with parents. This is closely followed by relationship difficulties with friends, school and social isolation. The previous study highlights that only a minority of the individuals sampled has had a previous psychiatric diagnosis. In addition, only a minority has had a psychiatric diagnosis and has had previous treatment.

Reference: Hawton K, et al. (1996). Deliberate self-poisoning and self-injury in children and adolescents under 16 years of age in Oxford, 1976–1993. *Br J Psychiatry*, 169: 202–208.

Question 22 Answer: e, Striatum

Explanation: Recent research has demonstrated that there is an association between the alleles rs167771 single nucleotide polymorphism and the volume of striatal nucleus. It has been demonstrated that greater caudate nucleus volume correlated with stereotyped behaviour.

Reference: Staal WG, Langen M, van Dijk S, Mensen VT, Duston S (2015). DDR3 gene and striatum in autism spectrum disorder. *Br J Psychiatry*, May; 206(5): 431–2.

Question 23 Answer: d, Multimodal therapy

Explanation: Multimodal therapy is highly indicated for the treatment of children with conduct-related disorders. The National Institute for Health and Care Excellence (NICE) guidance also recommends parent management training. In addition, other modalities of therapy that might be helpful include family therapy, individual psychotherapy and environmental interventions.

References: Puri BK, Hall AD, Ho RC (2014). *Revision Notes in Psychiatry*. Boca Raton, FL: CRC Press, p. 639; Moretti MM et al. (1997). The treatment of conduct disorder: Perspectives from across Canada. *Can J Psychiatry*, 42(6): 637–648.

Question 24 Answer: c, There is a weak association between suicidality and obsessive-compulsive disorder (OCD).

Explanation: OCD has a bimodal age of onset with peaks occurring between 12–14 and 20–22 years. Previous studies have highlighted that approximately 3% of adults and children are affected by this condition. It is true that the relief of the anxiety helps to bring about the vicious obsessive-compulsive cycle. Symptoms could range from mild-to-life-threatening symptoms. Previous research has demonstrated that a high proportion of individuals does demonstrate suicidal behaviours. There is moderate to high, significant association between suicidality and OCD. Most patients, irrespective of symptoms, severity, respond to treatment with graded exposure or with serotonin reuptake inhibitors, but some continue with a chronic or chronic relapsing course requiring ongoing psychiatric input and specialist interventions.

References: Angelakis I, Gooding P, Tarrier N, Panagioti M. (2015). Suicidality in obsessive-compulsive disorder (OCD): A systematic review and meta-analysis. *Clin Psychol Rev*, 39: 1–15; Lynne D (2013). Obsessive-compulsive disorder – in 100 words. *Br J Psychiatry*, 203: 416.

Question 25 Answer: c, Suicide in schizophrenia usually occurs late into the illness.

Explanation: It is true that approximately 10% of schizophrenics do commit suicide, and they tend to do so early in the course of their illness. Suicide is more common in the young, in males and those who are unemployed and having chronic illness and who have once had high educational attainment. Those who are recently discharged from the inpatient care are also at risk. Violence in schizophrenics is uncommon, but they tend to be at higher risk compared with that of the general population. The prevalence of recent aggressive behaviour amongst outpatients is 5%. Verbal aggression is the commonest type of aggression, amounting to 45% of all aggression.

Reference: Puri BK, Hall AD, Ho RC (2014). *Revision Notes in Psychiatry*. Boca Raton, FL: CRC Press, p. 370.

Question 26 Answer: a, Cholinergic agent

Explanation: Recent research has demonstrated the clinical efficacy of addition of cholinergic medications. They are believed to be associated with marginal improvements in both verbal learning and memory, as well as bringing about moderate improvements in spatial learning and memory.

There is a current lack of evidence to demonstrate the clinical efficacy of glutamatergic and serotonergic medications for improving cognition.

Reference: Choi KH et al. (2013). Adjunctive pharmacotherapy for cognitive deficits in schizophrenia: Meta-analytical investigation of efficacy. *Br J Psychiatry*, 203: 172–178.

Question 27 Answer: e, Bipolar disorder
Explanation: Previous studies have found that ADHD in childhood and adolescence is associated with an increased risk of major depression and bipolar disorder in later life. Recent studies have demonstrated that adolescents and young adults who had major depression with ADHD comorbidity had an increased incidence of subsequent bipolar disorder (18.9% compared with 11.2%).

References: Larsson H et al. (2013). Risk of bipolar disorder and schizophrenia in relatives of people with attention-deficit hyperactivity disorder. *Br J Psychiatry*, 203: 103–106; Chen MH et al. (2015). Comorbidity of ADHD and subsequent bipolar disorder among adolescent and young adults with major depression: A nationwide longitudinal study. *Bipolar Disord*, 17(3): 315–322.

Question 28 Answer: e, Dependence is common in patients who continue methylphenidate long-term.
Explanation: Most patients do not develop dependence on methylphenidate if the stimulant is used over the long term. Electrocardiogram should be checked before prescribing methylphenidate and clonidine. Methylphenidate is also indicated for narcolepsy.

Reference: Semple D, Smyth R, Burns J, Darjee R, McIntosh (2005). *Oxford Handbook of Psychiatry*. Oxford, UK: Oxford University Press.

Question 29 Answer: b, Post-schizophrenia depression
Explanation: The most likely diagnosis is post-schizophrenia depression. Schizoaffective disorder is unlikely because she is free of psychotic features. Due to the background of schizophrenia, she cannot be diagnosed with reactive depression. Complication schizophrenia and schizophrenia with negative symptoms are not established diagnostic entities.

Reference: Puri BK, Hall AD, Ho RC (2014). *Revision Notes in Psychiatry*. Boca Raton, FL: CRC Press, p. 354.

Question 30 Answer: b, History of right-sided brain injuries
Explanation: There are biological as well as psychosocial factors predisposing an individual towards Parkinson's disease depression. Biological factors include having a family history of depression, history of left-brain injury (memory aide: 'nothing LEFT to live for' left-sided brain lesions are more likely to be associated

with depression), hypo-metabolism in striatal-thalamic-frontal circuits and low dopamine levels in the mesolimbic system. Psychosocial factors include psychiatric history of depression, presence of cognitive impairments and loss of functional independence.

Both apathy and depression are associated with poor cognition in patients with Parkinson's disease. On neuropsychological testing, patients with apathy and depression performed worse than controls, mainly on speed-based measures.

References: Puri BK, Hall AD, Ho RC (2014). *Revision Notes in Psychiatry*. Boca Raton, FL: CRC Press, p. 489; Cohen ML, Aita S, Mari Z, Brandt J (2015). The unique and combined effects of apathy and depression on cognition in Parkinson's disease. *J Parkinson Dis*, [Epub ahead of print].

Question 31 Answer: b, Obsessive-compulsive disorder
Explanation: The child has Prader–Willi syndrome, and the most common comorbidity is that of OCD.

Reference: Puri BK, Hall AD, Ho RC (2014). *Revision Notes in Psychiatry*. Boca Raton, FL: CRC Press, p. 675.

Question 32 Answer: b, 3%–5%
Explanation: People with learning disability have higher prevalence of schizophrenia, ranging from 3.7%–5.2%. The prevalence of schizophrenia is inversely related to IQ. Schizophrenia cannot be diagnosed reliably if IQ is less than 45. It is possible to make reliable diagnoses of early-onset schizophrenia in people with mental retardation, provided the assessment system is carefully structured and based on other important sources of information.

References: Puri BK, Hall AD, Ho RC (2014). *Revision Notes in Psychiatry*. Boca Raton, FL: CRC Press, p. 674; Vera A Morgan, et al. (2008). Intellectual disability co-occurring with schizophrenia and other psychiatric illness: Population-based study. *Br J Psych*, 193(5): 364–372.

Question 33 Answer: c, Monoamine oxidase A (MAO-A) promoter gene
Explanation: Previous studies have demonstrated that amongst those diagnosed with antisocial personality disorder, there are MAO-A and serotonergic dysregulation. Previous studies have demonstrated that there is a reduction in the expression of enolase gene (ENO2) in autistic children. Hypermethylation of the serotonin transporter (5HTT) gene has been associated with bipolar disorder.

References: Checknita D et al. (2015). Monoamine oxidase A gene promoter methylation and transcriptional downregulation in an offender population with antisocial personality disorder. *Br J Psychiatry*, 206(3): 216–222; Yu Wang et al. (2014). Hypermethylation of the enolase gene (ENO2) in autism. *Eur J Pediatrics*, 173(9): 1233–1244; Sugawara H et al. (2011). Hypermethylation of serotonin transporter gene in bipolar disorder detected by epigenome analysis of discordant monozygotic twins. *Transl Psychiatry*, 26(1): e24.

Question 34 Answer: c, 3%
Explanation: Depressive disorder affect between 10% and 15% of those who are over 65. Out of which, almost 3% suffer from major depressive disorder. First admissions for elderly woman admitting for affective illness peak at the age of 80 years and then fall off. The first admissions for elderly men continue to climb until the end of the life, overtaking women at the age of 85 years. It is of importance to recognize that the prevalence of depression falls with the advancing age. This might be because of a survivor effect with fewer depressed adults surviving to old age.

Reference: Puri BK, Hall AD, Ho RC (2014). *Revision Notes in Psychiatry*. Boca Raton, FL: CRC Press, p. 709.

Question 35 Answer: c, Representational role reversal
Explanation: There are two role reversal techniques: reciprocal and representational. The former is role reversal between the self and another person, and the latter is amongst objects, roles or parts of the self. Role reversal is used to gain information, understand the role of the other, heighten spontaneity and increase empathy. Cognitive restructuring and psychoeducation are components of cognitive behavioural therapy (CBT); free association is part of psychodynamic therapy, and systematic desensitization is a behavioural therapy technique.

References: International Association for the Study of Attachment (IASA). Introduction to Psychodrama Workshop for IASA Conference, Cambridge, 2010. Available at: www.iasa-dmm.org/images/uploads/Chip%20Chimera%20and%20Clark%20 Baim%20Workshop%20on%20Psychodrama.pdf; Puri BK, Treasaden I (eds) (2010). *Psychiatry: An Evidence-Based Text*. London: Hodder Arnold, pp. 934–946.

Question 36 Answer: b, Acting out
Explanation: Acting out is a less subtle form of resistance. Resistance represents a kind of retaliation in favour of the status quo and may take many forms both inside the therapeutic sessions and between them. Patients are said to 'act out' when, instead of disclosing their thoughts and feelings to their therapist, they respond to invitations to contact their inner feelings by enacting their conflicts and distress outside of therapeutic sessions. Acting out may take the form of dramatic appeals for help from other people and incidents of self-harm. It is also possible to enact distress, rather than articulating it, during therapeutic sessions, behaviour that is sometimes referred to as 'acting in'. Regression refers to the tendency, when placed under stress, to revert to ways of coping belonging to an earlier stage of life, for example, becoming more child-like and dependent on the therapist. Transference is an unconscious process in which the patient transfers to the therapist feelings, emotions and attitudes that were experienced and/or desired in the patient's childhood, usually in relation to parents and siblings.

Reference: Puri BK, Treasaden I (eds) (2010). *Psychiatry: An Evidence-Based Text*. London: Hodder Arnold, pp. 940, 948–949.

Question 37 Answer: e, It is a measure of the variability of the observations.
Explanation: The standard error of the mean (SEM), which is often shortened to standard error, is a measure of the precision of the sample mean as an estimate of the population mean. It is the SD of the sample mean. The more observations one sample has, the smaller the SEM will be – that is, the more likely it is that the sample mean reflects the true mean value of a parameter in the general population. SEM can be used to assess the sampling error by indicating how close a sample mean is to the population mean it is estimating. Option E refers to SD.

References: Lewis GH, Sheringham J, Kalim K, Crayford TJ (2008). *Mastering Public Health*. London: Royal Society of Medicine Press p. 81; Gosall N, Gosall G (2012). *The Doctor's Guide to Critical Appraisal*. Cheshire, UK: PasTest, pp. 117–119.

Question 38 Answer: c, Independent sample *t*-test is used to compare the effects of two drugs on a particular patient at different points in time.
Explanation: A student's *t*-test is any statistical hypothesis test that follows a student's *t* distribution if the null hypothesis is supported. It can be used to determine whether two sets of data are significantly different from each other and is most commonly applied when the test statistic would follow a normal distribution if the value of a scaling term in the test statistic were known. When the scaling term is unknown and is replaced by an estimate based on the data, the test statistic (under certain conditions) follows a student's *t* distribution. Student's *t*-test is used to compare the means of two samples. Student's *t*-test can be used when you have one nominal variable and one measurement variable, and you want to compare the mean values of the measurement variable. It assumes that the observations within each group are normally distributed, and the variances are equal in the two groups. A paired *t*-test is used to compare the effects of two drugs on a particular patient at different points in time.

Reference: Lewis GH, Sheringham J, Kalim K, Crayford TJ (2008). *Mastering Public Health*. London: Royal Society of Medicine Press, pp. 88–92.

Question 39 Answer: d, Snowball sampling
Explanation: Snowball sampling is a method of survey sample selection that is often used to locate rare or difficult-to-find populations. The procedure usually involves two stages: (i) identification of a sample of respondents with a particular characteristic and (ii) asking initial sample members to provide names of other potential sample members. Although this method is relatively low cost and often effective for locating hard-to-find individuals, little is known about the statistical properties of the resulting samples.

Reference: Everitt BS (2006). *Medical Statistics from A to Z* (2nd edition). Cambridge, UK: Cambridge University Press, p. 218.

Question 40 Answer: a, Constipation
Explanation: Tolerance for opioid is more pronounced for some effects than for others. Tolerance occurs slowly to the effects on mood, itching, urinary retention and respiratory depression but occurs more quickly than the analgesia and other

physical side effects. However, tolerance does not develop to constipation; thus, a laxative might be needed.

References: Collett BJ (1998). Opioid tolerance: The clinical perspective. *Br J Anaesth*, 81: 58–68; Puri BK, Treasaden I (eds) (2010). *Psychiatry: An Evidence-Based Text*. London: Hodder Arnold, pp. 877–878; McCarberg, B. (2013). Overview and treatment of opioid-induced constipation. *Postgraduate Medicine*, 125(4): 7–17.

Question 41 Answer: e, Lysergic acid diethylamide (LSD)
Explanation: LSD is a hallucinogen that is available in tablet form or absorbed on to paper. Minute amounts (≤100 μg) produce marked psychoactive effects. These peak at 2–4 hours and subside after 12 hours. It is taken orally. The onset of the 'trip' occurs very rapidly with oral ingestion (15 minutes). Tolerance develops rapidly, but sensitivity to its effects returns rapidly with abstinence. Psychological effects include the heightening of perceptions, with perceptual distortion of shape, intensification of colour and sound, apparent movement of stationary objects and changes in sense of time and place. Hallucinations may occur but are relatively rare. The user usually retains insight into the nature and the experiences. Physical withdrawal symptoms do not occur following the abrupt discontinuation of LSD. Withdrawal of stimulants may cause physical symptoms such as lethargy.

Reference and Further Reading: Puri BK, Hall AD, Ho RC (2014). *Revision Notes in Psychiatry*. Boca Raton, FL: CRC Press, p. 546; Puri BK, Treasaden I (eds) (2010). *Psychiatry: An Evidence-Based Text*. London: Hodder Arnold, pp. 1021–1046.

Question 42 Answer: e, Bupropion
Explanation: A recent meta-analysis of randomized controlled trials has indicated that bupropion is associated with a lower rate of treatment-emergent sexual dysfunction than usually seen with escitalopram, fluoxetine, paroxetine or sertraline.

In addition, the current evidence does suggests that antidepressants can be divided into high-risk (selective serotonin reuptake inhibitors, serotonin-norepinephrine reuptake inhibitors, tricyclic antidepressants and MAO inhibitors) and low-risk (agomelatine, bupropion, moclobemide and reboxetine) categories with regard to their potential for antidepressant-induced sexual dysfunction.

References: Baldwin DS, Thomas F (2013). Antidepressant drugs and sexual dysfunction. *Br J Psychiatry*, 202: 396–397; Keks NA, Hope J, Culhane C (2014). Management of antidepressant-induced sexual dysfunction. *Australas Psychiatry*, 22(6): 525–528.

Question 43 Answer: a, Premature delivery
Explanation: A recent study compared the offspring of mothers with schizophrenia who are exposed to first-generation antipsychotic with the offspring of mothers who were unexposed. It has been found that the offspring of those exposed are more susceptible towards premature delivery. Association has not been found for options B, C, D and E.

Reference: Lin Hc et al. (2010). Maternal schizophrenia and pregnancy outcome: Does the use of antipsychotics make a difference? *Schizophr Res,* 116: 55–60.

Question 44 Answer: b, Dopamine transporter (DAT1) gene
Explanation: It has been found that a polymorphism of the DAT-1 (10-repeat) is associated with hyperkinetic disorder, and this polymorphism has also been found to be associated with enhanced response to methylphenidate. One of the features of inattention in hyperkinetic disorder is that of a subtle left-sided inattention. This subtle sign has been found to be associated with the DAT-1 genotype. In a group of children with this DAT-1 allele, it has been demonstrated that methylphenidate is effective for them, as it helps to improve a DAT-1-induced hypodopaminergic state.

Reference: Bellgrove MA et al. (2005). Association between dopamine transporter (DAT-1) genotype, left-sided inattention and an enhanced response to methylphenidate in ADHD. *Neuropsychopharmacology*, 30: 2290–2297.

Question 45 Answer: d, Fluoxetine
Explanation: The condition that she has is restless leg syndrome. The DSM-5 states that, for the diagnosis to be made, it has to fulfil the following criteria: there must be an urge to move the leg as a result of unpleasant sensations, worsening of symptoms during rest and at night and no relief of the symptoms by movement. Very often, it is associated with underlying medical disorders such as autoimmune thyroid disorders and iron deficiency. Medications that help with the underlying disorders might bring relief to her symptoms. Other medications could be considered if the symptoms are impairing sleep for more than two nights per week. These medications include clonazepam, gabapentin and levodopa.

Recent research has suggested that restless leg syndrome is associated with enhanced risk of nocturnal hypertension, as well as cardiovascular events, and it has also a consequential effect on a patient's sleep. There are currently two major theories that have been developed with regard to the pathophysiology of this syndrome – the first concerns the central nervous system dopamine imbalance, and the second one concerns intracellular iron dysregulation.

References: Puri BK, Hall AD, Ho RC (2014). *Revision Notes in Psychiatry*. Boca Raton, FL: CRC Press, pp. 614–615; Einollahi B, Izadianmehr N (2014). Restlesss leg syndrome: A neglected diagnosis. *Nephrourol Mon*, 5;6(5): e22009.

Question 46 Answer: d, Paranoid personality disorder
Explanation: Apart from genetic factors that would predispose individuals towards schizophrenia, other factors such as personality do play a role. In a subset of paraphrenic patients, there is a history of those who have long-standing paranoid personalities, which are thought to predispose to the development of this condition in the older age.

Reference: Puri BK, Hall AD, Ho RC (2014). *Revision Notes in Psychiatry*. Boca Raton, FL: CRC Press, p. 708.

Question 47 Answer: b, Visual hallucinations
Explanation: Psychotic-like state results from acute or chronic ingestion. It leads to paranoia, hallucinations and sometimes a delirium-like state. The effect usually lasts for 3–4 days. In contrast to paranoid schizophrenia, amphetamine-induced psychosis is associated with visual hallucinations, appropriate affect, hyperactivity, hyper-sexuality and confusion. Thought disorder and alogia are not found in amphetamine-induced psychosis. It usually resolves with abstinence but may continue for some months. In the withdrawal state, the person will develop fatigue, hypersomnia, hyper-phagia, depression and nightmare.

Reference: Puri BK, Hall AD, Ho RC (2014). *Revision Notes in Psychiatry*. Boca Raton, FL: CRC Press, p. 538.

Question 48 Answer: e, Neither supervised injectable heroin treatment nor supervised injectable methadone treatment showed benefits over optimized oral methadone in health and social outcomes.
Explanation: Recent research demonstrated that supervised heroin treatment and supervised injectable methadone treatment did not differ in terms of outcomes compared with oral methadone. However, with treatment, there has been a reduction in the wider drug usage, crime, physical and mental health within a 6-month period. The rationale for the trial was that heroin addicts do persistently fail to benefit from conventional treatments. Hence, the trial was set out to compare the effectiveness of supervised injectable treatment with medical heroin against that of supervised injectable methadone, with further comparisons with optimized oral methadone.

Reference: Metrebian N, Groshkova T, Hellier J et al. (2015). Drug use, health and social outcomes of hard to treat heroin addicts receiving supervised injectable opiate treatment: Secondary outcomes from the Randomized Injectable Opioid Treatment Trial (RIOTT). *Addiction*, 110(3): 479–490.

Question 49 Answer: c, Number needed to treat (NNT) is the NNT to get one bad outcome.
Explanation: NNT is defined as the NNT to get one good outcome or prevent one additional adverse event by treatment. It is the reciprocal of the absolute risk reduction between two interventions. If the value of NNT is lower, it is better. The minimum value of NNT is 1, and the maximum value is infinity. NNTs are easy to interpret, but comparisons between them can only be made if the baseline risks are the same. There is no cutoff level for guidance. The number should be rounded up to the next whole number.

References: Lewis GH, Sheringham J, Kalim K, Crayford TJ (2008). *Mastering Public Health*. London: Royal Society of Medicine Press, p. 42; Gosall N, Gosall G (2012). *The Doctor's Guide to Critical Appraisal*. Cheshire, UK: PasTest, p. 97.

Question 50 Answer: a, They are not ideal for rare diseases/outcomes.
Explanation: Case–control studies are ideal for studying rare diseases/outcomes. They are also known as 'case comparison' or 'retrospective' studies. They are used

to investigate the causes of outcomes. They are particularly useful in situations where there is a long time period between exposure and outcome, as there is no waiting involved. Such studies are usually quick and cheap to do because few subjects are required, but it can be difficult to recruit a matching control group. There is also risk of recall bias, as subjects need to recall the risk factors to which they have been exposed. The temporal relationship between exposure and outcome can be difficult to establish.

References: Lewis GH, Sheringham J, Kalim K, Crayford TJ (2008). *Mastering Public Health*. London: Royal Society of Medicine Press Ltd, p. 53; Gosall N, Gosall G (2012). *The Doctor's Guide to Critical Appraisal*. Cheshire, UK: PasTest, p. 26.

Question 51 Answer: a, How well a category appears to describe an illness.
Explanation: Face validity is defined as the extent to which the test, on superficial consideration, measures what it is supposed to measure. Option B refers to reliability – how consistent a test is on repeated measurements; option C refers to predictive validity – the extent to which test is able to predict something it should theoretically be able to predict; option D refers to inter-rater reliability – measures the level of agreement between assessments made by two or more raters at the same time and option E refers to construct validity – the extent to which the test measures a theoretical construct by a specific measuring device or procedure.

References: Puri BK, Hall A, Ho R (2014). *Revision Notes in Psychiatry* (3rd edition). Boca-Raton, FL: CRC Press, p. 318; Gosall N, Gosall G (2012). *The Doctor's Guide to Critical Appraisal*. Cheshire, UK: PasTest, pp. 72–75.

Question 52 Answer: b, It indicates the internal consistency of the test.
Explanation: Cronbach's alpha gives a measure of the average correlation between all the items when assessing split-half reliability. If it is >0.5, there is moderate agreement and if it is >0.8, there is excellent agreement. It thereby indicates the internal consistency of the test. Option A is the definition of validity – the extent to which a test measures what it is supposed to measure; option C is the definition of predictive validity – the extent to which test is able to predict something it should theoretically be able to predict; option D is the definition of inter-rater reliability – measures the level of agreement between assessments made by two or more raters at the same time and option E is the definition of the kappa statistic – measures the level of agreement between assessments made by two or more raters at the same time where responses can fall into categories.

References: Puri BK, Hall A, Ho RC (2014). *Revision Notes in Psychiatry* (3rd edition). Boca-Raton, FL: CRC Press, pp. 316–318; Gosall N, Gosall G (2012). *The Doctor's Guide to Critical Appraisal*. Cheshire, UK: PasTest, pp. 74–75.

Question 53 Answer: a, Atrial fibrillation
Explanation: A prolonged QTc interval mainly affects the ventricles but not the atrium. Tosade de pointes is a form of irregular heartbeat that originates from the

ventricles and causes ventricular fibrillation. A prolonged QTc interval is also associated with palpitations, sudden cardiac death and ventricular fibrillation.

A recent review has compared the comparative cardiac effects of haloperidol against that of quetiapine. It has been suggested that haloperidol is associated with QTc prolongation more than that of quetiapine.

References: Howland RH. The comparative cardiac effects of haloperidol and quetiapine: Parsing a review. *J Psychosoc Nurs Ment Health Serv*, 52(6): 23–26; Howlan RH (2015). Psychiatric medications and sudden cardiac death: Putting the risk in perspective. *J Psychosoc Nurs Ment Health Serv*, 53(2): 34–35.

Question 54 Answer: e, Sleep disturbances
Explanation: With regard to the depressive symptoms, both young and old patients demonstrate sleep disturbances (such as frequent early morning awakening, frequent awakening and poor sleep quality). The common symptoms also include poor appetite and weight loss. The following features of depression are more common in the elderly: behavioural disturbances, complaints of loneliness, depressive pseudodementia, irritability and anger, loss of interest, psychomotor retardation and paranoid or delusional ideations.

Reference: Puri BK, Hall AD, Ho RC (2014). *Revision Notes in Psychiatry*. Boca Raton, FL: CRC Press, p. 710.

Question 55 Answer: b, Tricyclic antidepressants are absolutely contraindicated in old people.
Explanation: Newer antidepressants such as SSRIs and serotonin-norepinephrine reuptake inhibitors (SNRIs) are the treatment of choice, as they are better tolerated than the older tricyclic antidepressants. Old people tend to be sensitive and might develop hyponatraemia; hence, baseline laboratory tests should be done. Tricyclic antidepressants are not absolutely contraindicated, and some elderly patients do well with lofepramine. ECT remains to be the most effective treatment for depression and is the treatment of choice in those with life-threatening depression. Around two-thirds of patients who are resistant to first line therapy do well with lithium augmentation.

Reference: Puri BK, Hall AD, Ho RC (2014). *Revision Notes in Psychiatry*. Boca Raton, FL: CRC Press, p. 711.

Question 56 Answer: a, Female gender
Explanation: Seventy percent of elderly people with depression recover within a year, but around 20% of them would have a relapse. Only 10%–15% of elderly people are considered to have suffered from treatment-resistant depression. Chronicity in late-life depression is more common in the following: male gender, those with active medical illness or poor physical health, high severity and frequent episode of depression, atypical features of depression, history of dysthymia, delusions, cognitive impairments and morphological brain abnormalities.

Reference: Puri BK, Hall AD, Ho RC (2014). *Revision Notes in Psychiatry*. Boca Raton, FL: CRC Press, p. 711.

Question 57 Answer: b, Down syndrome

Explanation: Down syndrome is the most common cause of mental retardation, with the risk increasing with maternal age. It accounts for 30% of all children with mental retardation. The IQ of people with Down syndrome is between 40 and 45. IQ less than 50 is found in approximately 85% of cases. Verbal processing is better than auditory processing. In contrast, fragile X syndrome is the most common inherited cause of mental retardation. Women with fragile X syndrome suffer from mild learning disability, while men suffer from moderate-to-severe learning disability (in 80% of male patients, IQ is less than 70). Verbal IQ is better than performance IQ.

In addition, compared with other form of mental retardation, Down syndrome has been associated with increased prevalence of psychosis not otherwise specified (NOS) or depression with psychotic features.

References: Puri BK, Hall AD, Ho RC (2014). *Revision Notes in Psychiatry*. Boca Raton, FL: CRC Press, pp. 663–665; Dykens EM, Shah B, Davis B, Baker C, Fife T, Fitzpatrick J (2015). Psychiatric disorders in adolescents and young adults with Down syndrome and other intellectual disabilities. *J Neurodev Disord*, 7(1): 9.

Question 58 Answer: d, 60%

Explanation: People with Down syndrome are at higher risk of developing Alzheimer disease. Over the age of 40 years, there is a high incidence of neurofibrillary tangles and plaques in people with Down syndrome, with the increase in P300 latency. They are at higher risk of developing Alzheimer disease (36%–40% at 50–59 years and 55% at 60–69 years). Because people with Down syndrome live, on average, 55–60 years, they are more likely to develop younger-onset Alzheimer's disease (occurring before age 65) than older-onset Alzheimer's disease (occurring at age 65 or older).

Reference: Puri BK, Hall AD, Ho RC (2014). *Revision Notes in Psychiatry*. Boca Raton, FL: CRC Press, p. 665.

Question 59 Answer: b, Autosomal recessive

Explanation: Wilson disease is an autosomal-recessive disorder of copper metabolism in the liver. The incidence is 1 in 200,000. The gene responsible for the disorder has been located on chromosome 13 and encodes a copper-binding, membrane-spanning protein with ATPase that regulates metal transport proteins. Pharmacological treatment does not involve the usage of antidepressant and antipsychotic. Pharmacological treatment usually includes D-penicillamine, an oral zinc. Liver transplantation is indicated for patients with fulminant hepatitis or advanced cirrhosis.

A recent case report has described a child with zinc deficiency as the main presenting symptoms of Wilson disease. This was confirmed genetically as there was found to be two mutations within the ATP7B gene and an increased amount of copper excretion.

References: Puri BK, Hall AD, Ho RC (2014). *Revision Notes in Psychiatry*. Boca Raton, FL: CRC Press, p. 475; Van Biervliet S, Kury S, De Bruyne R, Vanakker OM, Schmitt S, Vande Velde S, Blouin E, Bezieau S (2015). Clinical zinc deficiency as early presentation of Wilson disease. *J Pediatr Gastroenterol Nutr*, 60(4): 457–459.

Question 60 Answer: d, Interleukin-10 (IL-10)
Explanation: Acute stress and loneliness may increase the risk of coronary artery disease (CAD) through moderating inflammation and immune activation. Stress is associated with increase in natural killer cell counts in the circulation. Acute psychological stressor increases proinflamatory cytokines including mononuclear cell IL-1β gene expression and plasma IL-6. IL-10 is an anti-inflammatory cytokine and is less likely to be involved in the pathogenesis between stress and CAD. Acute psychological stress also increases haemostatic factors such as the von Willebrand factors and fibrinogen. This will increase the risk of atherosclerosis.

After an acute myocardial infarction, major depression predicts mortality in the first 6 months. The impact of a depressive episode is equivalent to the impact of a previous infarct. Twenty percent of patients suffering from ischaemic heart disease (IHD) have comorbid depression, and major depressive disorder is an independent risk factor for IHD. Depression also affects compliance to cardiac treatment and causes autonomic disturbance due to underlying serotonin dysfunction addition; a recent study has demonstrated that depression is associated with a prolonged QTc interval, CAD and coronary vasospasm in female patients with chest pain. This may suggest a possible mechanism by which depressive mood may be in turn linked to coronary endothelial dysfunction and atherosclerosis.

References: Puri BK, Hall AD, Ho RC (2014). *Revision Notes in Psychiatry*. Boca Raton, FL: CRC Press, p. 472; Cho KI, Shim WJ, Park SM, Kim MA, Kim HL, Son JW, Hong KS (2015). Association of depression with coronary artery disease and QTc interval prolongation in women with chest pain: Data from the KoRean wOmen'S chest pain Registry study. *Physio Behav*, 1(143): 45–50; Ho RC, Neo LF, Chua AN, Cheak AA, Mak A (2010). Research on psychoneuroimmunology: Does stress influence immunity and cause coronary artery disease? *Ann Acad Med Singapore*, 39(3): 191–196.

Question 61 Answer: b, Patients with schizophrenia have higher rates of offending compared with the general population.
Explanation: Patients with schizophrenia have similar rates of offending compared with the general population. They are more likely to commit violent offences compared with the general population. There is an increased incidence of violence with comorbid substance use. They usually assault a known person, but if they assault a stranger, the arresting police officer is the most common target. The delusional ideas often motivate the violent behaviours, and the patients usually admit to experiencing command hallucinations after the violent offence. Those with negative symptoms commit violent offences inadvertently and neglectfully. However, violence in patients with schizophrenia is not always due to psychosis.

A recent study published by Witt et al. (2015) in the *British Journal of Psychiatry* has found that amongst patients with schizophrenia, criminal history factors most strongly associated with subsequent violence for both men and women were that of a previous conviction for a violent offence, assault, illegal threats, intimidation and imprisonment.

References: Puri BK, Hall AD, Ho RC (2014). *Revision Notes in Psychiatry*. Boca Raton, FL: CRC Press, p. 724; Witt K, Lichtenstein P, Fazel S (2015). Improving risk assessment in schizophrenia: Epidemiological investigation of criminal history factors. *Br J Psychiatry*, 5.

Question 62 Answer: b, Offending in epileptics is usually during the ictal phase of the illness.
Explanation: The prevalence of violence amongst patients with epilepsy can vary according to the definition of violent behaviour, epilepsy subtypes and the origin of the study population. For example, temporal lobe epilepsy has been reported to be related to a high rate of about 7% of violent acts. Offending in patients with epilepsis is rarely ictal. Most violent crimes take place during interictal periods, and diverse medical conditions, including inebriation, psychosis and low intelligence, are associated with violent crimes amongst patients with epilepsis. The increase in prevalence of epilepsy in prisoners (about two times that of the general population) is a result of common social and biological adversity leading to both epilepsy and crime.

References: Puri BK, Hall AD, Ho RC (2014). *Revision Notes in Psychiatry*. Boca Raton, FL: CRC Press, p. 724; Kim JM, Chu K, Jung KH, Lee ST, Choi SS et al. (2011). Characteristics of epilepsy patients who committed violent crimes: Report from the National Forensic Hospital. *J Epilepsy Res*, 30;1(1): 13–18.

Question 63 Answer: d, 50%
Explanation: The most common comorbid disorder is that of learning disability. Approximately 70% of children with autism have mental retardation, with 30% of them having mild-to-moderate mental retardation, and another 50% of them having severe-to-profound mental retardation. Other associated conditions are that of academic learning problems, as well as ADHD, OCD, tics or Tourette's syndrome, anxiety disorder and even depression.

Reference: Puri BK, Hall AD, Ho RC (2014). *Revision Notes in Psychiatry*. Boca Raton, FL: CRC Press, p. 627.

Question 64 Answer: e, Low testosterone
Explanation: Conduct disorder usually begins earlier in males (10–12 years) compared with girls (14–16 years). In terms of genetic factors, it has been previously shown that conduct disorder is associated with inheritance of antisocial traits from parents who demonstrate criminal behaviours. Biological factors that have been implicated include low plasma serotonin level, low plasma dopamine level, low cholesterol, excess testosterone, greater right frontal EEG activity, abnormal prefrontal cortex, history of head injury and neurological impairment.

Reference: Puri BK, Hall AD, Ho RC (2014). *Revision Notes in Psychiatry*. Boca Raton, FL: CRC Press, p. 635.

Question 65 Answer: e, Presence of first-rank symptoms
Explanation: The classical clinical features include odd affect, being withdrawn, being distracted by auditory hallucinations, being incompetent, confused, catatonic; or alternatively being elated, labile, rambling in speech, agitated or excessively active. Women with childbearing-related onset psychosis frequently experienced cognitive disorganization and unusual psychotic symptoms. These were often mood-incongruent delusions of reference, persecution, jealousy and grandiosity, along with visual, tactile or olfactory hallucinations that suggest an organic syndrome.

Reference: Dorothy SIT et al. (2006). A review of postpartum psychosis. *J Womens Health (Lachmt)*, 15(4): 352–368.

Question 66 Answer: c, Fire Setting
Explanation: Fire-associated crimes are common amongst individuals diagnosed with Asperger syndrome. A previous study done by Siponmaa et al. reported that approximately 63% of such crimes were committed by individuals with Asperger syndrome.

In addition, unique characteristics of these individuals would predispose them to forensic issues. Theory of mind deficits and a predilection for intense narrow interests, when coupled with deficient social awareness of salient interpersonal and social constraints on behaviour, can result in criminal acts.

References: Siponmaa L et al. (2001). Juvenile and young mentally disordered offenders: The role of child neuropsychiatric disorders. *J Am Acad Psychiatry Law*, 29: 420–426; Haskins BG, Silva JA (2006). Asperger's disorder and criminal behavior: Forensic-psychiatric considerations. *J Am Acad Psychiatry Law*, 34(3): 374–384.

Question 67 Answer: b, Two times increment
Explanation: There were four groups in the Multimodal Treatment Study. It includes medication only, psycho-education, combined reduction and psychosocial treatment and community control group. The four treatment groups demonstrated reduction in ADHD symptoms. The combined medication and psychosocial treatment group showed the most reduction in ADHD symptoms. The study also showed that children with ADHD continue to show higher than normal rates of delinquency (four times) and substance use (two times).

Reference: Puri BK, Hall AD, Ho RC (2014). *Revision Notes in Psychiatry*. Boca Raton, FL: CRC Press, p. 635.

Question 68 Answer: e, Venlafaxine
Explanation: The concurrent usage of tamoxifen with potent CYP2D6-inhibitor antidepressants paroxetine and fluoxetine is associated with a significant reduction in circulating endoxifen levels in some women. Based on current research, the psychotropic medications that are the strongest CYP2D6 inhibitors include

paroxetine, fluoxetine, bupropion, duloxetine, while sertraline, escitalopram and doxepin are moderate inhibitors, and venlafaxine is a weak inhibitor.

Venlafaxine has little or no effect on the metabolism of tamoxifen and hence may be considered the safest choice of antidepressants. Des-venlafaxine is not metabolized by the P450 system and hence may be considered to be another option.

References: Jin Y et al. (2005). CYP2D6 genotype, antidepressant use, and tamoxifen metabolism during adjuvant breast cancer treatment. *J Natl Cancer Inst*, 5;97(1): 30–39; Desmarais JE, Looper KJ (2009). Interactions between tamoxifen and antidepressants via cytochrome P450 2D6. *J Clin Psychiatry*, 70(12): 1688–1697.

Question 69 Answer: d, Reduction in suicidal ideations
Explanation: Khat is derived from a flowering plant from Africa and contains a monoamine alkaloid called cathinone, which is related to amphetamine. Hence, an acute ingestion of khat would cause symptoms such as excitement, loss of appetite and euphoria. The typical long-term effects include depression, infrequent hallucinations, impaired inhibition, diminished sexual drive, psychosis, increased risk of myocardial infarction and oral cancer. The usage is often associated with an increase in suicidal ideations.

References: Al-Mugahed L (2008). Khat chewing in Yemen: Turning over a new leaf: Khat chewing is on the rise in Yemen, raising concerns about the health and social consequences. *Bull World Health Organization*, 86(10): 741–742; Richard H et al. (2010). Khat use and neurobehavioral functions: Suggestions for future studies. *J Ethnopharmacol*, 132(3): 554–563.

Question 70 Answer: e, The multiple endocrine neoplasia type 1 (MEN 1) syndrome involves parathyroid tumour, pituitary adenoma and phaeochromocytoma.
Explanation: MEN 1 syndrome involves hyperparathyroidism, pituitary adenoma and pancreatic islet cell tumour.

Reference: Marini F, Falchetti A, Del Monte F, Carbonell Sala S et al. (2006). Multiple endocrine neoplasia type 1. *Orphanet Journal of Rare Diseases*, 1:38.

Question 71 Answer: a, It refers to predictive and concurrent validity together.
Explanation: Criterion validity is used to demonstrate the accuracy of a measure or procedure by comparing it with another measure or procedure that has been demonstrated to be valid. It refers to predictive and concurrent validity together. Predictive validity is the extent to which test is able to predict something it should theoretically be able to predict. Concurrent validity is the extent to which the test correlates with a measure that has been previously validated.

References: Puri BK, Hall A, Ho R (2014). *Revision Notes in Psychiatry* (3rd edition). Boca-Raton, FL: CRC Press, p. 318; Gosall N, Gosall G (2012). *The Doctor's Guide to Critical Appraisal*. Cheshire, UK: PasTest, pp. 72–73.

Question 72 Answer: e, Cluster randomization

Explanation: Cluster trials using cluster randomization techniques are often used to prevent contamination between intervention and control groups. Cluster trials are usually very much larger than individually randomized trials and can be susceptible to recruitment bias. The problem of contamination could be overcome if the sample size is increased.

Reference: David JT (2001). Contamination in trials: Is cluster randomization the answer? *BMJ*, 322(7282): 355–357.

Question 73 Answer: d, Meta-analysis

Explanation: Figure 1.1 is a forest plot and reports the odd ratio to develop attention deficit and hyperactivity in people suffering from Internet addiction (IA) compared with healthy controls. Forest plot is produced by meta-analysis, and it demonstrates the pooled effect size after combining data from different studies. Cochrane review performs meta-analyses only related to intervention. This forest plot does not evaluate any intervention, and it would not be published by Cochrane review. Data-mining, qualitative study and systemic review do not produce a forest plot.

Question 74 Answer: e, Yen et al. (2009)

Explanation: In the forest plot, the size of the square is proportional to the sample size. On inspection, the study by Yen et al. (2009) has the largest square, and the sample size is estimated to be the largest amongst all studies. The actual sample size is listed as follows: Ko et al. (2008) = 216 participants, Ko et al. (2009) = 1,848 participants, Yoo et al. (2004) = 535 participants and Yen et al. (2009) = 2,619 participants.

Question 75 Answer: d, (The number of IA participants with ADHD times the number of controls without ADHD)/(The number of controls with ADHD times the number of IA without ADHD).

Explanation: The candidate should construct the following table before answering the question.

	IA	Controls
ADHD	A	B
No ADHD	C	D

Odds ratio = (A times D)/(B times C), which means that (The number of IA participants with ADHD times the number of controls without ADHD)/(The number of controls with ADHD times the number of IA without ADHD).

Question 76 Answer: c, 95% confidence interval (CI) of the odds ratio

Explanation: The horizontal line represents 95% CI (1.759–6.117) of the odds ratio (3.280) in the study conducted by Yoo et al. (2009).

Question 77 Answer: b, There is no heterogeneity.

Explanation: The candidate can assess heterogeneity in the forest plot by drawing a line to check whether it can intersect each of the 95% confidence. If yes, there is no heterogeneity. If not, there is potential heterogeneity at a statistically significant level. The candidate cannot decide on the level of heterogeneity by looking at the forest plot. The level of between-study heterogeneity is assessed with the I^2 statistic (not shown in the forest plot), which describes the percentage of variability amongst effect estimates beyond that expected by chance. As a reference, I^2 value of 25% is considered low, 50% moderate and 75% high heterogeneity.

Reference: Ho RC, Zhang MW, Tsang TY, Toh AH, Pan F, Lu Y, Cheng C, Yip PS, Lam LT, Lai CM, Watanabe H, Mak KK (2014). The association between Internet addiction and psychiatric co-morbidity: A meta-analysis. *BMC Psychiatry*, 20(14): 183.

Question 78 Answer: d, People suffering from IA are more likely to develop ADHD compared with controls.
Explanation: The lower part of Figure F shows that the odds of developing ADHD favour the IA group. The odds ratio is 2.847 (95% CI = 2.147–3.774, $p < 0.001$). The forest plot does not state IA favours the ADHD group. As a result, option B is incorrect.

Question 79 Answer: b, Blurting things out without censoring them.
Explanation: No matter how willing and co-operative the patient may be consciously in attempting to free associate, the signs of resistance are apparent throughout the course of every analysis. Signs of resistance in psychotherapy include abrupt pausing, correcting themselves, remaining silent, asking unrelated questions, intellectualizing things, fidgeting, being late for appointments, finding excuses for not keeping appointments, offering critical evaluations of the rationale underlying the treatment method and censoring thoughts and ideas. Resistance tends to emerge more in the middle phase of the analysis, in which regressive emergence of the transference is a central concern.

Reference: Sadock BJ, Sadock VA, Ruiz P et al. (2009). *Kaplan and Sadock's Comprehensive Textbook of Psychiatry* (9th edition). Philadelphia, PA: Lippincott Williams & Wilkins, pp. 835–836.

Question 80 Answer: a, Anticipation
Explanation: Psychological defence mechanisms can be grouped hierarchically according to the relative degree of maturity associated with them. Narcissistic defences are the most primitive and appear in children and persons who are psychologically disturbed. Immature defences are seen in adolescents and some nonpsychotic patients. Neurotic defences are encountered in obsessive-compulsive and hysterical patients as well as in adults under stress. Mature defence mechanisms include altruism (using constructive and instinctually gratifying service to others to undergo a vicarious experience), anticipation (realistically anticipating or planning for future inner discomfort), humour (using comedy to overtly express feelings and thoughts without personal discomfort or immobilization and without producing an unpleasant effect on others), sublimation (achieving impulse gratification and the retention of goals but altering a socially objectionable aim or object to a socially acceptable one) and asceticism (eliminating the pleasurable effects of experiences).

Reference: Sadock BJ, Sadock VA (2003). *Kaplan and Sadock's Synopsis of Psychiatry* (9th edition). Philadelphia, PA: Lippincott Williams & Wilkins, pp. 205–208.

Question 81 Answer: c, Memory deficits are often reported by others.
Explanation: The onset of pseudo-dementia is usually acute. There is the presence of the lack of motivation and attempt to answer questions. Individuals usually give the answer 'I don't know' to the questions. Memory deficits are usually reported by the patients themselves, instead of their relatives and friends. Compared with dementia, there are intact arithmetic skills, paired associate learning and visual-spatial organization.

Current outcome studies and ongoing research have shown that cognitive deficits in cases of depression commonly cannot be full reversed, and it might indicate and signify the presence of an underlying progressive dementing disorder.

References: Puri BK, Hall AD, Ho RC (2014). *Revision Notes in Psychiatry*. Boca Raton, FL: CRC Press, p. 710; Snowdon J (2011). Pseudodementia, a term for its time: The impact of Leslie Kiloh's 1961 paper. *Australas Psychiatry*, 19(5): 391–397.

Question 82 Answer: a, Rapid flight of idea
Explanation: Elderly patients with mania tend not to show flight of ideas. They may have slow flight of ideas. Other common clinical features include speech being more circumstantial and less disorganized, more paranoid delusions, less hyper-activity, more cognitive impairment, irritability instead of euphoria and mixed affective states. They are also noted to have longer duration and higher frequency of acute episodes and the presence of neurological abnormalities, especially in elderly men with mania.

Reference: Puri BK, Hall AD, Ho RC (2014). *Revision Notes in Psychiatry*. Boca Raton, FL: CRC Press, p. 712.

Question 83 Answer: e, Lyonization
Explanation: Lyonization, also known as X-inactivation, is the process by which one of the two copies of the X chromosome present in the female is inactivated.

Reference: Jiang J, Jing Y, Gregory JC et al. (2013). Translating dosage compensation to trisomy 21. *Nature*, Aug 15:500(7462): 296–300.

Question 84 Answer: b, Hypertrophic feet
Explanation: Patients suffering from Rett syndrome usually have small hands and feet. Rett syndrome is predominantly a female disorder, but males with clinical features similar to Rett syndrome have been described. It involves mutation in the transcription regulatory gene methyl CpG binding protein 2 (MECP2) at chromo-some Xq28. The prevalence rate is between 1 in 15,000 and 1 in 22,000 females. The incidence of sudden and unexpected death is around 2%. Treatment involves anticonvulsant medication for seizure control, behaviour therapy to control self-injurious behaviour and physiotherapy to prevent muscular dysfunction and regulate breathing.

In addition, current research findings suggest that early truncating mutations or large deletions are usually associated with much greater severity. Early regression was also associated with a more severe disorder. All three are associated with lower current abilities. Epilepsy and weight, gastrointestinal and bowel problems have been known to be common comorbidities. Participants with classic variant also tend to have greater health-related problems compared with those with atypical variant.

References: Puri BK, Hall AD, Ho RC (2014). *Revision Notes in Psychiatry*. Boca Raton, FL: CRC Press, pp. 629–630; Clanfaglione R, Clarke A, Kerr M, Hastings RP, Oliver C, Felce D (2015). A national survey of Rett syndrome: Age, clinical characteristics, current abilities and health. *Am J Med Genet A*, Mar 28.

Question 85 Answer: c, Depression and post-traumatic stress
Explanation: Lange et al. (2014) reported that the combination depression and post-traumatic stress were most strongly associated with post-concussion symptoms compared with combination of other factors including severity of body injury and injury that occurred during military operation.

Post-concussion symptoms are common after a head injury and the prevalence rate of 50% after 2 months of head injury and 12% after 1 year of head injury. Depression and anxiety conditions are common as well. Secondary mania occurs in 9% of head injury victims. Schizophreniform disorder occurs in 2.5% of head injury victims. Paranoid psychosis occurs in 2%, and psychotic depression occurs in 1% of head injury victims.

References: Silverberg ND, Gardner AJ, Brubacher JR, Panenka WJ, Li JJ, Iverson GL (2015). Systematic review of multivariable prognostic models for mild traumatic brain injury. *J Neurotrauma*, 32(8): 517–526; Puri BK, Hall AD, Ho RC (2014). *Revision Notes in Psychiatry*. Boca Raton, FL: CRC Press, p. 498.

Question 86 Answer: a, 1%
Explanation: In the United Kingdom, the rate of deliberate self-harm (DSH) is raised, especially amongst Asian women. A history of DSH is a long-term predictor of suicide, and the risk of suicide is 100 times greater than that of the general population. One percent of patients eventually kill themselves in the year following the DSH. Approximately, 3%–5% of patients kill themselves in 5–10 years following DSH.

Reference: Puri BK, Hall AD, Ho RC (2014). *Revision Notes in Psychiatry*. Boca Raton, FL: CRC Press, p. 289.

Question 87 Answer: e, Testosterone
Explanation: The aim of pharmacological treatment of sex offenders is to reduce sexual libido and thus prevent future sexual offences, especially in sex offenders who have failed to respond to psychological treatment, including a Sex Offender Treatment Programme (SOTP). Cyproterone and medroxyprogesterone are antilibidinal and can be used to reduce sexual drive. Cyproterone is a testosterone antagonist. It is contraindicated in patients with chronic liver disease and thromboembolic diseases. Medroxyprogesterone provides negative feedback inhibition to the production of

follicle-stimulating hormone (FSH) and luteinizing hormone (LH), thus reducing testerone production. It is also contraindicated in patients suffering from chronic liver disease and thromboembolic disorders. SSRIs are also effective in the management of sex offenders where preoccupation and rumination over paraphilic behaviour are apparent.

Reference: Puri BK, Hall AD, Ho RC (2014). *Revision Notes in Psychiatry*. Boca Raton, FL: CRC Press, pp. 607–608.

Question 88 Answer: b, Sociopathic rapist
Explanation: Option (b) is correct. Usually these individuals tend to have poor social adjustment with criminality, poor work record, have previously used substances and have unstable relationships. For them, rape is often impulsive with immediate gratification and little regard to the consequences. Threats of violence are common.

Reference: Puri BK, Hall AD, Ho RC (2014). *Revision Notes in Psychiatry*. Boca Raton, FL: CRC Press, p. 606.

Question 89 Answer: c, 8 years of age
Explanation: Based on the Isle of Wight study, the prevalence of ODD has been estimated to be between 6% and 16%. The age of onset of ODD is usually before the age of 8 years. This differs from that of conduct disorder: the age of onset of conduct disorder begins earlier in boys (10–12 years) compared with girls (14–16 years). Approximately, 5%–10% of children suffer from problems that result from a mixture of ODD and conduct disorder.

Reference: Puri BK, Hall AD, Ho RC (2014). *Revision Notes in Psychiatry*. Boca Raton, FL: CRC Press, p. 635.

Question 90 Answer: d, Risperidone
Explanation: For conduct disorder, aggression and conduct problems are a major source of disability and are risk factors predisposing towards poor longer-term outcomes. Previous systematic review and meta-analysis have evaluated randomized controlled trials with regard to the usage of antipsychotics as well as anticonvulsants. Of note, only risperidone has been supported by current evidences to be effective.

Reference: Pringsheim T et al. (2015). The pharmacological management of oppositional behaviour, conduct problems, and aggression in children and adolescents with attention-deficit hyperactivity disorder, oppositional defiant disorder, and conduct disorder: A systematic review and meta-analysis. Part 2: Antipsychotics and traditional mood stabilizers. *Can J Psychiatry*, 60(2): 52–61.

Question 91 Answer: e, Language delay
Explanation: Young people with Asperger's syndrome usually do not have language delay.

Further Reading: Puri BK, Treasaden I (eds.) (2010). *Psychiatry: An Evidence-Based Text*, London: Hodder Arnold, p. 1099.

Question 92 Answer: b, Predominance of phobic ruminative ideas, with the absence of compulsions.
Explanation: Option (b) is actually a favourable prognostic factor. Other favourable prognostic factors include mild symptoms, short duration of symptoms and no childhood symptoms or abnormal personality traits.

Reference: Puri BK, Hall AD, Ho RC (2014). *Revision Notes in Psychiatry*. Boca Raton, FL: CRC Press, p. 418.

Question 93 Answer: b, Middle social class
Explanation: Suicide accounts for approximately 1% of all deaths in the United Kingdom. The male-to-female gender ratio is 3:1, and the rate in women is rising. There is higher risk in the low and high social classes and lower risk in the middle social class. Suicide rates in the divorced and widowed are higher than that of people who are married. Unemployment, low socioeconomic status and certain occupations such as bar owners, doctors, pharmacists and farmers are risk factors. Suicide attempts occurring after significant life events are common amongst people with poor social support and living alone.

Reference: Puri BK, Hall AD, Ho RC (2014). *Revision Notes in Psychiatry*. Boca Raton, FL: CRC Press, p. 289.

Question 94 Answer: e, Tuberous sclerosis
Explanation: Tuberous sclerosis is an autosomal disorder with 100% penetrance. Clinical features include skin depigmentation that is especially noted under ultraviolet light, hypomelanotic macules, intractable epilepsy and tumours in the spleen, lungs and kidneys. Psychiatric features include autism (in 75% of cases), hyperactivity, impulsivity, aggression, self-injurious behaviours and sleep disturbance. Thirty percent of sufferers have a normal IQ. If learning disability is present, it is usually profound. The initial presentation is usually infantile spasms.

Recent research has found that the presence of severe, early onset epilepsy may impair intellectual development in this condition. Hence there needs to be early, prompt and effective treatment or the active prevention of epilepsy in patients with this condition.

References: Puri BK, Hall AD, Ho RC (2014). *Revision Notes in Psychiatry*. Boca Raton, FL: CRC Press, pp. 671–672; Bolton PF, Clifford M, Tye C et al. (2015 Apr). Intellectual abilities in tuberous sclerosis complex: Risk factors and correlates from the Tuberous Sclerosis 2000 study. *Psychol Med* 1: 1–11.

Question 95 Answer: b, 5%
Explanation: For the elderly population, the onset of the first manic episode is bimodal in distribution, with peaks at the age of 37 and also at the age of 73. Mania has been noted to be relatively uncommon in the elderly and comprises about 5% of all elderly psychiatric admissions.

Reference: Puri BK, Hall AD, Ho RC (2014). *Revision Notes in Psychiatry*. Boca Raton, FL: CRC Press, p. 711.

Question 96 Answer: d, Sudden removal of symptoms by suggestion under hypnosis can lead to rebound depression and anxiety.

Explanation: Hypnosis is not commonly used in psychiatry and currently not recommended in NICE guidelines. It is not found to be superior to other psychological treatments. It has been used, with varying degrees of success, to control obesity and substance-related disorders such as alcohol abuse and nicotine dependence. It has also been applied to managing pain, asthma, warts, pruritus, aphonia and conversion disorder. Patients in hypnotic trances can recall memories that are unavailable to consciousness in the non-hypnotic state. Clinicians should be aware that bringing repressed memory into consciousness quickly may be hazardous and may overwhelm the patient with anxiety.

Reference: Sadock BJ, Sadock VA (2003). *Kaplan and Sadock's Synopsis of Psychiatry* (9th edition). Philadelphia, PA: Lippincott Williams & Wilkins, p. 964.

Question 97 Answer: d, Student's *t*-test

Explanation: Student's *t*-test is a significance test used to compare the means of two independent different sample populations; often one group is the experimental group and the other is the control. It is a parametric test that assumes the samples are normally distributed. Paired *t*-test is used for matched studies (e.g. case–control trials and matched-pair randomized controlled trials). In *Z*-test, an observation from a population may be converted into a standard normal deviate (also called a *z*-score), which is the number of SDs that separates the observation from the mean of the population. In one-way analysis of variance (ANOVA), a sample of individuals from a number of different populations is compared with some outcome measure of interest. The total variance in the observations is partitioned into a part due to differences between the group means and a part due to differences between subjects in the same group. The results of this division are usually arranged in an ANOVA table.

Reference: Lewis GH, Sheringham J, Kalim K, Crayford TJ (2008). *Mastering Public Health: A Postgraduate Guide to Examination and Revalidation*. London: Royal Society of Medicine Press, pp. 89–91.

Question 98 Answer: e, Poor impulse control with persistent preoccupation with eating and an irresistible craving for food

Explanation: The main characteristic features of bulimia nervosa are that individuals have a persistent preoccupation with eating and an irresistible craving for good, with episodes of overeating in which large amounts of food are consumed in short periods. They make attempts to counteract the fattening effects of food by one or more of the following: self-induced vomiting, purgative abuse, alternating periods of starvation and use of drugs. They also have a morbid dread of fatness. Patients set weight thresholds well below healthy weight. There is often a previous history of anorexia nervosa.

Reference: Puri BK, Hall AD, Ho RC (2014). *Revision Notes in Psychiatry*. Boca Raton, FL: CRC Press, p. 581.

Question 99 Answer: c, Crossover study

Explanation: A crossover study is a longitudinal study in which subjects are allocated to sequences of treatment with the purpose of studying differences between individual treatments. Random allocation is used to determine the order in which the treatments are received. They receive different treatments over the course of the study, so that all subjects will eventually receive all the same treatments. The analysis of such study design is complicated by the possible presence of carry-over effects – the results from a given period for a given patient may reflect not only the effect of the current treatment but also the effect of the previous treatment.

Reference: Everitt BS (2006). *Medical Statistics from A to Z* (2nd edition). Cambridge, UK: Cambridge University Press, p. 65.

Question 100 Answer: e, Duloxetine

Explanation: Based on the current literature, all the above medications are indicated, with the exception of (e). Indications for the usage of non-stimulant include inability to tolerate side effects, unsatisfactory treatment responses to two types of stimulant, history of stimulant abuse and the presence of comorbid conditions.

Reference: Puri BK, Hall AD, Ho RC (2014). *Revision Notes in Psychiatry*. Boca Raton, FL: CRC Press, p. 633.

Question 101 Answer: d, 40%

Explanation: 40% of young people with conduct disorder develop dissocial personality disorder in adulthood. Borderline IQ, mental retardation and family history of dissocial personality disorder are predictive factors.

Reference: Puri BK, Hall AD, Ho RC (2014). *Revision Notes in Psychiatry*. Boca Raton, FL: CRC Press, p. 639.

Question 102 Answer: b, Depression

Explanation: Cushing syndrome is most commonly caused by exogenous administration of corticosteroids. Other causes include adrenocorticotropic hormone (ACTH) dependent, ectopic ACTH-producing tumours, non-ACTH dependent and alcohol-dependent pseudo-Cushing syndrome. Approximately 50%–80% of patients suffer from depression with moderate-to-severe symptoms. Depression will usually resolve with control of the underlying medical condition. Cognitive impairment such as amnesia and attentional deficit is common.

Reference: Puri BK, Hall AD, Ho RC (2014). *Revision Notes in Psychiatry*. Boca Raton, FL: CRC Press, p. 476.

Question 103 Answer: c, Mild-to-moderate learning disability

Explanation: The prevalence of Cornelia De Lang syndrome is 1 in 40,000 to 1 in 100,000, with equal prevalence in both sexes. It is due to mutations on chromosome 5p, the production of plasma protein A (PAPPA) and is associated with infertility. Patients with Cornelia De Lange syndrome have severe-to-profound learning disability, feeding difficulties, stereotypic movements, microcephaly and short stature. Psychiatric features include autistic behaviour, self-injury, language delays, limited speech in severe cases, feeding difficulties, avoidance of being held, stereotypic movements, temper tantrums and mood disorders.

Reference: Puri BK, Hall AD, Ho RC (2014). *Revision Notes in Psychiatry*. Boca Raton, FL: CRC Press, p. 679.

Question 104 Answer: e, Violence Risk Appraisal Guide (VRAG)
Explanation: VRAG is an actuarial violence risk assessment tool and does not predict sex offender recidivism. Sexual offender recidivism is best predicted by either static or highly stable dynamic factors. The strongest predictors of risk are related to deviant sexual interests and victim choices, such as boys and strangers. The risk of recidivism is increased for offenders who have committed prior sexual offences, engaged in a range of sexual crimes and began offending sexually at a young age.

References: Hanson RK, Thornton D (2000). Improving risk assessments for sex offenders: A comparison of three actuarial scales. *Law Hum Behav*, 24: 119–136; Hanson RK, Bussière MT (1998). Predicting relapse: A meta-analysis of sexual offender recidivism studies. *J Consulting Clin Stud*, 66: 2.

Question 105 Answer: e, 600 mg/day
Explanation: P rior to the commencement of treatment, the old-age psychiatrist needs to check the potential drug interactions from existing medications such as diuretic and non-steroidal anti-inflammatory drugs (NSAIDs). Treatment is usually with lithium and antipsychotics. Lithium should be started at 150 mg daily, especially if the old person is frail, and the total dose is increased by 150 mg per week. The maximum total daily dose is recommended to be 600 mg/day. The blood lithium level is aimed between 0.6 and 0.9 mmol/L during acute mania and between 0.4 and 0.6 mmol/L during maintenance treatment.

Reference: Puri BK, Hall AD, Ho RC (2014). *Revision Notes in Psychiatry*. Boca Raton, FL: CRC Press, p. 712.

Question 106 Answer: a, Eclectic family therapy
Explanation: Eclectic family therapy concentrates on the present situation of the family and examines how family members communicate with one another. It is flexible and allows time for the family to work together on problems raised in the treatment. It is commonly used for adolescents and their families. The goals of family therapy include to resolve or reduce pathogenic conflict and anxiety within the matrix of interpersonal relationships, to enhance the perception and fulfilment by family members of one another's emotional needs, to promote appropriate role relationships between the sexes and generations, to strengthen the capacity of individual members and the family as a whole to cope with destructive forces inside and outside the surrounding environment and to influence family identity and values so that members are oriented towards health and growth.

Reference: Sadock BJ, Sadock VA (2003). *Kaplan and Sadock's Synopsis of Psychiatry* (9th edition). Philadelphia, PA: Lippincott Williams & Wilkins, pp. 941–946.

Question 107 Answer: b, Naltrexone

Explanation: A previous study, involving a total of 169 alcohol-dependent subjects, demonstrated the efficacy of naltrexone compared with acamprosate for patients whose craving was high. Acamprosate, only when in combination with counselling, may also be helpful in maintaining abstinence. It should be started as soon as possible after the achievement of abstinence. It should be maintained if a relapse occurs. For patients on acamprosate, they are allowed to have only one relapse.

Recent research has found that patients receiving the extended-release version of naltrexone tend to have longer duration of staying well and were more likely to be abstinent, compared with oral naltrexone and other medications and psychosocial treatment.

References: Richardson K et al. (2008). Do acamprosate or naltrexone have an effect on daily drinking by reducing craving for alcohol? *Addiction*, 103(6): 953–959; Crits-Christoph P, Lundy C, Stringer M, Gallop R, Gastfriend DR (2015). Extended-release naltrexone for alcohol and opioid problems in Missouri parolees and probationers. *J Subst Abuse Treat*, Mar 25.

Question 108 Answer: c, Cocaine

Explanation: Cocaine is a psychostimulant, which produces an intense euphoric state and may be accompanied by confusion, convulsions and cardiovascular problems. Acute psychotic episodes are a relatively common psychiatric presentation. Use of stimulants may lead to exhaustion, depression and weight loss. A paranoid or confused state may also occur. Hypertension, cardiac arrhythmias, stroke, hepatic and renal damage and abscesses can result from heavy use, especially if the drug is injected. Violent and aggressive behaviour may ensue. Snorting cocaine leads to nasal septal perforation and damage to the nasal passages.

Reference: Puri BK, Treasaden I (eds) (2010). *Psychiatry: An Evidence-Based Text*. London: Hodder Arnold, pp. 1021–1046.

Question 109 Answer: c, Repression

Explanation: Repression, isolation and displacement are defence mechanisms commonly associated with phobias. Repression is the pushing away of unacceptable ideas, affects, emotions, memories and drives, relegating them to the unconscious. When successful, no trace remains in the consciousness, but some affective excitation does remain. In isolation, thoughts, affects and behaviours are isolated so that their links with other thoughts or memories are broken. Isolation is a defence mechanism found in OCD. For displacement, emotions, ideas and wishes are transferred from their original object to a less threatening substitute.

Reference: Puri BK, Hall AD, Ho RC (2014). *Revision Notes in Psychiatry*. Boca Raton, FL: CRC Press, pp. 136–137, 336.

Question 110 Answer: c, Fluoxetine

Explanation: SSRIs do not need to be discontinued before the administration of ECT. Bupropion and clozapine may increase the risk of prolonged seizures. Lithium may increase the risk of delirium or prolonged seizures. Benzodiazepine has anticonvulsant activity and may decrease the efficacy of ECT. If there is a need for benzodiazepine before ECT, choose a short-acting benzodiazepine such as alprazolam and lorazepam.

Reference: Steffens DC, Blazer DG, Busse EW (2004). *The American Psychiatric Publishing Textbook of Geriatric Psychiatry* (3rd edition). Arlington, VA: American Psychiatric Press Inc., p. 421.

Question 111 Answer: b, Attention-deficit hyperactivity disorder

Explanation: Amongst a large number of existing neurotransmitter systems, serotonin system dysfunction has been implicated in many psychiatric disorders; the therapeutic efficacy of many drugs is also thought to be based on modulation of serotonin. 5HTT gene polymorphism is one of the most extensively studied polymorphisms in psychiatric behavioural genetics. Strong evidence supports the roles of 5HTT gene polymorphism in the following psychiatric disorders: mood disorders, post-traumatic stress disorder, suicide, OCD and autism. ADHD has not been found to be associated with 5HTT gene polymorphism.

Reference: Margoob MA, Mushtaq D (2011). Serotonin transporter gene polymorphism and psychiatric disorders: Is there a link? *Indian J Psychiatry*, 53(4): 289–299.

Question 112 Answer: b, Basal ganglia

Explanation: Several researchers suggest that OCD may be the result of frontal lobe–limbic–basal ganglia dysfunction. Injury in the basal ganglia from brain injury tumours has been reported to be related to onset of OCD. Brain-imaging techniques show morphological changes of basal ganglia structures in OCD. Frontostriatal abnormality is present. Functional neuroimaging studies show increased blood flow in the basal ganglia and orbital, prefrontal and anterior cingulate cortex. Caudate metabolic rate is reduced after treatment with drugs or behavioural therapy in those responsive to treatment, with the percentage change in symptom severity correlating significantly with the change in metabolic rate in right caudate nucleus.

A recent meta-analysis published in the *British Journal of Psychiatry* pooled the data on serum and cerebrospinal fluid anti-basal ganglia antibody (ABGA) positivity and has determined that a significant greater proportion of those with primary OCD were noted to have ABGA positivity compared with that of controls.

References: Puri BK, Hall AD, Ho RC (2014). *Revision Notes in Psychiatry*. Boca Raton, FL: CRC Press, pp. 416–417; Pearlman DM, Vora HS, Marquis BG, Najjar S, Dudley LA (2014). Anti-basal ganglia antibodies in primary obsessive-compulsive disorder: Systematic review and meta-analysis. *Br J Psychiatry*, 205(1): 8–16.

Question 113 Answer: a, Case–control study
Explanation: A case–control study analyses an outcome (in this case schizophrenia) and looks back in time to assess exposure (in this case, cannabis). In this type of study, individuals with the outcome of interest (cases) are matched with individuals who do not have the outcome of interest (controls). The strengths of such study are that it is rapid and cheap and ideal for rare disease/outcomes; useful for diseases with long latent periods and can simultaneously examine a large number of potential exposures. The weaknesses are that it is prone to selection bias, temporal relationships may be difficult to establish, it is a poor method for rare exposures and it does not compare incidence rates.

Reference: Lewis GH, Sheringham J, Kalim K, Crayford TJ (2008). *Mastering Public Health: A Postgraduate Guide to Examination and Revalidation*. London: Royal Society of Medicine Press, p. 37.

Question 114 Answer: a, 8%
Explanation: The 1-year prevalence of somatoform pain disorder is 8%, and the lifetime prevalence is around 12.7%. This condition usually presents with persistent, severe, distressing pain, not explained by physical disorder. Pain occurs in association with emotional conflict and results in increased support and attention. The onset of somatoform pain disorder is usually between 40 and 50 years. The female-to-male ratio is 2:1. Acute pain is associated with anxiety disorder. Chronic pain (more than 6 months) is associated with depressive disorder. The onset of somatoform pain disorder is usually abrupt. Treatment involves antidepressants, gradual withdrawal of analgesics, CBT and relaxation techniques. In general, acute pain carries a better prognosis than chronic pain.

Reference: Puri BK, Hall AD, Ho RC (2014). *Revision Notes in Psychiatry*. Boca Raton, FL: CRC Press, p. 466.

Question 115 Answer: b, CBT is more effective than interpersonal psychotherapy (IPT).
Explanation: Studies have shown that CBT is more effective than IPT in treating people with depression and comorbid personality disorders. Patients higher on attachment avoidance show significantly greater reduction in depression severity and greater likelihood of symptom remission with CBT compared with IPT, even after controlling for OCD and avoidant personality disorder symptoms.

Reference: Eagle MN. Attachment as moderator of treatment outcome in major depression: A randomized control trial of interpersonal psychotherapy versus cognitive behavior therapy. *J Consult Clin Psychol*, 74: 1086–1097.

Question 116 Answer: a, Memory impairment
Explanation: It has been estimated that the cause in approximately 75% of cases of adrenocortical insufficiency is Addison disease. The female-to-male ratio has been estimated to be 2:1. Fatigue, weakness and apathy are common in the early stages. Ninety percent of patients with this condition present with psychiatric symptoms.

Memory impairment is considered to be the most common condition. Depression, anxiety and paranoia tend to have a fluctuating course with occasional symptom-free intervals. Psychosis occurs in 20% of patients. An adrenal crisis might lead to the onset of delirium.

Patients with adrenal insufficiency would need to replace the glucocorticoids and mineral corticoids, as both these receptors are highly expressed in the hippocampus and are closely associated with cognitive abilities.

References: Puri BK, Hall AD, Ho RC (2014). *Revision Notes in Psychiatry*. Boca Raton, FL: CRC Press, p. 477; Schultebraucks K, Wingenfeld K, Hemles J, Quinker M, Otte C (2015). Cognitive function in patients with primary adrenal insufficiency (Addison's disease). *Psychoneuroendocrinology*, 55: 1–7.

Extended-Matching Items

Theme: Adult Psychiatry – Personality Disorders

Question 117 Answer: g, Narcissistic personality disorder
Explanation: This is defined as a pervasive pattern of grandiosity, a need for admiration and lack of empathy, beginning by early adulthood and presenting in a variety of contexts. Diagnostic criteria are five or more of the following: grandiose sense of self-importance; fantasies of unlimited success, power, brilliance, beauty, or ideal love; beliefs that he or she is 'special' and unique and can only be understood by, or should associate with, other special or high-status people; requires excessive admiration; has a sense of entitlement; is interpersonally exploitative; lacks empathy; is often envious of others or believes others are envious of him or her and shows arrogant, haughty behaviours or attitudes.

Question 118 Answer: f, Histrionic personality disorder
Explanation: Histrionic personality disorder is characterized by at least three of the following: self-dramatization; theatricality; exaggerated expression of emotions; suggestibility; easily influenced by others or by circumstances; shallow and labile affectivity; continual seeking of excitement and activities in which the patient is the centre of attention; inappropriate seductiveness in appearance or behaviour and over-concern with physical attractiveness. The individual is egocentric, self-indulgent and longing for appreciation. They are manipulative and have their feelings easily hurt.

Question 119 Answer: e, Emotionally unstable personality disorder, borderline type
Explanation: There is emotional instability. Self-image, aims and internal preferences are often unclear or disturbed. There are chronic feelings of emptiness. Intense unstable relationships cause repeated emotional crises, and there are associated excessive efforts to avoid abandonment, such as suicide threats or deliberate self-harm.

References: Puri BK, Treasaden I (eds) (2010). *Psychiatry: An Evidence-Based Text*. London: Hodder Arnold, pp. 704–714; Puri BK, Hall AD, Ho RC (2014). *Revision Notes in Psychiatry*. Boca Raton, FL: CRC Press, pp. 437–458.

Theme: Psychotherapy

Question 120 Answer: b, Catharsis

Explanation: Yalom identified 11 therapeutic factors in group therapy, including universality, imitative behaviour and catharsis. The experience of finding that one is not a unique, irreparably damaged, repulsive or unworthy individual (universality) helps raise self-esteem. The shared expression of deep feeling (catharsis) and the realization that everyone is to some degree alone, will struggle in life and will die (existential factors) is especially poignant and meaningful in group psychotherapy. The other factors are altruism, instillation of hope, imparting information, corrective recapitulation of the primary family experience, development of socializing techniques, imitative behaviour, cohesiveness, existential factors, catharsis, interpersonal learning and self-understanding.

Question 121 Answer: f, Foulkes

Explanation: Foulkes propounded the clinical theory that fundamentally located the individual within group relationships: the social matrix. From Foulkes' perspective, there is no such thing as an abstract individual apart from his or her groups. The concepts of individual and group (society) are totally interrelated; they mutually constitute one another. Through cultural transmission, group norms are profoundly active inside individuals and make up their identities, moulding the forms of physical, temperament, emotional and behavioural expression.

Question 122 Answer: d, Dependency

Explanation: In 1961, Bion introduced two concepts. The basic assumption group refers to the set of assumptions underlying the behaviours of those in the group. This poses a threat to the group. In contrast, the work group is rational, purposeful and cooperative. Bion's three basic assumptions are dependency, fight–flight and pairing. These will lead to individual disappointment, pessimism and antagonism of therapist.

Reference: Puri BK, Hall AD, Ho RC (2014). *Revision Notes in Psychiatry*. Boca Raton, FL: CRC Press, pp. 973–983.

Theme: Research Methodology

Question 123 Answer: a, Continuous scale

Explanation: A continuous scale refers to data with no break in values and includes all possible data. It is a measurement not restricted to particular values, and this is restricted by the accuracy of the measuring instrument. Common examples include weight, height and blood pressure. For such a variable, equal-sized differences on different parts of the scale are equivalent.

Question 124 Answer: b, Interval scale

Explanation: An interval scale refers to a scale without an absolute zero. There are meaningful intervals between measurements, for example, age groups 0–4, 5–9, 10–14, …, 90+. It is typically displayed as a table or histogram.

Question 125 Answer: c, Norminal scale

Explanation: A nominal scale refers to classification of observations into unordered qualitative categories. Nominal data have no order and thus only give names or labels to various categories, for example, ABO blood group (A, B, AB, O), names of colour (red, yellow, pink, etc.) and types of hospital ward (surgery, medical, rehabilitation).

Question 126 Answer: e, Ratio scale

Explanation: A ratio scale is an interval scale with a true zero point. Ratio data are the most flexible data to work with, since they contain the most information of any data type. Ratio data are ideal for use as outcome variables in regression.

Question 127 Answer: d, Ordinal scale

Explanation: An ordinal scale refers to classification of data into ranked categories. Ordinal data have order, but the interval between measurements is not meaningful. Although ordinal data should not be used for calculations, it is not uncommon to find averages calculated from data collected of the type: strongly disagree, disagree, neither agree nor disagree, agree and strongly agree.

References: Everitt BS (2006). *Medical Statistics from A to Z* (2nd edition). Cambridge, UK: Cambridge University Press, p. 58; Lewis GH, Sheringham J, Kalim K, Crayford T JB. (2008). *Mastering Public Health: A Postgraduate Guide to Examination and Revalidation*. London: Royal Society of Medicine Press, p. 10.

Theme: Research Methodology

Question 128 Answer: g, Volunteer bias

Explanation: Volunteer bias occurs because those who agree to participate in the study tend to be both healthier and more compliant than those who do not. This is a type of selection bias.

Question 129 Answer: f, Selection bias

Explanation: Selection bias occurs when the presence or absence of exposure influences either allocation to particular study groups or participation in the study. In this case, treatment is chosen by the personnel involved and bypasses randomization.

Question 130 Answer: a, Ascertainment bias

Explanation: Ascertainment bias occurs if the collection of data from one group is more accurate or complete than that from the other; the longer the follow-up time, the higher the propensity to ascertainment bias. It is a particular problem when the outcome being measured is subjective. This occurs in retrospective studies and when describing a relationship between risk factors and diseases.

Reference: Lewis GH, Sheringham J, Kalim K, Crayford T JB. (2008). *Mastering Public Health: A Postgraduate Guide to Examination and Revalidation*. London: Royal Society of Medicine Press, pp. 30–31.

Theme: Substance Abuse

Question 131 Answer: e, 8 days

Explanation: For phencyclidine, the length of time detected in urine is 8 days. It is a dissociative anaesthetic agent, as the person remains conscious during the anaesthetized state. It is taken by smoking, snorting and injecting. It produces stimulant, anaesthetic and hallucinogenic effects. At low doses, it induces euphoria and a feeling of weightlessness. At high doses, visual hallucinations and synaesthesia occur. Psychosis, violence, paranoia and depression can occur following a single dose. Physical effects include incoordination, slurred speech, blurred vision, convulsions, coma and respiratory arrest.

Question 132 Answer: c, 48 hours

Explanation: For ecstasy, the length of time detected in urine is 48 hours. It is a designer drug and serotonin neurotoxin. It possesses both stimulant and mild hallucinogenic properties. It is taken orally or intranasally. When taken orally, its effects last 4–6 hours. Tolerance develops rapidly, and subsequent doses have less potency. It causes a feeling of closeness to other people, altered sensual and emotional overtones and increase in empathy and extroversion. There is also accelerated thinking, impaired decision-making and memory impairment with chronic use.

Question 133 Answer: c, 48 hours

Explanation: For amphetamine, the length of time detected in urine is 48 hours. It is a long-acting stimulant with a half-life of 10 hours. Amphetamine abuse occurs in all socioeconomic groups and increases amongst white professionals. It is administered orally and intravenously. Psychotic-like state results from acute or chronic ingestion. It leads to paranoia, hallucination and sometimes a delirium-like state. The effect usually lasts 3–4 days.

Question 134 Answer: b, 24 hours

Explanation: For LSD, the length of time detected in urine is 12–24 hours. It is a 5-hydroxytryptamine (serotonin) 2A (5-HT2A) agonist and the most potent hallucinogen. It is available in tablets or absorbed onto paper. The onset of action occurs within an hour, peaks in 2–4 hours and lasts 8–12 hours. Intravenous use is not common because the onset of the trip is very rapid with oral ingestion (15 minutes). Tolerance develops rapidly, but sensitivity to its effects returns rapidly with abstinence. It leads to psychic effects that include heightening of perceptions with perceptual distortion of shape, intensification of colour and sound, apparent movement of stationary objects and changes in sense of time and place.

Reference: Puri BK, Hall AD, Ho RC (2014). *Revision Notes in Psychiatry*. Boca Raton, FL: CRC Press, p. 529.

Theme: Old-Age Psychiatry

Question 135 Answer: c, Dopamine transporter (DAT) single photon emission computerized tomography

Explanation: This patient suffers from Lewy body dementia (LBD). Striatal dopamine transporter (DaT) visualization using single photon emission computed tomography, which involves injection solution of ioflupane (123I) and is used for the diagnosis of LBD and Parkinson disease. Dopamine is a transmitter the brain uses to stimulate movement and is diminished in individuals with Parkinson disease and LBD. DaTSCAN detects changes in the DAT responsible for allowing brain cells to take up dopamine.

Question 136 Answer: d, Perfusion hexamethylpropyleneamine oxime (HMPAO) single photon emission computed tomography (SPECT)

Explanation: This person suffers from vascular dementia. Hexamethylpropyleneamine oxime (HMPAO) single-photon emission computed tomography (SPECT) is indicated to differentiate vascular dementia from Alzheimer disease and frontotemporal dementia. It is least useful in differentiating between Alzheimer disease and Lewy body disease and between vascular dementia, frontotemporal dementia and progressive aphasia. It is also used for locating cerebral ischaemia acutely and demonstrates high sensitivity and specificity within the first 48 hours for the localization of the vascular territory of cerebral infarction. It is most sensitive for cortical ischaemia but is limited by its resolution in the subcortex, particularly of white-matter perfusion changes.

Question 137 Answer: b, Magnetic resonance imaging (MRI) brain scan

Explanation: This patient suffers from MS, and an MRI scan of the brain is recommended to look for focal white-matter lesions. MS is a relapsing and remitting autoimmune disorder with diverse neurological signs as a result of plaques of demyelination and degenerative axonal loss throughout the white matter except peripheral nerves. It also involves focal blood–brain barrier disruption. Psychiatric manifestations include fatigue, depression, anxiety, elation, mania or hypomania, pathological laughter and crying, suicide and schizophreniform psychosis.

References: Kaufman DM, Milstein MJ (2013). *Kaufman's Clinical Neurology for Psychiatrists* (7th edition). Philadelphia, PA: Saunders, pp. 122–123, 335; National Institute for Health and Care Excellence. Dementia. Supporting People with Dementia and their Carers in Health and Social Care. NICE Clinical Guideline 42. NICE, 2006. Available at: http://www.nice.org.uk/nicemedia/pdf/cg042niceguideline.pdf; Talbot P, Lloyd J, Snowden J, Neary D, Testa H (1998). A clinical role for 99mTc-HMPAO SPECT in the investigation of dementia? *J Neurol Neurosurg Psychiatry*, 64(3): 306–313.

Theme: Learning Disability

Question 138 Answer: f, Flapping hand movements

Explanation: Angelman syndrome is also known as happy puppet syndrome. It is characterized by paroxysms of laughter, cheerful disposition and ataxia. There is axial hypotonia, jerky movements and flapping hand movements. Other clinical features include epilepsy and gastrointestinal problems.

Question 139 Answer: l, Simian crease with almond-shaped eyes
Explanation: Down syndrome is the most common chromosomal (cyto-) genetic cause of learning disability. It is due to trisomy of chromosome 21. It is characterized by small round head with flat back of skull, almond-shaped eyes slanting laterally upwards, brushfield spots on the iris, prominent epicanthic folds, low-set simple external ears, hearing impairment, nuchal swelling due to excess skin in the neck, atlanto-axial instability, short fingers with curved little fingers and transverse palmer creases, reduced muscle tone in infancy, hyperextensible joints and increased rates of congenital heart disease, especially involving defects of the endocardial cushion.

Question 140 Answer: a, Cat-like cry
Explanation: Cri du chat is a microdeletion syndrome involving the short arm of chromosome 5. It is characterized by severe mental retardation, microcephaly, severe psychomotor and growth retardation, slanting palpebral fissures, broad flat nose, low set ears, cardiac abnormalities, gastrointestinal abnormalities, infantile cat cry, hyperactivity and stereotypes.

Question 141 Answer: j, Self-hugging and a hoarse voice
Explanation: Smith–Magenis syndrome involves the complete or partial deletion of chromosome 17p11.2. It is characterized by hearing problems, hoarse and deep voice, renal problems, inguinal and umbilical hernias, hypospadias, short broad hands and small toes, hypotonia, hyperextensible fingers and stereotyped self-hugging.

Question 142 Answer: h, Overlapping of fingers over thumb
Explanation: Patau syndrome is the result of trisomy 13. It is characterized by microcephaly, structural eye defects, meningo-myelocele, polydactyly, low-set ears, overlapping of fingers over thumb, cleft palate and kidney and heart defects.

Question 143 Answer: e, Elfin-like features with social disinhibition
Explanation: Williams syndrome involves a small deletion of one elastin allele at chromosome 7q11.23. It is characterized by short stature, hypercalcaemia, microcephaly, supravalvular aortic stenosis, kidney and bladder complications, elfin facial appearance, obsessions, compulsions and impulsive behaviour.

Question 144 Answer: m, Short stature, webbed neck
Explanation: Turner syndrome involves nondisjunction of paternal XY chromosomes resulting in sex chromosomal monosomy (karyotype 45 XO, phenotypically female). It is characterized by short stature, low hairline, shield-shaped thorax, widely spaced nipples, poor breast development, elbow deformity, abnormality of the wrist known as madelung deformity and brown spots (naevi). Learning disability is rare.

Question 145 Answer: g, Hamartomatous tumours
Explanation: Tuberous sclerosis is autosomal dominant with 100% penetrance. Spontaneous mutation occurs in 70% of cases. It is characterized by skin depigmentation that is especially noted under ultraviolet light (most common feature), hypomelanotic macules, intractable epilepsy, facial angiofibromas in butterfly distribution, gingival fibromata, tumours in the lungs, spleen and kidneys and hamartomas.

Question 146 Answer: b, Cleft palate with cardiac problems
Explanation: DiGeorge (velocardiofacial) syndrome involves microdeletion in involving chromosome 22q11.2. It is characterized by microcephaly, long face, minor ear abnormalities, small mouth, prominent tubular nose, bulbous nasal tip, cardiac abnormalities that include, in 75% of such cases, Fallot's tetralogy and also ventricular septal defect, interrupted aortic arch and pulmonary atresia, hypocalcaemia, seizures and short stature.

Question 147 Answer: i, Rocker bottom feet
Explanation: Edwards syndrome is also known as trisomy 18. It is characterized by structural heart abnormalities, kidney malformations, omphalocoele, oesophageal atresia, breathing and feeding difficulties, microcephaly, micrognathia, cleft lip and palate, widely spaced eyes, ptosis, underdeveloped thumbs and/or nails, absent radius, webbing of the second and third toes, clubfoot or rocker bottom feet.

Question 148 Answer: k, Self mutilation, dystonia and writhing movements
Explanation: Lesch–Nyhan syndrome is an X-linked recessive condition involving a mutation on the hypoxanthine-guanine phosphoribosyltransferase (HPRT) gene on the short arm of chromosome Xq26-27, leading to hyperuricaemia. It is characterized by microcephaly, orange uricosuric acid sand that is found in the nappy during infancy, hypotonia followed by spastic choreoathetosis, dysphagia and dysarthria, self-injurious behaviour and generalized aggression with tantrums directed against objects and people.

Question 149 Answer: n, Tall with small testicles
Explanation: Klinefelter syndrome (XXY) occurs in 1 in 1000 males. Newborn boys are clinically normal. Individuals are usually passive and compliant in childhood. While the median IQ is around 90, there is a skewed distribution to the 60–70 range, with difficulty particularly noted in acquiring verbal skills. Tall stature, slightly feminized physique, tendency to lose chest hair, female-type pubic hair pattern, gynaecomastia, osteoporosis, testicular atrophy and infertility also characteristically occur.

Question 150 Answer: d, Excessive weight gain and skin pricking
Explanation: Prader–Willi syndrome is an autosomal-dominant condition involving microdeletion of chromosome 15q11-13 of paternal origin. It is characterized by hypotonia leading to feeding difficulties and failure to thrive in infancy. There is also a triangular mouth that causes feeding and swallowing problems. In childhood, orthopaedic problems such as congenital hip dislocation and scoliosis are common. In adolescence, behavioural problems such as overeating and obesity, self-injurious

behaviour, compulsive behaviour, aggression, excessive daytime sleepiness, skin pricking and hoarding are seen.

Question 151 Answer: c, Down-turned fishlike mouth with Greek warrior helmet face
Explanation: Wolf–Hirschhorn syndrome results from a partial deletion of chromosomal material on the short arm of chromosome 4. It is characterized by microcephaly, micrognathia, down-turned fishlike mouth with Greek warrior helmet face, short philtrum, prominent glabella, ocular hypertelorism, dysplastic ears and periauricular tags, growth retardation, severe learning disability, muscle hypotonia, seizures, congenital heart defects, hypospadias, colobomata of the iris, renal anomalies and deafness. Such individuals may survive into adulthood.

Reference: Puri BK, Hall AD, Ho RC (2014). *Revision Notes in Psychiatry*. Boca Raton, FL: CRC Press, pp. 663–680.

Theme: Learning Disability

Question 152 Answer: j
Explanation: According to ICD-10 criteria for mental retardation, the IQ range is 50–69, with a mental age of 9–12 years. About 85% of those with learning disability have mild mental retardation. There is delayed understanding and use of language, possible difficulties in gaining independence, but work is possible, especially in practical occupations.

Question 153 Answer: h, 35
Explanation: According to ICD-10 criteria for mental retardation, for moderate mental retardation, the IQ range is 35–49, with a mental age of 6–9 years. It accounts for about 10% of those with learning disability. It is often associated with epilepsy, neurological abnormalities or other disabilities. There is delay in achievement of self-care; simple practical work is possible, but independent living is rarely achieved.

Question 154 Answer: f, 20
Explanation: According to ICD-10 criteria for mental retardation, in severe mental retardation, the IQ range is 20–34, with a mental age of 3–6 years. This accounts for 3% of those with learning disability.

Reference: Puri BK, Hall AD, Ho RC (2014). *Revision Notes in Psychiatry*. Boca Raton, FL: CRC Press, p. 663.

Theme: Genetic Risk of Schizophrenia

Question 155 Answer: c, 10%–14%
Explanation: The risk of developing schizophrenia in children if one parent has schizophrenia reaches a lifetime risk of about 13%.

Question 156 Answer: h, 35%–50%
Explanation: The risk of developing schizophrenia in children is very much higher (36%–50%) if both parents have schizophrenia.

Question 157 Answer: e, 20%–24%
Explanation: Velocardiofacial syndrome, which is also known as Di George syndrome, is caused by small interstitial deletions of chromosome 22q11. People with this syndrome show characteristic cranio-facial dysmorphology, cleft palate, congenital heart disease, learning difficulties and have an increased risk of psychosis. In a study by Murphy et al. (1999), about 24% met the criteria for schizophrenia.

Question 158 Answer: a, 0%–4%
Explanation: The risk of acquiring schizophrenia in half-siblings is about 4.2%.

Question 159 Answer: a, 0%–4%
Explanation: The risk of acquiring schizophrenia in cousins is about 2.4%.

Question 160 Answer: a, 0%–4%
Explanation: The risk of acquiring schizophrenia in nephews and nieces is about 3%.

Question 161 Answer: a, 0%–4%
Explanation: The risk of acquiring schizophrenia in a biological uncle and aunt is about 2.4%.

Question 162 Answer: k, 80%–85%
Explanation: The percentage of people with schizophrenia who smoke cigarettes is about 85%. The reasons for this are multifactorial and include smoking as a means of self-medication to feel better, including because smoking lowers antipsychotic levels and thus reduces side effects.

Question 163 Answer: j, 70%–75%
Explanation: Studies have shown that about 74% of people with schizophrenia do not continue antipsychotic medication after 1 year. Factors influencing antipsychotic adherence include patient related (number of episodes of illness, ethnicity, age, cognitive functioning, degree of insight, substance abuse and symptom constellation) and provider and system related (patient–provider relationship, complexity of medication regime and degree of family support).

References: Casey P (2007). Clinical features of personality and impulse control disorders, in Stein G, Wilkinson G (eds), *Seminars in General Adult Psychiatry*. London: Gaskell, pp. 206, 211; Sadock BJ, Sadock VA, Ruiz P (2009). *Kaplan and Sadock's Comprehensive Textbook of Psychiatry* (9th edition). Philadelphia, PA: Lippincott Williams & Wilkins, p. 1463; Olivier D1, Lubman DI, Fraser R (2007). Tobacco smoking within psychiatric inpatient settings: Biopsychosocial perspective. *Aust N Z J Psychiatry*, 41(7): 572–580; Valenstein M, Blow FC, Copeland LA, McCarthy JF et al. (2004). Poor antipsychotic adherence among patients with schizophrenia: Medication and patient factors. *Schizophr Bull*, 30(2): 255–264.

Theme: Obsessive-Compulsive Disorder

Question 164 Answer: a, Fear of contamination

Question 165 Answer: f, Checking

Question 166 Answer: e, Sexual or aggressive thoughts

Question 167 Answer: h, Counting
Explanation: Obsessions are defined as recurrent and intrusive thoughts, urges or images that cause marked anxiety. Compulsions are defined as repetitive behaviours or mental acts in response to an obsession. The most common obsession (in descending order) is fear of contamination (45%), doubting (42%), fear of illness, germs or bodily fears (36%), symmetry (31%) and sexual or aggressive thoughts (28%). The most common compulsions (in descending order) are checking (63%), washing (50%) and counting (36%).

Reference: Puri BK, Hall AD, Ho RC (2014). *Revision Notes in Psychiatry*. Boca Raton, FL: CRC Press, pp. 417–418.

Theme: Congenital Abnormalities and Medications

Question 168 Answer: a, Pulmonary hypertension, d, Reduction in gestational age, e, Reduction in birth weight, and f, Spontaneous abortion
Explanation: The usage of SSRIs could cause pulmonary hypertension (after 20 weeks) in the newborn. The usage of SSRIs is associated with reduction in gestational age, reduction in birth weight and spontaneous abortion.

Question 169 Answer: c, Foetal heart defects
Explanation: Paroxetine is associated with foetal heart defects in the first trimester and is less safe than other SSRIs. Sertraline, another SSRI antidepressant, can reduce the Apgar score.

Question 170 Answer: b, Agitation and irritability
Explanation: Neonates are likely to experience withdrawal (agitation and irritability), especially when paroxetine and venlafaxine have been used.

Question 171 Answer: c, Foetal heart defects
Explanation: The incidence of Ebstein's anomaly is between 0.05% and 0.1% after maternal exposure to lithium in the first trimester.

Question 172 Answer: g, Neural tube defects
Explanation: The incidence of foetal birth defect (mainly neural tube defect) has been estimated to be 1 in 100.

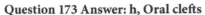

Question 173 Answer: h, Oral clefts
Explanation: Lamotrigine does require further evaluation as it is not routinely prescribed in pregnancy. It is believed to cause oral cleft (9 in 1000) and Stevens–Johnson syndrome in infants.

Reference: Puri BK, Hall AD, Ho RC (2014). *Revision Notes in Psychiatry*. Boca Raton, FL: CRC Press, p. 561.

Theme: Child Psychiatry

Question 174 Answer: d, Parent management training
Explanation: The NICE guidelines recommend group-based parent training and education programmes. When there are particular difficulties in engaging with the parents of family's needs that are too complex, individual-based parent training or education programmes are recommended. Training should be structured and have a curriculum informed by principles of social learning theory. It includes relationship-enhancing strategies and role-playing sessions. Eight to twelve sessions to maximize the possible benefits for participants.

Question 175 Answer: g, Risperidone
Explanation: To control for the aggression and the behavioural problems, antipsychotics such as risperidon and olanzapine could be used.

**Question 176 Answer: b, Duty to inform the police if not reported yet.
c, Obtain informed consent from the child and his or her parents.**
Explanation: Juvenile delinquency is defined as law-breaking behaviour by 10- to 21-year-olds. The aetiology is usually multifactorial and is not associated with any established psychiatric disorder. Factors associated include unsatisfactory child rearing, low intelligence quotient, conduct disorder in childhood, parental criminality and large family size. Approximately 50% of children would have stopped their behaviour by the age of 19 years.

Question 177 Answer: a, Multisystemic therapy
Explanation: In this form of therapy, it is multimodal and multidisciplinary in nature. It involves parent management training, family therapy, individual psychotherapy (problem solving, anger management and social skills training) as well as environmental interventions.

Question 178 Answer: d, Parent management training, and e, Family therapy
Explanation: Family therapy and parent management training are both possible treatments for ODD.

Reference: Puri BK, Hall AD, Ho RC (2014). *Revision Notes in Psychiatry*. Boca Raton, FL: CRC Press, pp. 635–639.

Theme: Old-Age Psychiatry and Neuroimaging

Question 179 Answer: c, Dopaminergic iodine-123-radiolabelled 2β carbomethoxy-3β (4-iodophenyl)-N-(3-fluoropropyl) nortropane (FP-CIT) SPECT or DaTSCAN

Explanation: This is a case of LBD, and DaTSCAN involves injecting solution of ioflupane (123I) into a living test subject for the diagnosis of Parkinson's disease (PKD) and LBD.

Question 180 Answer: d, Perfusion HMPAO SPECT

Explanation: This is a case of vascular dementia (VaD), and HMPAO SPECT is indicated to differentiate VaD from DAT and frontal temporal lobe dementia (FTLD).

Question 181 Answer: b, MRI brain scan

Explanation: This is a case of MS, and MRI is used to look for focal white-matter lesions.

Reference: Puri BK, Hall AD, Ho RC (2014). *Revision Notes in Psychiatry*. Boca Raton, FL: CRC Press, pp. 205, 681.

Theme: Psychotherapy

Question 182 Answer: f, Latent learning

Explanation: Latent learning shows that learning can take place in the absence of reinforcement.

Reference and Further Reading: Puri BK, Treasaden I (eds) (2010). *Psychiatry: An Evidence-Based Text*, London: Hodder Arnold, pp. 207, 222.

Question 183 Answer: b, Chaining

Explanation: This phenomenon is known as chaining.

Question 184 Answer: g, Penalty

Explanation: Penalty refers to the removal of a pleasant stimulus following undesirable behaviour. It is different from punishment that gives an unpleasant outcome, for example, caning.

Reference: Puri BK, Hall AD, Ho RC (2014). *Revision Notes in Psychiatry*. Boca Raton, FL: CRC Press, pp. 25–31.

Theme: General Adult Psychiatry – Prevention and Treatment

Question 185 Answer: d, Follow-up studies

Explanation: Longitudinal evidence includes follow-up studies or epidemiological surveys indicating a reduction in specific negative outcomes for the interventions was originally designed.

Question 186 Answer: e, Prevalence rate
Explanation: Prevalence rates and associated factors in a specific target group such as age, sex, race, family history, economic status and geographic locations.

Question 187 Answer: g, Skill training, h, Stress management
Explanation: Education, skill training, stress management and social problem – solving training are strategies used to enhance coping capacity of a population.

Question 188 Answer: b, Changing the settings
Explanation: Changing setting may reduce environmental risks.

Reference: Paykel ES, Jenkins R (1994). *Prevention in Psychiatry*. London: Gaskell.

Theme: Substance Abuse and Addictions

Question 189 Answer: a, Advertising controls, e, Educational efforts
Explanation: Advertising controls and educational efforts are preventive measures to reduce demand.

Question 190 Answer: h, Safe drinking limit
Explanation: Harm reduction includes establishment of safe drinking limit.

Question 191 Answer: c, Controls on prescribed drugs, d, Crop-control measures, f, Interception and interdiction measures, i, Taxation and legislative controls on tobacco and alcohol
Explanation: Crop-control measures, interception and interdiction measures, controls on prescribed drugs and taxation and legislative controls on tobacco and alcohol include supply or availability reduction.

Reference: Paykel ES, Jenkins R (1994). *Prevention in Psychiatry*. London: Gaskell.

MRCPYSCH PAPER B MOCK EXAMINATION 2: QUESTIONS

GET THROUGH MRCPSYCH PAPER B MOCK EXAMINATION

Total number of questions: 193 (110 MCQs, 83 EMIs)
Total time provided: 180 minutes

Question 1
Which of the following is not associated with increased risk of suicide in patients with cancer?
 a. Delirium with poor impulse control
 b. Extreme need for control
 c. Male gender
 d. Social isolation
 e. Decreased need for control

Question 2
Which of the following statements about first-rank and second-rank symptoms is incorrect?
 a. First-rank symptoms include auditory hallucinations that are in the third person.
 b. First-rank symptoms include delusions such as made feelings, impulses and actions.
 c. First-rank symptoms include somatic passivity.
 d. First-rank symptoms are pathognomonic of schizophrenia.
 e. Second-rank symptoms include emotional blunting.

Question 3
Which of the following is not a psychiatric feature of Smith–Magenis syndrome?
 a. Aggression
 b. Inappropriate affect
 c. Obsessive-compulsive behaviour
 d. Schizophrenia-like psychosis
 e. Sleep disturbance

Question 4

Which of the following parameters on the Violence Risk Appraisal Guide (VRAG) has the strongest correlation with violent recidivism?

a. Alcohol abuse
b. Female victim
c. History of non-violent offence
d. Psychopathy Checklist – Revised (PCL-R) score
e. Separated from parents before age of 16 years

Question 5

What is the increase in risk of a 17-year-old male adolescent of acquiring alcohol disorder if his father has been diagnosed with chronic alcoholism?

a. Twofold
b. Threefold
c. Fourfold
d. Fivefold
e. Sixfold

Question 6

A 55-year-old woman is concerned about developing dementia and consults you on supplementation that she can use to prevent dementia. Which of the following medications or supplements would you recommend?

a. Non-steroidal anti-inflammatory drugs (NSAIDs).
b. Vitamin E.
c. Statin.
d. Hormone replacement therapy.
e. Do not recommend any of the above.

Question 7

A 45-year-old man, who was treated by his psychiatrist for alcohol dependence, is brought in to the emergency department for drunk driving and rowdy behaviour. He denies drinking alcohol and claims that he has abstained from alcohol for the past 6 months. Which of the following tests would you perform to confirm that he is drinking again?

a. Gamma-glutamyl transferase (GGT)
b. Haematocrit
c. Mean corpuscular volume (MCV)
d. Serum alcohol level
e. Serum albumin level

Question 8

A researcher wants to know the prevalence of various psychiatric illnesses in the country. He selects a representative sample and surveys them about their psychiatric history. What type of study is this?

a. Case–control study
b. Cohort study
c. Crossover study

d. Cross-sectional study
e. Randomized control trial

Question 9
Which of the following is not a measure of internal validity of a randomized controlled trial (RCT)?
a. Instruments used
b. Research setting
c. Research design
d. Reliability of study results
e. Sample size computation

Question 10
Which of the following statements regarding meta-analysis is false?
a. Combining results of RCTs and open-label trials in one forest plot is appropriate.
b. Publication bias may skew results because of the tendency to publish studies with positive results.
c. Meta-analysis offers greater precision as a result of larger sample size.
d. The Cochrane Collaboration produces and disseminates systematic reviews of healthcare interventions and promotes the search for evidence in the form of clinical trials and other studies of the effects of interventions.
e. Systematic review of RCTs is level 1A evidence.

Question 11
Which of the following medical complications is not routinely associated with anorexia nervosa?
a. Decreased bone mineral density
b. Leukopenia
c. Mitral valve prolapse
d. Decreased growth hormone
e. Pancreatitis

Question 12
A 55-year-old shopkeeper presented to the Accident and Emergency Department with memory loss. You are the psychiatric specialist trainee on call tonight. Which of the following features do not suggest transient global amnesia?
a. He cannot remember the events that occurred in the afternoon.
b. He cannot recall the name of his shop.
c. He is disorientated in time and place.
d. He demonstrates anterograde amnesia after admission to the ward.
e. He demonstrates retrograde amnesia for variable durations.

Question 13
Which of the following statements regarding narcolepsy is false?
a. Genotype HLA-DQB1*0602 is present in nearly 99% of people suffering from narcolepsy.
b. Hypnopompic hallucinations are commoner than hypnagogic hallucination.

c. Loss of hypocretin cells in the hypothalamus is an aetiological factor.

d. Modafinil is useful to treat this condition.

e. Nocturnal sleep polysomnography shows rapid eye movement (REM) sleep latency less than or equal to 15 min.

Question 14

A 55-year-old man presents to the outpatient service with a history of rapidly progressive dementia. In addition, on clinical examination, there were multiple pyramidal and extra-pyramidal deficits noted. Collateral history from his family members revealed that prior to the onset of the rapidly progressing memory losses, there was a brief period of anxiety and depression. Which of the following disorders is he likely to be suffering from?

a. Vascular dementia

b. Fronto-temporal dementia

c. Lewy body dementia

d. Human immunodeficiency virus (HIV) dementia

e. Creutzfeldt–Jakob disease

Question 15

A 72-year-old woman with a background of cerebrovascular accident 2 years ago presents to the emergency department with seizure attacks. This is the third time she has had seizures over the last year. Which of the following statements regarding seizures in the elderly is false?

a. A high percentage of people with seizure may have normal electroencephalogram (EEG) findings.

b. Alzheimer's disease dementia is not a risk factor for refractory seizures.

c. Strokes or tumours are common causes of seizures in the elderly.

d. Recurrent seizures are common.

e. The incidence of seizures is high.

Question 16

Based on previous studies, the diagnosis of very-late-onset psychosis should be made only if the individual is above which of the following ages?

a. 40 years old

b. 50 years old

c. 55 years old

d. 60 years old

e. 65 years old

Question 17

A 42-year-old woman says that she has repeated thoughts that her table is dirty and she has to snap her fingers five times to dispel these thoughts. Which one of the following defence mechanisms is this?

a. Displacement

b. Intellectualization

c. Repression

d. Suppression
e. Undoing

Question 18
Which of the following defence mechanisms is most often seen in people with phobias?
a. Denial/displacement
b. Denial/introjection
c. Isolation/displacement
d. Splitting/projection
e. Undoing/projection

Question 19
For an antipsychotic to be effective, it has to achieve what percentage blockage of the dopaminergic receptors?
a. 50%
b. 56%
c. 68%
d. 90%
e. 95%

Question 20
The male-to-female gender ratio for conduct disorder is which of the following?
a. 2:1
b. 3:1
c. 4:1
d. 5:1
e. 6:1

Question 21
Which of the following is the most common neuropsychiatric disorder in patients with systemic lupus erythematosus (SLE)?
a. Anxiety disorder
b. Cognitive dysfunction
c. Delirium
d. Mood disorder
e. Psychosis

Question 22
Which of the following assessment toolkits best predicts the needs for support services for an elderly patient with dementia?
a. Mini Mental State Examination (MMSE)
b. Clifton assessment procedures for the elderly
c. Kew cognitive map
d. Wechsler adult intelligence scale (WAIS)
e. National adult reading test

Question 23

A 40-year-old man has been diagnosed with HIV/acquired immune deficiency syndrome (AIDS) 10 years ago. Lately, he has developed delirium, and his CD4 counts are less than 200. He was thus admitted to the medical ward 6 weeks ago. He came today to the emergency service complaining of low mood and loss of interest for the past month or so. The core trainee has discussed the case with the consultant on call. The consultant on call has recommended that the patient be commenced on a course of antidepressant. Which of the following antidepressants is better to be avoided?

a. Fluoxetine
b. Paroxetine
c. Venlafaxine
d. Bupropion
e. Mirtazapine

Question 24

A 30-year-old man has been diagnosed with schizophrenia since young. His symptoms have been more stable over the past 2 years after he has been maintained on both an oral antipsychotic and a depot antipsychotic injection. He is here for his routine outpatient follow-up today and expresses concerns about his sexual functioning. The effects of his antipsychotics on which of the following receptors would have resulted in his current symptoms of sexual dysfunction?

a. D2 partial agonist
b. 5-hydroxytryptamine A (5-ht1A) partial agonist
c. 5-HT2A antagonist
d. Histamine antagonist
e. Muscarinic antagonist

Question 25

Regarding the course of illness for autistic disorder, which of the following symptoms do not improve across time?

a. Lack of reciprocal social interactions
b. Abnormal communication
c. Restricted, stereotyped and repetitive behaviour
d. Phobias
e. Sleeping and eating disturbances

Question 26

An 11-year-old child has been referred by his family general practitioner (GP) to the Child and Adolescent Mental Health Services (CAMHS) for assessment. He has never had bed-wetting before but currently has symptoms of it. Which of the following has not been found to be associated with nocturnal enuresis?

a. Family history of enuresis
b. Neurological abnormalities
c. Recurrence after withdrawal of tricyclic
d. Male gender
e. Tall stature

Question 27

Which of the following statements regarding the impact of divorce on children is incorrect?
a. Children of divorced parents are sexually active at a younger age.
b. If the mother remarries, her son has a better relationship with the step-father compared with her daughter.
c. The mother–daughter bond is more affected than the mother–son bond if the mother remarries.
d. Divorce causes more anxiety in children than parental death.
e. On average, girls are more distressed than boys by the divorce.

Question 28

Which of the following statements regarding reading disorder is incorrect?
a. The prevalence of dyslexia in the United Kingdom is 5%.
b. The prevalence of genuine dyslexia and mild dyslexia is 10%.
c. In the United States, 17%–20% of elementary school children are estimated to suffer from reading disabilities.
d. In the United States, 17%–20% of the population display a reading disability.
e. A survey conducted across Japan, Taiwan and the United States concluded that using more than one criterion, the percentage of children who were reading disabled were 8% in Japan, 8% in Taiwan and 7% in the United States.

Question 29

Personality disturbances are common among individuals with eating disorders. A 28-year-old woman with bulimia nervosa has been referred to the psychologist for a personality test. The psychologist has administered the Minnesota Multiphasic Personality Inventory (MMPI) for her. In which domains would she have elevated scores compared with the anorexics?
a. Neuroticism
b. Depression
c. Social introversion
d. Psychopathic deviant
e. Paranoia

Question 30

Which of the following offences is the most common first presentation of conduct disorder?
a. Fire-setting
b. Shoplifting
c. Robbery
d. Assaulting someone
e. Molesting someone

Question 31

In the United Kingdom, the elderly account for almost 25% of all completed suicide. Approximately 5% of them attempted suicide. It has been noted that suicide rates tend to increase with age until old age. All the following statements about suicide in the elderly are true, with the exception of which?

a. Males tend to have a higher rate of suicide compared with females, and they tend to use a more lethal method.
b. Presence of symptoms such as hopelessness, guilt, insomnia and delusions of guilt predispose elderly individuals to suicide.
c. Individuals are at enhanced risk if they suffer a recent loss or during anniversaries.
d. Individuals are at enhanced risk in the first few weeks after the commencement of antidepressant therapy.
e. Most elderly individuals who have committed suicide tend not to have sought consultation prior to their act.

Question 32
Which of the following statements about aging and its effects on memory is incorrect?

a. Short-term memory as tested by digit span does not change with age.
b. Memory tasks requiring monitoring or complex decision making are usually performed more poorly in the elderly.
c. Retrieval of information in the elderly is impaired, and in particular, cued recall is affected.
d. Older subjects tend to be less likely to code at the semantic level for memories.
e. Memory performance is best if the meaning is easily extracted.

Question 33
Approximately what percentage of patients with late-onset psychosis have at least one first-rank symptom?

a. 10%
b. 25%
c. 35%
d. 45%
e. 55%

Question 34
A 25-year-old patient was diagnosed with schizophrenia and Gilles de la Tourette's syndrome. The consultant would like to clarify the diagnosis further. He asks, Which of the following features is the most suggestive of the diagnosis of Gilles de la Tourette's syndrome?

a. Frequent handwashing
b. Age of onset is 19 years
c. Repeated purposeless movements
d. Not responding to clozapine
e. Shouting at the voices

Question 35
Which of the following is not an example of objective personality measure?

a. Million Behavioural Health Inventory (MBHI)
b. Million Clinical Multiaxial Inventory (MCMI)

c. Personality Assessment Inventory (PAI)
d. Rorschach Inkblot Test (RIT)
e. Minnesota Multiphasic Personality Inventory (MMPI)

Question 36

Which of the following measures is not part of the Halstead–Reitan Neuropsychological Test Battery (HRNTB)?
a. Abstraction
b. Input measures
c. Output measures
d. Sensory input
e. Verbal abilities

Question 37

Which of the following neurotransmitters is least likely to be involved in the modulation of aggression?
a. Adrenaline
b. Dopamine
c. Acetylcholine
d. Noradrenaline
e. Serotonin

Question 38

With regard to enuresis and encopresis, which of the following statements is incorrect?
a. Seventy percent of enuresis is caused by organic causes.
b. Regressive encopresis is associated with a good prognosis.
c. Encopresis is associated with aggression and a short attention span.
d. Diurnal enuresis is more common in females.
e. If a child presents with both enuresis and encopresis, enuresis should be treated first.

Question 39

Which of the following regarding the water deprivation test is false?
a. In normal subjects, urine osmolality rises as urine volume falls.
b. In patients with cranial diabetes insipidus, urine osmolality fails to rise, and a relative diuresis continues despite the increasing plasma osmolality.
c. In patients with nephrogenic diabetes insipidus, the urine concentrates normally in response to desmopressin.
d. With primary polydipsia, excessive fluid intake prior to the test may result in an apparent continued diuresis despite fluid restriction.
e. With primary polydipsia, plasma osmolality remains below 295 mosmol/kg after fluid restriction.

Question 40

You have designed a research project that investigates the effects of three different antipsychotics on the metabolic syndrome. Which one of the following

statistical tests would you use to demonstrate differences between the three antipsychotics?
   a. Analysis of variance (ANOVA)
   b. Chi-square test
   c. Kruskal–Wallis test
   d. Mann–Whitney U-test
   e. t-test

Question 41
Which of the following statements is the correct definition of type one error?
   a. The probability that the false null hypothesis will be rejected.
   b. The probability of accepting the null hypothesis when it is false.
   c. The probability of rejecting the null hypothesis when it is true.
   d. The probability that the study lacks power.
   e. The probability that the null hypothesis will be accepted.

Question 42
Upon the release of a new antidepressant to the market, you want to find out the proportion of patients who develop gastric side effects from this new medication compared with those using fluoxetine. Which of the following statistical tests would you use to help you in this comparison?
   a. ANOVA
   b. Chi-square
   c. Mann–Whitney U-test
   d. Paired t-test
   e. Kruskal–Wallis

Question 43
A researcher is designing an epidemiological study and is planning to use mailed questionnaires as a means of collecting data. The researcher is concerned that response rates will be low. Which of the following is most likely to increase response rates?
   a. Conducting face-to-face interviews at the participants' homes
   b. Getting informed consent
   c. Monetary incentives
   d. Sending reminders
   e. Using shorter questionnaires

Question 44
Which of the following is the primary mechanism of action of cocaine?
   a. It blocks activity of monoamine oxidase.
   b. It blocks dopamine D2 receptor.
   c. It blocks reuptake of dopamine.
   d. It blocks reuptake of noradrenaline.
   e. It causes release of dopamine into synapses.

Question 45
Apart from detoxification, pharmacological treatment has been recommended as an alternative for individuals with alcohol dependence. Based on your knowledge, which of the following medications commonly used in alcohol dependence works via the inhibition of a critical step in the breakdown of alcohol?
a. Naltrexone
b. Naloxone
c. Acamprosate
d. Disulfiram
e. Lorazepam

Question 46
Which of the following is a serious side effect of 3,4-methylenedioxy-N-methylam-phetamine (MDMA)?
a. Disinhibition
b. Hallucinations
c. Hyperthermia
d. Paranoia
e. Respiratory depression

Question 47
Which of the following is not a symptom of cocaine withdrawal?
a. Fatigue
b. Insomnia
c. Loss of appetite
d. Nightmares
e. Psychomotor retardation

Question 48
Based on recent studies, what percentage of people convicted of homicide in England and Wales were assessed to have abnormal mental state at the time of the offence?
a. 5
b. 10
c. 15
d. 20
e. 25

Question 49
Which of the following personality disorders is most common in female prisoners in England?
a. Antisocial
b. Borderline
c. Dependent
d. Histrionic
e. Paranoid

Question 50

Which of the following statements regarding the Historical, Clinical and Risk Management Questionnaire (HCR-20) is false?
a. It does not consider protective factors in the assessment.
b. It does not require formal training.
c. It consists of 20 items.
d. It focuses on violence towards people and property.
e. It cannot be used to measure dangerousness.

Question 51

Which of the following environmental factors is not a risk factor for inpatient violence?
a. High levels of staff–patient interaction
b. High use of temporary staff
c. Lack of privacy
d. Overcrowding
e. Poor physical facilities

Question 52

Which of the following statements is false regarding homocystinuria?
a. Administration of vitamin B6 facilitates metabolism of homocysteine and reduces levels of homocysteine and methionine.
b. Elevated serum homocysteine level is a risk factor for stroke.
c. It is attributed to mutation on chromosome 22.
d. Patients have mental retardation, personality disorders and obsessive-compulsive symptoms.
e. There is malformation of multiple organs.

Question 53

A 4-year-old child has been referred to the CAMHS for delayed speech. The psychologist who saw him suspected that he suffered from autistic disorder initially, as he has gaze aversion as well as social avoidance. The psychometric test showed that his intelligence quotient (IQ) was that of 60. The core trainee has done a physical examination, which revealed that he has enlarged testes, large ears, long face and flat feet. Of note, there was marked preservation of words on mental state examination. Behaviours such as hand flapping were also noted. Which of the following is the most likely diagnosis?
a. Foetal alcohol syndrome
b. Fragile X syndrome
c. Turner syndrome
d. XXY syndrome
e. Hurler's syndrome

Question 54

The prevalence of mental retardation is approximately 1% of the population, with males being affected more than females. Which of the following is the most common cause of mental retardation?

a. Down syndrome
b. Exposure to toxins in utero
c. Fragile X syndrome
d. Idiopathic or unknown
e. Lead intoxication

Question 55
A 5-year-old boy presents with autism. Which of the following is false?
a. Attachments tend to be rigid.
b. There is a tendency to echolalia and pronoun reversal.
c. Stimulants can relieve the stereotyped behaviours.
d. IQ is the most important prognostic factor.
e. He may suffer from fragile X syndrome or tuberous sclerosis.

Question 56
A 20-year-old female university student suffers from bulimia nervosa. She finds medication ineffective and requests psychotherapy. Choose the most appropriate psychotherapy for her.
a. Psychodynamic psychotherapy
b. Interpersonal psychotherapy
c. Cognitive analytical therapy
d. Mentalization-based therapy
e. Dialectical behavioural therapy

Question 57
Previous research has noted that paranoid patients are at heightened risk of committing suicide compared with non-paranoid individuals. What is the estimated increment in the risk?
a. 2 times
b. 3 times
c. 4 times
d. 5 times
e. 10 times

Question 58
A 20-year-old woman with a history of bulimia nervosa presents to the mental health service with depressed mood, marked loss in interest and active suicidal ideations. The core trainee has obtained further information and has informed the on-call consultant about the case. The consultant advises the core trainee to start an appropriate antidepressant. Which of the antidepressant choices is contraindicated?
a. Fluoxetine
b. Sertraline
c. Clomipramine
d. Mirtazapine
e. Bupropion

Question 59

A 65-year-old man has been having memory impairments. A computed tomography (CT) scan was done which revealed the presence of markedly enlarged ventricles secondary to infarction in the hemispheric white matter. The infarcts seemed to have affected the periventricular and central white matter. On examination, there are noted to be neurological signs. Which of the following clinical signs or symptoms should be expected as well?

a. Bulbar palsy
b. Pseudobulbar palsy
c. Incontinence
d. Diplopia
e. Aphasia

Question 60

A 72-year-old woman has been diagnosed with Alzheimer's dementia 1 year ago. She has been having difficult behavioural and psychological symptoms lately. The geriatric psychiatrist has recommended non-pharmacological treatments to help her with her condition. He tries to explain a treatment that involves the 'here and now' and find meaning in the behaviour of the patient. Which of the following therapies is he referring to?

a. Reality orientation
b. Resolution therapy
c. Reminiscent therapy
d. Validation therapy
e. Snoezelen therapy

Question 61

Which of the following is not a characteristic neurotransmitter change in Alzheimer's dementia?

a. Decreased dopamine levels
b. Decreased noradrenaline levels
c. Increased serotonin in the cortex
d. Low cortical cholinergic activity
e. Reduced choline acetyl transferase

Question 62

Which of the following factors is not associated with higher rates of panic disorder among people seeking treatment for chest pain in emergency rooms?

a. Atypical quality of chest pain
b. Female gender
c. High level of self-reported anxiety
d. Presence of coronary artery disease
e. Younger age

Question 63

Which of the following statements regarding hypochondriasis is false?

a. Antidepressants are useful in treatment.
b. It is associated with lower socio-economic status and a history of medical illness.

c. Onset is most common in early adulthood.
d. The presence of comorbid medical illness is a poor prognostic factor.
e. Somatization disorder is a common comorbid diagnosis.

Question 64

A 74-year-old woman has been going to various dermatologists requesting examination of her skin. She complains that there are worms crawling under her skin, causing her to feel a weird tingling sensation over her limbs. Despite all investigations being negative, she is not reassured and insists that the worms are real. Which of the following statements regarding her condition is true?
   a. Antidepressants are helpful to remove the ruminations.
   b. Patients are usually keen for psychiatric consultation.
   c. Patients typically have experienced an actual infestation or exposure to organisms in the past.
   d. Patients are usually keen to receive psychiatric treatment as they have retained insight into their condition.
   e. There is usually no specific precipitating event.

Question 65

Which of the following is not a common comorbid psychiatric disorder of patients suffering from trichotillomania?
   a. Anxiety disorder
   b. Dependent personality disorder
   c. Eating disorder
   d. Substance abuse
   e. Depressive disorder

Question 66

Which of the following mood stabilizers would you least likely to consider in a patient who is concerned about cognitive side effects?
   a. Carbamazepine
   b. Gabapentin
   c. Lamotrigine
   d. Topiramate
   e. Valproate

Question 67

Referring to Table 3.1, which of the following best describes the above study?
   a. Cost–benefit analysis
   b. Cost-effectiveness analysis
   c. Cost-minimization analysis
   d. Cost–performance analysis
   e. Cost–utility analysis

Table 3.1 Annual direct and indirect costs of patients with mild, moderate and severe depressive disorder

	Mild (n = 12)	Moderate (n = 32)	Severe (n = 5)	p-Value	df
Mean HAMD score over 1 year					
Mean ± SD	7.00 ± 1.67	14.57 ± 2.94	24.55 ± 3.02	<0.01**	2
Median	7.25	13.50	25.00		
IQR	2	6	6		
Health-related quality of life: mental health					
Mean ± SD	44.22 ± 8.92	47.93 ± 8.10	52.48 ± 4.41	0.208	2
Median	44.79	47.95	51.54		
IQR	17.13	13.13	8.25		
Total direct costs (US$)					
Mean ± SD	590.12 ± 389.02	1179.17 ± 1112.73	5251.96 ± 3469.76	0.001**	2
Median	589.15	892.55	3661.83		
IQR	729.54	970.18	4950.76		
95% CI of mean	342.96–837.29	777.98–1580.34	943.13–9560.17		
Total indirect costs (US$)					
Mean ± SD	1534.75 ± 3742.41	4760.58 ± 11,987.72	26,509.17 ± 30,901.76	0.032*	2
Median	0	306.95	21,543.39		
IQR	954.92	5,665.74	48,862.00		
95% CI of mean	0–3912.54	438.54–908.25	0–3912.54		
Total cost					
Mean ± SD	2124.88 ± 3888.93	5939.75 ± 12,245.28	31,761.14 ± 34,122.95	0.004**	2
Median	736.69	1225.28	26,483.07		
IQR	1575.59	7427.88	52,374.48		
95% CI of mean	0–4595.75	1524.84–10354.56	0–74129.78		

Source: Ho RC, Mak KK, Chua AN, Ho CS, Mak A (2013). The effect of severity of depressive disorder on economic burden in a university hospital in Singapore. *Expert Rev Pharmacoecon Outcomes Res,* 13(4): 549–559.

Notes: Comparisons were made using chi-square test; *p < 0.05 and **p < 0.01. All other comparisons using Kruskal–Wallis test.

Abbreviations: CI, confidence interval; df, degrees of freedom; HAMD, Hamilton depression rating scale; IQR, interquartile range; SD, standard deviation.

Question 68

Which of the following is not considered to be a direct cost related to depressive disorder?

a. Cost of consultation with GP related to depressive disorder
b. Cost of hospitalization related to depressive disorder
c. Cost of psychotherapy to treat depression

d. Cost of sick leave related to depressive disorder
e. Cost of thyroid function tests to rule out underlying organic cause for depression

Question 69
Referring to Table 3.2, which of the following factors is the most important predictor of indirect cost for depressive disorder in Singapore?
a. Age
b. Gender
c. Education level
d. Mean HAMD score over 1 year
e. Number of suicide attempts in 1 year

Table 3.2 Univariate analyses and multivariate linear regression analyses of cost predictors for depressive disorder in Singapore

	Univariate analysis		Multivariate analysis			Collinearity statistics
	β-Standardized coefficient	p-Value	β-Standardized coefficient	p-Value	R^2	Tolerance
Direct cost						
Age	0.111	0.449	0.134	0.207		0.971
Gender	−0.197	0.174	−0.188	0.097		0.859
Education level	0.262	0.069	0.278	0.015		0.886
SF-12 PH	0.031	0.836	0.161	0.272		0.505
SF-12 MH	0.164	0.275	0.076	0.628	0.601	0.430
Mean HAMD score over 1 year	0.616	<0.01	0.569	<0.01		0.724
Number of suicide attempts in 1 year	0.328	0.021	0.254	0.024		0.903
Indirect cost						
Age	0.233	0.107	0.212	0.098		0.971
Gender	−0.291	0.042	−0.233	0.089		0.859
Education level	0.237	0.101	0.254	0.061		0.886
SF-12 PH	0.173	0.250	0.248	0.162		0.505
SF-12 MH	−0.009	0.952	−0.15	0.937	0.420	0.430
Mean HAMD score over 1 year	0.409	0.004	0.451	0.004		0.724
Number of suicide attempts in 1 year	0.140	0.336	0.042	0.747		0.903

Abbreviations: HAMD, Hamilton depression rating scale; SF-12 MH, ShortForm-12 mental health; SF-12 PH, ShortForm-12 physical health.

Question 70

Based on Table 3.3, which of the following statements is incorrect?

a. The higher scores on the DFIQ correlate with poorer HRQOL in the children, and the correlation is significant.

b. The higher scores on the DFIQ correlate with poorer physical health (i.e. SF-12 PH) and mental health (i.e. SF-12 MH). The correlations are significant.

c. The later age of onset correlates with better mental health, and the correlation is significant.

d. The severity of atopic dermatitis (i.e. SCORAD) correlates with older age of the child, and the correlation is significant.

e. The severity of atopic dermatitis (i.e. SCORAD) correlates with poorer physical health (i.e. SF-12 PH), and the correlation is significant.

Question 71

A 45-year-old man with a long-standing history of multiple substance abuse presents with cognitive impairment. Which of the following drugs is most likely to be responsible?

a. Amphetamine

b. Cannabis

c. Cocaine

d. Lysergic acid diethylamide (LSD)

e. An inhalant

Question 72

Henry is a 40-year-old unemployed man who has been dependent on alcohol for 20 years. He wants to find out from you the risk of his 14-year-old son developing

Table 3.3. Correlations among demographic, SCORAD and HRQOL variables ($n = 104$)

	Age of child	Onset age	HRQOL (children)	SCORAD	SF-12 PH	SF-12 MH	DFIQ
Age of child	1.00						
Onset age	0.62**	1.00					
HRQOL (children)	0.15	0.03	1.00				
SCORAD	0.24*	0.08	0.51**	1.00			
SF-12 PH	0.03	−0.27	−0.10	−0.22*	1.00		
SF-12 MH	0.18	0.25*	−0.31**	−0.24*	0.05	1.00	
DFIQ	−0.96	−0.38	0.48**	0.35**	−0.24*	−0.52**	1.00

Note: *$p < 0.05$ and **$p < 0.01$.

Source: Ho RC, Giam YC, Ng TP, Mak A, Goh D, Zhang MW, Cheak A, Van Bever HP (2010). The influence of childhood atopic dermatitis on health of mothers, and its impact on Asian families. *Pediatr Allergy Immunol*, 21(3):501–507.

Abbreviations: HRQOL, heath-related quality-of-life; SCORAD, Severity Scoring of Atopic Dermatitis; SF-12, 12-item Short-Form health survey; PH, physical health; MH, mental health; DFIQ, Dermatitis Family Impact Scale; HRQOL (patients) = scores from IDQOL (Infant's Dermatitis Quality of Life Index) or CDLQI (Children's Dermatology Life Quality Index).

alcohol dependence compared with those adolescents whose biological fathers do not drink. His son has been adopted by a family who do not drink. What would you tell him?

a. Two times
b. Three times
c. Four times
d. Five times
e. Six times

Question 73

A 20-year-old man has been using inhalant as a stimulant for the past couple of years. The core trainee is trying to engage the patient via motivational interviewing. During an episode of usage, which of the following leads to the greatest risk of death?

a. Cardiac arrest
b. Burns to the throat and lungs
c. Liver damage
d. Renal damage
e. Persistent cerebellar syndrome and peripheral neuropathy

Question 74

A 35-year-old drug dealer is stopped by the police. During urine drug test, he was found to have haematuria and difficulty passing urine. He seems to be incoherent and violent. Which of the following illicit substances has he consumed?

a. Amphetamine
b. Cocaine
c. Methylenedioxymethamphetamine
d. Heroin
e. Ketamine

Question 75

A 23-year-old woman has just been admitted to the emergency department. The medical core trainee who has assessed her found her to be having tachycardia. In addition, she is confused and reported feelings of closeness to others. Her friends who accompanied her mentioned that she was offered some pills at the party that they have just attended. Which of the following could she be intoxicated on?

a. Benzodiazepines
b. Ketamine
c. Opioid
d. Morphine
e. Methylenedioxymethamphetamine

Question 76

What is the lifetime prevalence rate of schizophrenia in all perpetrators of homicide?

a. 5%
b. 10%

c. 15%

d. 20%

e. 25%

Question 77

A 20-year-old university student has been admitted to the inpatient unit, and he has been diagnosed with first-episode psychosis. He has been started on a trial of olanzapine, to which, unfortunately, precipitated a neuroleptic malignant syndrome. He is now currently managed in the medical unit, and his antipsychotics have been stopped. His father is here and wants an update. One of his concerns pertains to the percentage of individuals diagnosed with first-episode psychosis that would eventually have schizophrenia. Which of the following is true?

a. 5%

b. 15%

c. 20%

d. 25%

e. 35%

Question 78

Which of the following is the strongest predictor of sexual recidivism?

a. Alcohol and opioid misuse

b. Diagnosis of bipolar disorder

c. Low remorse and victim blaming

d. Three previous convictions for sexual offending

e. Young age of first sexual offence conviction

Question 79

A 24-year-old married man with a background of mild learning disability has been referred to you. He has fertility problems. On physical examination, he is found to have gynaecomastia and small testes. He is diagnosed to have Klinefelter syndrome. Which one of the following best describes the inheritance pattern of this syndrome?

a. Autosomal dominant

b. Autosomal recessive

c. Sporadic

d. X-linked dominant

e. X-linked recessive

Question 80

Adults with Down syndrome are not at increased risk of which of the following?

a. Hearing loss

b. Hypothyroidism

c. Leukaemia

d. Obstructive sleep apnoea

e. Vascular dementia

Question 81

Cri du chat syndrome is a genetic syndrome that involves a de novo deletion of the short arm of chromosome 5 (in 85% of the cases). Which of the following is not a characteristic feature of this condition?

a. Hyperactivity
b. Cardiac abnormalities
c. Gastro-intestinal abnormalities
d. Moderate mental retardation
e. Severe psychomotor retardation

Question 82

Which of the following statements is true regarding fragile X syndrome?

a. Symptoms tend to be much more severe in females than in males.
b. It occurs secondary to mutations in the fragile mental retardation 2 (FMR2) gene on the long arm of chromosome X.
c. It occurs in expansion of CGG trinucleotide repeats of over 200 triplets.
d. There is atrophy of the caudate nucleus and hippocampus.
e. Those with permutations are not at risk of developing fragile X–associated tremor/ataxia syndrome (FXTAS).

Question 83

A 35-year-old man is charged for molesting a woman in her house. The defendant was known to the woman and her husband. He was invited to stay in their house as a guest after a drink in the pub. The defendant suffered from somnambulism, and he walked into the couple's room at night. He removed her underwear and was discovered by her husband. Concerning the defence of 'not guilty by reason of insanity' in this case, which of the following statements is true?

a. Somnambulism is classified as sane automatism.
b. Somnambulism is classified as insane automatism.
c. There is a fixed maximum punishment for legal automatisms.
d. Voluntary intoxication with alcohol is classified as sane automatism.
e. Voluntary intoxication with alcohol is classified as insane automatism.

Question 84

Which of the following statements regarding melatonin is incorrect?

a. If an adolescent takes melatonin and the oral contraceptive pill concurrently, melatonin has less propensity to cause drug interactions.
b. A prolonged-release formulation of melatonin is licensed for the short-term treatment of insomnia in children in the United Kingdom.
c. Meta-analyses of small RCTs comparing melatonin with placebo in children with insomnia show consistent improvement in sleep, with earlier sleep onset and increased total sleep duration.
d. Melatonin can worsen asthma and seizure in the short term.
e. The optimal dose of melatonin in the treatment of insomnia in children and adolescents is unknown.

Question 85

An advanced practice nurse wants to incorporate a structured interview to assess both substance misuse and psychiatric disorders among the service users. Which of the following could be recommended?

a. Assessment of Lifestyle Instrument (DALI)
b. Chemical Use, Abuse and Dependence (CUAD) survey
c. Inventory of Substance Abuse Treatment Services (SATS)
d. Psychiatric Research Interview for Substance and Mental Disorders (PRISM)
e. Stages of Change Readiness and Treatment Eagerness Scale (SOCRATES)

Question 86

Which of the following statements is false regarding the General Health Questionnaire (GHQ)?

a. It is a self-administered questionnaire.
b. It primarily identifies non-psychotic psychiatric illness and assesses its severity.
c. It focuses on functioning over the past 2 weeks.
d. It uses a four-point scale ranging from 'much more than usual' to 'less than usual'.
e. It has four versions.

Question 87

Which of the following statements is true about the Montgomery and Asberg Depression Rating Scale (MADRS)?

a. It is a self-administered questionnaire.
b. It is not a sensitive measure of change in symptom severity during treatment.
c. It is useful for people with concurrent physical illness, as it places less emphasis on somatic symptoms.
d. A score of 7–25 is indicative of mild depression.
e. It cannot be used for assessing patients who are likely to experience side effects from medication.

Question 88

Which of the following statements is false regarding the Hamilton Depression Scale?

a. It assesses symptoms in the last 7 days.
b. It monitors changes in the severity of the symptoms during treatment.
c. It should only be used on patients with an established diagnosis of depression, as it is not a diagnostic instrument.
d. Its validity is affected if the person has concurrent physical illness.
e. One of its strengths is that behavioural symptoms and somatic complaints are preferred over self-reported distress.

Question 89

Which of the following statements regarding differences between parametric and non-parametric tests is correct?

a. ANOVA is used for non-parametric data.
b. Mann–Whitney U is used for parametric data.

c. Non-parametric data follows a normal distribution but not for parametric data.
d. Sample size for parametric data is preferably >30, but for non-parametric, it is best for <50 data cases.
e. The confidence interval calculation for parametric data is more difficult than for non-parametric data.

Question 90
Which of the following statistical tests would you use for measuring differences in education level among different ethnic groups (Caucasians, African Caribbean, Southern and Eastern Asians)?
a. ANOVA
b. Chi-square
c. Kruskal–Wallis test
d. Mann–Whitney U test
e. Spearman correlation

Question 91
Which of the following statistical methods is used for correlation analysis in ranked or skewed data?
a. Kappa correlation
b. McNemar test
c. Pearson correlation
d. Spearman correlation
e. Wilcoxon signed-rank

Question 92
Which of the following statements is false for confidence interval (CI)?
a. A 99% CI is wider than a 95% CI.
b. A 95% CI means that one is 95% confident that the interval contains the true population mean.
c. For relative risk or odds ratio, if the CI contains 1, then the results are not different.
d. The CI is the interval that true statistics believes to be found within a given population with a known probability.
e. Width of the CI is dependent on sample size: a larger sample generates wider CI.

Question 93
Which of the following statements regarding hoarding is false?
a. Hoarding is most commonly found in people with obsessive-compulsive disorder (OCD).
b. It shows an autosomal dominant inheritance pattern.
c. Schizophrenia is a psychiatric comorbidity.
d. There is lower activity in the dorsal anterior cingulate gyrus and occipital cortex of people with hoarding and OCD.
e. Treatment involves selective serotonin reuptake inhibitors (SSRIs).

Question 94
Which of the following statements regarding immune function in depressed patients is false?
   a. A syndrome of 'sickness behaviour' that resembles major depression can occur with the administration of interferons.
   b. Peripheral blood shows decreased lymphocyte number and increased neutrophil number.
   c. There are decreased levels of interleukin (IL)-6 and IL-1-beta.
   d. There are increased acute phase proteins.
   e. There is increased level of tumour necrosis factor (TNF)-alpha compared with non-depressed individuals.

Question 95
Based on the P50 auditory-evoked potential, which chromosome is implicated in the failure of sensory gating phenomenon in schizophrenia?
   a. 10
   b. 12
   c. 15
   d. 16
   e. 20

Question 96
A 32-year-old woman, who has been diagnosed with schizophrenia since she was 25, returns for her regular outpatient follow-up appointment. She shared with you that she has already seen the neurologist, who has ruled out an organic aetiology for the cause of her raised prolactin levels. You are aware that she has been on long-term oral Risperidone as well as intramuscular Risperidone Consta. Based on your understanding, what percentage of dopaminergic blockage would result in symptoms of elevated prolactin?
   a. 48%
   b. 56%
   c. 68%
   d. 72%
   e. 78%

Question 97
Which of the following is a not common biological abnormality shared by both schizophrenia and schizotypal disorder?
   a. Dopamine dysregulation
   b. Impaired smooth pursuit eye movements
   c. Impaired test of executive functioning
   d. Reduction in temporal lobe volumes
   e. Acetylcholine dysregulation

Question 98
In this form of depression, it should be noted that depressed mood is not always the chief complaint. Somatic symptoms might be the main concern. In addition,

this variant of depression tends to be more common in undeveloped world. Which of the following is the correct diagnosis?
a. Endogenous depression
b. Reactive depression
c. Double depression
d. Recurrent brief depression
e. Masked depression

Question 99
Dialectical behavioural therapy was developed for patients with borderline personality disorder. Which of the following is not a core component of dialectical behavioural therapy?
a. Dialectical thinking
b. Mindfulness skills
c. Life-skills training
d. Behavioural therapy
e. Analysis of communication

Question 100
The Cambridge Mental Disorders of the Elderly Examination (CAMDEX) includes all the following, with the exception of which one?
a. MMSE
b. Blessed Rating Scale
c. National Adult Rating Scale
d. National Adult Reading Test
e. Tower of London Test

Question 101
A 65-year-old man has been diagnosed with Parkinson's disease 3 years ago. He has been regularly with his follow-ups with his neurologist. Of late, he has been having marked neurological manifestation of his Parkinson's disease, and his neurologist have been giving him dopamine agonist treatment. It is believed that dopamine agonist treatment might give rise to which of the following symptoms?
a. Auditory hallucinations
b. Visual hallucinations
c. Olfactory hallucinations
d. Tactile hallucinations
e. Haptic hallucinations

Question 102
A 23-year-old man has been diagnosed with schizophrenia. The core trainee has taken a history from him and noted that he has an abrupt onset of his illness. In addition, his core symptoms were that of paranoia. The core trainee could not elicit any history of negative symptoms or any cognitive deficits currently. The patient has been living with his family currently and is not in any relationship. He does

have a family history of mood disorder. Which of the following is a negative prognostic factor for his condition?
a. Abrupt onset of his illness
b. Being unmarried
c. Family history of mood disorders
d. Marked paranoid symptoms
e. Lack of negative symptoms

Question 103
Which of the following interventions would be more appropriate for a man who is dependent on alcohol but currently in the contemplation stage of change?
a. Cognitive behavioural therapy
b. Follow-up in 1 month
c. Intensive outpatient therapy
d. Motivating interviewing
e. Twelve-step facilitation

Question 104
Which of the following statements about Rett syndrome is incorrect?
a. The incidence of sudden and unexpected death is usually around 5%.
b. The condition has been predominantly a female disorder.
c. The deterioration usually occurs between 7 and 24 months.
d. Anticonvulsant treatment is helpful with seizure control.
e. Behaviour therapy is helpful for controlling self-injurious behaviour.

Question 105
Childhood disintegrative disorder has a prevalence of 1.7 per 1000 individuals. There is noted to be a male predominance. Normal development occurs for up to how many years after birth?
a. 1 year
b. 2 years
c. 3 years
d. 4 years
e. 5 years

Question 106
A 12-year-old boy is here with his mother for an assessment after being referred by their GP. The GP has noted mother's concerns about him having abnormal movement. To make the diagnosis of a possible Tourette's syndrome, you should look out for which of the following symptoms, as it is usually the first to appear in Tourette's syndrome?
a. Motor tics
b. Vocal tics
c. Facial dystonia
d. Trunk dystonia
e. Tremors

Question 107

To make a diagnosis of attention deficit hyperactivity disorder (ADHD), questionnaires such as the Connors' rating scale is commonly used. The Connors' rating scale includes all the following components, with the exception of
a. ADHD symptoms
b. Social problems
c. Anxiety symptoms
d. Depressive symptoms
e. Cognitive symptoms

Question 108

What is the relapse rate for non-psychotic depression for those who have had one prior episode of post-partum depression?
a. One in two
b. One in three
c. One in four
d. One in five
e. One in six

Question 109

The risk of psychosis recurring in a subsequent pregnancy after one episode of post-partum psychosis has been estimated to be which of the following?
a. One in two
b. One in three
c. One in seven
d. One in ten
e. None of the above

Question 110

Which of the following statements about the usage of psychotropic medications in breast feeding is incorrect?
a. For bipolar disorder, valproate can be used, but the mother should be advised to ensure adequate contraception to prevent pregnancy.
b. For bipolar disorder, lithium, at low doses, can be used and is safe for neonates.
c. For depressive disorder, the recommended medications are those of paroxetine and sertraline.
d. For schizophrenia, only olanzapine and sulpiride have been recommended.
e. Methadone is not contraindicated for usage in mothers who are breastfeeding.

Extended Match Items

Theme: Psychotherapy

Options:
a. Acting out
b. Denial
c. Displacement

d. Intellectualization
e. Projection
f. Rationalization
g. Repression
h. Sublimation

Lead in: A 55-year-old man who was working in a multinational company as manager, with a background of poorly controlled diabetes, underwent a right below-knee amputation 3 months ago because of complications of his diabetes. Since then, he has been feeling depressed with passive thoughts of suicide.

Select the one most appropriate defence mechanism for each of the following situations. Each option may be used once, more than once or not at all.

Question 111
He denies being depressed and says that everything is fine. When the psychiatrist asks him how he feels about the amputation, he always evades the question and talks about something else. (Choose one option.)

Question 112
He becomes angry with the psychiatrist for asking him questions about his work and family situation. He says that the psychiatrist deliberately makes his mood worse, and there is nothing that can be done to help him. (Choose one option.)

Question 113
He is made to resign from work, as he cannot keep up to the demands of his job. He overhears colleagues passing sarcastic remarks about him. When at home, he scolds his wife badly for a trivial matter. (Choose one option.)

Question 114
Two months later, after adequate pharmacological and psychotherapy treatment, he appears to be coping well and tells his psychiatrist that he has decided to help out in a volunteer social service catering to support the disabled. (Choose one option.)

Theme: Psychotherapy
Options:
a. Acting out
b. Idealization
c. Identification
d. Intellectualization
e. Isolation of affect
f. Projective identification
g. Rationalization
h. Regression
i. Suppression
j. Undoing

Lead in: A 23-year-old woman with a psychiatric diagnosis of borderline personality disorder is admitted to the ward for deliberate self-harm. She has a history of physical abuse by her parents when she was young.

Select the one most appropriate defence mechanism for each of the following situations. Each option may be used once, more than once or not at all.

Question 115
The nurse asks her to change out of her own clothing and wear hospital attire. She becomes upset and tries to hit the nurse. During a psychotherapy session, she realizes that her desire to hit the nurse was related to her father hitting her when she was a child. (Choose one option.)

Question 116
She mentions that she has been trying to block memories about her past abuse from entering her mind. (Choose one option.)

Question 117
She says that she cut herself on the arm with a penknife to externalize her pain and ease her stress in life. She feels that self-cutting is an acceptable way of coping and that it has benefits in making her mind clearer and stabilizing her emotions. (Choose one option.)

Question 118
She refers to abstract philosophy to explain her current plight. (Choose one option.)

Question 119
After speaking to the ward doctor for 20 min, she believes that he is the best doctor she has ever seen. She demands to be seen only by the ward doctor. (Choose one option.)

Question 120
She is noted to be lying flat on the floor, clutching a teddy bear and crying loudly. When the nurse asks what happened, she replies, in a child-like manner, that the other patients bullied her. (Choose one option.)

Question 121
Her brother mentions that she had tried to separate herself from her emotions ever since her aunt, with whom she was close, passed away a few months ago. (Choose one option.)

Question 122
She tries to take on the quality of her aunt, who had passed away a few months ago, by behaving like her. (Choose one option.)

Theme: Research Methodology

Options:
- a. Kruskal–Wallis
- b. McNemar test
- c. One-way ANOVA
- d. Paired *t*-test
- e. Wilcoxon rank sum test
- g. Two-way ANOVA

Lead in: Match one statistical test to each of the following scenarios. Each option may be used once, more than once or not at all.

Question 123
A study was conducted to evaluate the effects of antidepressants on immunological function. Thirty depressed patients were treated with SSRIs and placebo in a cross-over design with a wash-out period in-between. Cytokine levels were measured during treatment and placebo. (Choose one option.)

Question 124
A researcher wants to find out which type of antidepressants (tricyclic antidepressants, SSRIs and serotonin–norepinephrine reuptake inhibitors) leads to better quality of life in depressed patients. The patients fill up SF-36, which assesses their health-related quality of life, and the doctor independently assesses the global assessment of functioning (GAF) score. Both SF-36 and GAF scores are normally distributed. The researcher will compare the SF-12 and GAF scores of patients receiving the three types of antidepressants. (Choose one option.)

Question 125
In an undergraduate examination that follows the closed marking system (candidates usually score the marks between 4 and 7, where 4 = fail, 5 = pass, 7 = distinction), the chief examiner wants to compare the median examination score between local and immigrant doctors. (Choose one option.)

Theme: Research Methodology

Options:
- a. Level 1A
- b. Level 1B
- c. Level 1C
- d. Level 2A
- e. Level 2B
- f. Level 2C
- g. Level 3A
- h. Level 3B
- i. Level 4
- j. Level 5

Lead in: Match one correct hierarchy of research evidence with each of the following study types. Each option may be used once, more than once or not at all.

Question 126
Case series. (Choose one option.)

Question 127
Ecological studies. (Choose one option.)

Question 128
Expert opinion. (Choose one option.)

Theme: Learning Disability
Options:
  a. 15
  b. 30
  c. 40
  d. 60
  e. 90

Lead in: Match one number to each of the following disabilities. Each option may be used once, more than once or not at all.
   Of all learning disability patients, what percentage suffers from each of the following:

Question 129
Mild learning disability. (Choose one option.)

Question 130
Moderate learning disability. (Choose one option.)

Question 131
Severe learning disability. (Choose one option.)

Question 132
Profound learning disability. (Choose one option.)

Theme: Old-Age Psychiatry
Options:
  a. MMSE
  b. Addenbrooke's cognitive assessment revised
  c. Montreal cognitive assessment
  d. Clinical dementia rating scale
  e. Dementia questionnaire for the mentally retarded
  f. Dementia scale for Down syndrome
  g. Cambridge Cognition Examination
  h. Blessed Dementia Rating Scale

i. Hachinski ischaemic score
   j. National adult reading test
   k. Kendrick object learning test
   l. Wisconsin card sorting test

Lead in: Match the questionnaires with each of the following questions. Each option may be used once, or more than once or not at all.

Question 133
Which of the following are considered as standardized instruments for formal cognitive testing? (Choose four options.)

Question 134
Which two of the above could be used for assessment of cognition for those with learning disabilities? (Choose two options.)

Question 135
The CAMDEX includes which of the above questionnaires? (Choose six options.)

Theme: Neuroimaging in the Elderly

Options:
   a. Cortical atrophy and ventricular enlargement
   b. Atrophy of the hippocampus
   c. Subcortical vascular encephalopathy
   d. Small, well-localized subcortical infarcts
   e. Anterior hypo-perfusion on functional imaging
   f. Gross atrophy in fronto-temporal regions

Lead in: Match one finding with each of the following questions. Each option may be used once, more than once or not at all.

Question 136
Which one of the above is one of the classical findings in Creutzfeldt–Jakob disease (CJD)? (Choose one option.)

Question 137
Which one is a classical neuro-imaging finding for frontotemporal dementia? (Choose one option.)

Question 138
Which two are characteristic findings for vascular dementia? (Choose one option.)

Question 139
Which two of the above are classical imaging findings for individuals with Alzheimer's dementia? (Choose one option.)

Theme: General Adult

Options:
  a. Conversion disorder
  b. Dissociative amnesia
  c. Factitious disorder
  d. Ganser syndrome
  e. Hypochondriasis
  f. Malingering
  g. Somatization disorder
  h. Trance and possession disorder

Lead in: Select one diagnosis for each of the following clinical descriptions. Each option may be used once, more than once or not at all.

Question 140
A 25-year-old woman with no medical history of note presents with sudden onset of blindness following the death of her mother. She is reviewed by both the neurologist and the ophthalmologist, but no physical cause is found for her symptoms. (Choose one option.)

Question 141
A 30-year-old man presents to the hospital complaining of abdominal pain and haemoptysis. He demands admission. He undergoes colonoscopy and blood investigations, which were all normal. He self-discharges when given the results of the investigations. This is his tenth admission in 8 months, each admission resulting in self-discharge. (Choose one option.)

Question 142
A 40-year-old woman comes to the hospital complaining of severe headache. She is very worried that she has a severe brain condition that will make her lose her mind. Her grandmother passed away from a brain tumour a few years ago. Despite repeated normal brain scans and reassurance from the doctors, she is not totally convinced. She decides to seek a consultation from another doctor, as she is concerned that her current doctor could have missed a serious medical condition causing her headache. (Choose one option.)

Question 143
A 17-year-old woman comes to the emergency department complaining of leg pain. She is noted to be joking with the friends who accompanied her, but she becomes tearful and demands to be given a sick note to rest at home when the doctor comes to review her. Her history and physical examination are inconsistent, and investigations are unremarkable. A staff nurse overhears the patient telling her friends that she is planning to go on a holiday for the next 3 days. (Choose one option.)

Theme: Forensic Psychiatry

Options:

a. 5%
b. 10%
c. 15%
d. 20%
e. 30%
f. 35%
h. 40%
i. 45%
j. 50%

Lead in: A 30-year-old man with schizophrenia has been admitted involuntarily to a psychiatric hospital after he was found to be agitated and had been violent towards family members.

Match one approximate percentage to each of the following acts of violence. Each option may be used once, more than once or not at all.

Question 144
Verbal aggression. (Choose one option.)

Question 145
Physical violence towards objects. (Choose one option.)

Question 146
Physical violence towards others. (Choose one option.)

Question 147
Self-directed violence. (Choose one option.)

Question 148
Family members involved in the assaults. (Choose one option.)

Question 149
Strangers being attacked in the assaults. (Choose one option.)

Theme: Hospital Liaison Psychiatry

Options:

a. Alzheimer's disease
b. Anxiety
c. Bipolar disorder
d. Catastrophic reaction
e. Depression
f. Emotional incongruity
g. Emotionalism
h. Mania
i. Psychotic depression
j. Vascular dementia

Lead in: Choose one psychiatric sequela for each of the following clinical scenarios. Each option may be used once, more than once or not at all.

Question 150
A 79-year-old man with right-sided hemiparesis presents with sudden episodes of uncontrollable crying. (Choose one option.)

Question 151
A 70-year-old woman with left opercular lesions presents with aggression and emotional outbursts when she is unable to express herself using language. (Choose one option.)

Question 152
A 73-year-old man with lacunar infarcts presents with hemiparesis, dysphasia, depression and cognitive impairment. (Choose one option.)

Question 153
A 68-year-old woman with a vascular insult to the basal ganglia presents with feelings of hopelessness, anhedonia, psychomotor retardation and hypersomnia. (Choose one option.)

Theme: Psychotropic Medications in Breastfeeding
Options:
  a. Valproate
  b. Lithium
  c. Paroxetine
  d. Sertraline
  e. Citalopram
  f. Fluoxetine
  g. Mirtazapine
  h. Sulpiride
  i. Olanzapine
  j. Clozapine
  k. Methadone

Lead in: Match the correct drugs to the following statements. Each option may be used once, more than once or not at all.

Question 154
If the mother develops a relapse of bipolar disorder immediately after pregnancy, which one of the commonly used mood stabilizers should not be used in view of her intending to still breastfeed her child? (Choose one option.)

Question 155
If the mother is depressed after pregnancy, which of the commonly used antidepressants could be used, if she is still keen to breastfeed her child? (Choose one option.)

Question 156

If the mother is psychotic after pregnancy, which one of the commonly used anti-psychotics should be avoided, in view of the fact that she is actively breastfeeding her child? (Choose one option.)

Question 157

Which medication is suitable for mothers who are using substances but who also want to breastfeed their newborn? (Choose one option.)

Theme: Cardiovascular Disease and Psychotropics

Options:
   a. Clozapine
   b. Olanzapine
   c. Aripiprazole
   d. Mirtazapine
   e. Tricyclic antidepressants
   f. Lithium
   g. Valproate
   h. Benzodiazepines
   i. Rivastigmine
   j. Donepezil

Lead in: For a patient diagnosed with atrial fibrillation, match the correct drugs to the following statements. Each option may be used once, more than once or not at all.

Question 158

Which antipsychotic medications are not indicated? (Choose two options.)

Question 159

Which antidepressant is safe for use in patients with atrial fibrillation? (Choose one option.)

Question 160

Which mood stabilizers are safe for use in patients with atrial fibrillation? (Choose two options.)

Question 161

Which medication for dementia is safe for patients with atrial fibrillation? (Choose one option.)

Theme: Research Methodology

Options:
   a. Concurrent validity
   b. Content validity
   c. Face validity
   d. Incremental validity
   e. Predictive validity

Lead in: Match one correct type of validity with each of the following definitions. Each option may be used once, more than once or not at all.

Question 162
It indicates whether the measurement being assessed is superior to other measurements in approaching true validity. (Choose one option.)

Question 163
It examines whether the specific measurements aimed for by the measuring instrument are assessing the content of the measurement in question. (Choose one option.)

Question 164
It compares the measure being assessed with an external valid yardstick at the same time. (Choose one option.)

Theme: Research Methodology

Options:
   a. Convenience
   b. Cluster
   c. Judgement
   d. Quota
   e. Random
   f. Snowball
   g. Stratified
   h. Systematic

Lead in: Match one correct type of sampling with each of the following methods. Each option may be used once, more than once or not at all.

Question 165
   Ask the subject to recommend acquaintances who meet the sample criteria. (Choose one option.)

Question 166
Subjects are chosen on basis of being readily available. (Choose one option.)

Question 167
Assign members of the population into relatively homogeneous subgroups (strata) before sampling. Then, draw random sample of subjects from within each strata. (Choose one option.)

Theme: Psychotherapy

Options:
   a. Balint
   b. Bowlby
   c. Carl Jung

d. Fairburn
   e. Heinz Kohut
   f. Margaret Mahler
   g. Melanie Klein
   h. Wilfred Bion
   i. Winnicott

Lead in: Match one person to each of the following correct theories. Each option may be used once, more than once or not at all.

Question 168
Concepts of projective identification and splitting in borderline personality disorder. (Choose one option.)

Question 169
Archetypes are representations of experiences in the collective unconscious that lead to conflicts and anxiety. (Choose one option.)

Question 170
Ocnophil (clingy and dependent) and philobat (grandiose and pseudo-independent) are two types of defensive strategies against separation anxiety. (Choose one option.)

Question 171
Autistic phase, symbiosis, separation-individuation. (Choose one option.)

Question 172
The therapist acts as container for the client's projections for exploration of feelings. (Choose one option.)

Question 173
Internal world is a substitute for a frustrating experience in external relationships and frustration often leads to aggression. (Choose one option.)

Question 174
A good-enough mother helps the child to progress from dependency to independence. (Choose one option.)

Question 175
Classified attachment based on the adult attachment interview into autonomous attachment, dismissive attachment, preoccupied attachment. (Choose one option.)

Question 176
Concept of self-psychology where self has a central and functional role in the mind. (Choose one option.)

Theme: Addictions and Mechanism of Actions

  a. Alcohol
  b. Opioid
  c. Cannabis
  d. Lysergic acid diethylamide
  e. Phencyclidine
  f. 3,4-methylenedioxy-methamphetamine

Lead in: Please match the following mechanism of actions with the appropriate drug of abuse.

Question 177
The main neurochemical effect is via the blockage of N-methyl-D-aspartate (NMDA) glutamate receptors.

Question 178
The mechanism of action of this particular drug of abuse is via serotonin neurotoxin.

Question 179
This leads to the activation of particular receptors, and this would inhibit adenylate cyclase.

Question 180
The binding of this particular drug to the mu receptors inhibits the release of gamma-aminobutyric acid (GABA) from the nerve terminal and this reducing the inhibitory effect of GABA on dopaminergic neurons.

Theme: Learning Disability and Clinical Phenotypes

  a. Primary prevention
  b. Secondary prevention
  c. Tertiary prevention

Lead in: Please match the levels of prevention in accordance to the following questions.

Question 181
In this form of prevention, it involves the reduction of birth-related trauma as well as the prevention of infection and the prevention of neural tube defects by taking folate during pregnancy.

Question 182
This involves typically active resettlement programs with expansion of support networks.

Question 183
This involves the typical prenatal diagnosis and maternal serum alpha foetoprotein screening.

Theme: Child Psychiatry

a. 1%
b. 3%
c. 5%
d. 7%
e. 10%

Lead in: Please match the correct percentage to the following questions.

Question 184
A mother who has one child with autism is currently expecting her second child. What is the estimated risk of her second child developing autism?

Question 185
A 12-year-old has been previously diagnosed with Tourette's syndrome. What is the estimated probability that he might have Asperger's syndrome as a comorbid?

Theme: Old-Age Psychiatry

a. Alzheimer's disease
b. Binswanger's disease
c. Cerebral autosomal-dominant arteriopathy with subcortical infarcts and leukoencephalopathy (CASDIL)
d. Frontal lobe dementia
e. Lewy body dementia
f. Psychogenic fugue
g. Pseudodementia
h. Vascular dementia
i. Vitamin B1 deficiency

Lead in: Please match the above diagnosis with each of the following clinical situations.

Question 186
An 80-year-old man presents with fluctuating, progressive memory loss and emotional incontinence. He has history of falls and is being treated for hypertension by his GP. His relatives say that his personality is preserved.

Question 187
A 65-year-old woman presents with memory loss following the death of her husband 4 months ago. She also complains of poor sleep, lack of energy and weight loss. During the cognitive assessment, she is not keen to answer the questions.

Question 188
A 75-year-old man presents with cognitive impairment and fluctuating levels of consciousness, particularly confusion and bizarre behaviour in the evenings. His daughter claims that he has been seeing ghosts and not able to turn in his bed. On physical examination, he is found to have hypertonia and hypersalivation. The score on MMSE is 15/30. These above symptoms worsen following the commencement of antipsychotic medication.

Question 189

A 40-year-old woman presents with a cognitive deterioration and mood changes. On physical examination, there are gait abnormalities. She has a past medical history of epilepsy and migraines with aura. She also has episodes of left-sided muscular weakness. On further inquiry, her aunt has similar problems.

Question 190

A 60-year-old woman was found wandering on the streets with some memory loss after the recent funeral of her husband. She was brought in by the police for psychiatric assessment. When you assess her, she is unable to recall her personal details. She is physically well, and all investigations are normal.

Question 191

A 60-year-old man who was previously a reserved and religious teacher began making out-of-character remarks, talking aloud about pornography and talking to strangers in the bus stop. He has been aggressive to his wife. When you ask him a new question, he gives you the answers to the previous questions.

Question 192

A 60-year-old woman with chronic hypertension presents with gradual reduction in memory, step-like intellectual decline and slowness in motor functions. Magnetic resonance imaging (MRI) shows periventricular lucencies, multiple microvascular infarcts in areas supplied by perforating vessels and white matter leukoaraiosis. Single-photon emission computed tomography (SPECT) scan shows bilateral reduction of blood flow in thalamus, basal ganglia and frontal lobes.

Question 193

A 30-year-old woman who is 10 weeks' pregnant was admitted to the obstetric ward after excessive vomiting. She has very poor oral intake and was given intravenous dextrose solution for fluid replacement. Subsequently, she develops memory problems. Neurological examination reveals horizontal diplopia and ataxia. Her husband mentions that she does not drink alcohol.

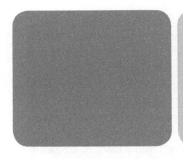

MRCPYSCH PAPER B MOCK EXAMINATION 2: ANSWERS

GET THROUGH MRCPSYCH PAPER B MOCK EXAMINATION

Question 1 Answer: e, Decreased need for control
Explanation: Increased risk of suicide in patients with cancer is associated with male gender, advanced stage of disease, poor prognosis, delirium with poor impulse control, poor pain control, depression, hopelessness, history of psychiatric illness, history of previous suicidal attempt, family history of suicide, substance or alcohol abuse, social isolation, advanced age, presence of fatigue and extreme need for control. Patients with cancer have twice the risk of committing suicide as the general population. Hopelessness is even a stronger predictive factor than depression itself. Patients with cancer usually commit suicide by overdosage with analgesics or sedative drugs prescribed by their doctors. Men use violent means, such as hanging or gunshot, more often than women.

References: Levenson JL (2004). *The American Psychiatric Publishing Textbook of Psychosomatic Medicine*. Arlington, VA: American Psychiatric Publishing, p. 519; Massie MJ, Gagnon P, Holland JC (1994). Depression and suicide in patients with cancer. *J Pain Symptom Manage*, 9(5): 325–340.

Question 2 Answer: d, First-rank symptoms are pathognomonic of schizophrenia
Explanation: The classical first-rank symptoms include auditory hallucinations (repeating the thoughts out loud, in third person, in the form of a running commentary), delusions of passivity (thought insertion, withdrawal and broadcasting and made feelings, impulses and actions) and somatic passivity and delusional perception. Second-rank symptoms include perplexity, emotional blunting, hallucinations and other delusions. It should be noted that first-rank symptoms could occur in other psychosis and, although highly suggestive of schizophrenia, are not pathognomonic of the condition.

Reference: Puri BK, Hall AD, Ho RC (2014). *Revision Notes in Psychiatry*. Boca Raton, FL: CRC Press, p. 350.

Question 3 Answer: c, Obsessive-Compulsive Behaviour
Explanation: Smith–Magenis syndrome is caused by the complete or partial deletion of chromosome 17p11.2. Its psychiatric features include schizophrenia-like psychosis, inappropriate affect, aggression, sleep disturbances and self-harming behaviour. Other clinical features include hearing problems, hoarse and deep voice, renal problems, inguinal/umbilical hernia, hypospadias (in 10% of male patients), short broad hands and small toes, hypotonia, hyperextensible fingers and moderate-to-severe learning disability. Naltrexone is useful in reducing self-injurious behaviour.

Clinically, they are given multiple diagnosis, ranging from autism to attention-deficit hyperactivity disorder (ADHD) and even obsessive-compulsive disorder (OCD) and mood disorders.

References: Puri BK, Hall AD, Ho RC (2014). *Revision Notes in Psychiatry*. Boca Raton, FL: CRC Press, pp. 678–679; Ann CM Smith et al. Smith-Magenis Syndrome. GeneReviews (https://ghr.nlm.nih.gov/condition/smith-magenis-syndrome).

Question 4 Answer: d, Psychopathy checklist – revised (PCL-R) score
Explanation: The Violence Risk Appraisal Guide (VRAG) is an actuarial violence risk assessment that is entirely reliant on historical factors. It is made up of 12 items and includes PCL-R as a subscale. The other items on VRAG include difficulties at primary school, personality disorder, younger age, never married, absence of schizophrenia, victim injury and failed conditional release/supervision order. The strongest correlate with violent recidivism is the PCL-R score with a positive correlation equivalent to explaining approximately 10% of the variance in violent reoffending.

Reference: Dolan M, Doyle M (2000). Violence risk prediction. Clinical and actuarial measures and the role of the psychopathy checklist. *Br J Psychiatr*, 177: 303–311.

Question 5 Answer: c, Fourfold
Explanation: There is an estimated fourfold increase in risk of alcohol dependency in first-degree relatives of alcoholics. Family members of alcoholics also have an increased risk of other substance-use disorders. However, there is also evidence of specificity of familial aggregation of the prominent drug of abuse, suggesting that there may be not only risk factors that are specific to the particular class of drug but also risk factors that underlie substance abuse in general. Adopted children of alcoholic parents have the same fourfold increased risk of alcohol dependency as children raised by their alcohol-dependent parents.

Reference: Puri BK, Treasaden I (eds) (2010). *Psychiatry: An Evidence-Based Text*. London: Hodder Arnold, pp. 480–481.

Question 6 Answer: e, Do not recommend any of the above
Explanation: The National Institute for Health and Care Excellence (NICE) guidelines advise not to use the above drugs as specific treatment for the primary prevention of dementia. If this question is changed and asks which medication may reduce the risk of dementia, the answer is selegiline, because it has an antioxidant effect.

Reference: Sano M, Ernesto C, Thomas RG et al. (1997). A controlled trial of selegi-line, alpha-tocopherol, or both as treatment for Alzheimer's disease. The Alzheimer's Disease Cooperative Study. *N Engl J Med*, 336: 1216–1222.

Question 7 Answer: a, Gamma-glutamyl transferase (GGT)

Explanation: GGT becomes elevated after acute or chronic alcohol use and remains elevated for 2–5 weeks afterwards. It is commonly used as an objective indicator of relapse. Other typical laboratory findings in people with alcohol abuse include increased serum carbohydrate-deficient transferrin, increased mean corpuscular volume, increased aspartate transaminase and alanine transaminase and lactate dehydrogenase and prolonged prothrombin time.

Reference: Levenson, JL (2004). *The American Psychiatric Publishing Textbook of Psychosomatic Medicine*. Arlington, VA: American Psychiatric Publishing, p. 397.

Question 8 Answer: d, Cross-sectional study

Explanation: Cross-sectional studies analyse a population (or a representative subset) at a single point in time and are used to assess disease prevalence. In this type of study, all of the variables (exposure and outcomes) are measured at the same time. They can be descriptive (description of the point prevalence of a disease in a population linked to health service usage data), analytical (comparison of several exposures with the outcome of interest) and ecological (neither exposure nor outcome is measured at the individual level). The strengths of this type of study include ability to study multiple exposures and outcomes, rapid, cheap and useful for rare disease. The weakness is that, because this type of study measures prevalence and not incidence, findings cannot differentiate the determinants of aetiology and survival.

Reference: Lewis GH, Sheringham J, Kalim K, Crayford TJ (2008). *Mastering Public Health: A Postgraduate Guide to Examination and Revalidation*. London: Royal Society of Medicine Press, p. 36.

Question 9 Answer: e, Sample size computation

Explanation: Internal validity is the extent to which the results of a study are true. That is, the intervention really did cause the change and that it is not caused by extraneous factors. Bias in randomized controlled trial (RCT) can affect the extent to which the results are true. It is usually not intentional but is pervasive and insidious. There are many specific types of bias associated with an RCT: selection, measurement and analysis bias. The result of bias in a clinical study is to over- or under-estimate the treatment effect as a result. Methods in clinical trials that are used to minimize bias include randomization, concealment allocation, blinding and intention-to-treat analysis.

References: Everitt BS (2006). *Medical Statistics from A to Z* (2nd edition). Cambridge, UK: Cambridge University Press, p. 241; Turlik M (2009). Evaluating the internal validity of a randomized controlled trial. *Foot Ankle Online J*, 2(3): 5.

Question 10 Answer: a, Combining results of RCTs and open label trials in one forest plot is appropriate
Explanation: Meta-analysis is a collection of techniques whereby the results of two or more independent studies are statistically combined to yield an overall answer to a question of interest. The rationale behind this approach is to provide a test with more power than is provided by the separate studies themselves. Either a fixed-effects or random-effects model is used to reach an overall estimate of effect size. In the meta-analysis, it is impossible to combine both types of trial (random control and open label trials) in one forest plot.

Reference: Everitt BS (2006). *Medical Statistics from A to Z* (2nd edition). Cambridge, UK: Cambridge University Press, p. 150.

Question 11 Answer: d, Decreased growth hormone
Explanation: Growth hormone is increased in patients suffering from anorexia nervosa. Bone mineral density is reduced; leukopaenia with relative lymphocytosis, mitral valve prolapse and pancreatitis can occur in patients with anorexia nervosa.

Reference: Puri BK, Hall AD, Ho RC (2014). *Revision Notes in Psychiatry*. Boca Raton, FL: CRC Press, pp. 578–579.

Question 12 Answer: d, He demonstrates anterograde amnesia after admission to the ward
Explanation: Transient global amnesia usually lasts for a few hours and seldom recurs. It will not lead to anterograde amnesia.

Reference: Puri BK, Treasaden I (eds) (2010). *Psychiatry: An Evidence-Based Text*. London: Hodder Arnold, pp. 95, 557.

Question 13 Answer: b, Hypnopompic hallucinations are commoner than hypnagogic hallucination
Explanation: Narcolepsy is caused by the loss of hypocretin cells in the hypothalamus. Hypocretin is a neurotransmitter that regulates arousal and wakefulness. Clinical features of narcolepsy include hypersomnia, sleep attacks, cataplexy, hypnagogic hallucinations and sleep paralysis. Stimulants such as modafinil and methylphenidate can reduce daytime sleepiness. Hypersomnia and cataplexy have stable course over time.

Hypnagogic hallucinations occur in 20%–40% of individuals. They are usually visual hallucinations or dream-like imagery. Hypnopompic hallucinations are less common compared with hypnagogic hallucinations.

Reference: Puri BK, Hall AD, Ho RC (2014). *Revision Notes in Psychiatry*. Boca Raton, FL: CRC Press, pp. 616–617.

Question 14 Answer: e, Creutzfeldt–Jakob disease
Explanation: Option (e) is correct. It is considered to be a very rare cause of rapidly progressive dementia. There might be a brief prodromal period of anxiety, depres-

sion or hallucinations. Sudden onset and rapid progression of dementia, pyramidal and extrapyramidal deficits are present.

Reference: Puri BK, Hall AD, Ho RC (2014). *Revision Notes in Psychiatry*. Boca Raton, FL: CRC Press, p. 705.

Question 15 Answer: b, Alzheimer's disease dementia is not a risk factor for refractory seizures

Explanation: Alzheimer's disease is a risk factor for refractory seizure in the elderly. About half of seizures in the elderly are related to strokes or tumours, while up to a quarter have unknown causes. As many as 80% of seizures become recurrent.

Reference: Blazer DG, Steffens DC, Busse EW (2004). *The American Psychiatric Publishing TextBook of Geriatric Psychiatry* (3rd edition). Arlington, VA: American Psychiatric Publishing, p. 67.

Question 16 Answer: d, 60 years old

Explanation: Paraphrenia was a term introduced in 1909 to describe a psychotic condition that has a relatively late age of onset, with the presence of chronic delusions and hallucinations but with the preservation of volition and lack of personality changes. The terminology of this condition lost favour until 1955, where it was once again reintroduced to describe a condition that has an age of first onset after 60 years old, with well-organized delusions with or without hallucinations and a well-preserved personality and affective response.

Early onset psychosis occurs before the age of 40 years. Late onset schizophrenia occurs after the age of 40 years, and very late onset occurs at the age of 60 years.

Reference: Puri BK, Hall AD, Ho RC (2014). *Revision Notes in Psychiatry*. Boca Raton, FL: CRC Press, p. 712.

Question 17 Answer: e, Undoing

Explanation: Undoing is an attempt to negate shameful, sexual or aggressive implications from a previous comment or behaviour by elaborating, clarifying or doing the opposite. This is often seen in patients with OCD. Other defence mechanisms often seen in OCD include projection and reaction formation. Projection involves perceiving and reacting to unacceptable inner impulses and their derivatives as although they were outside the self. Reaction formation involves transforming an unacceptable impulse into its opposite.

Reference: Sadock BJ, Sadock VA (2003). *Kaplan and Sadock's Synopsis of Psychiatry* (9th edition). Philadelphia, PA: Lippincott, Williams & Wilkins, pp. 207–208.

Question 18 Answer: c, Isolation/displacement

Explanation: In people with phobia, there is often isolation of unconscious fears and displacement of fear onto an external object. Denial/displacement is often seen in eating disorder, denial/introjection is often seen in depressive disorder, splitting/projection is often seen in schizophrenia and undoing/projection is often seen in OCD.

Reference: Gabbard GO (2014). *Psychodynamic Psychotherapy in Clinical Practice* (5th edition). Arlington, VA: American Psychiatric Press, pp. 268–273.

Question 19 Answer: c, 68%
Explanation: Based on a previous review article, neuroimaging studies have identified that approximately 65%–78% receptor blockade would help individuals to achieve the best benefits from the medications, while experiencing the least amount of side effects. However, it should be noted that clozapine do not conform to the typical therapeutic window.

Reference: Ginovart N, Kapur S (2012). Role of dopamine D(2) receptors for antipsychotic activity. *Handb Exp Pharmacol*, 212: 27–52.

Question 20 Answer: b, 3:1
Explanation: Based on previous epidemiological research data, the male-to-female gender ratio for conduct disorder is approximately 3:1 and for oppositional defiant disorder is also 3:1 before puberty but approaches 1:1 after puberty.

Reference: Puri BK, Hall AD, Ho RC (2014). *Revision Notes in Psychiatry*. Boca Raton, FL: CRC Press, p. 635.

Question 21 Answer: b, Cognitive dysfunction
Explanation: Neuropsychiatric systemic lupus erythematosus (NPSLE) is the least understood yet perhaps the most prevalent manifestation of lupus. It affects 14% to over 80% of adults and 22%–95% of children and can occur independently of active systemic disease and without serologic activity. NSPLE is associated with increased morbidity and mortality. Cognitive dysfunction is the most common neuropsychiatric disorder in patients with SLE, affecting up to 80%. Depression is the second-most-common disorder, occurring in about 50% of patients. It is estimated that 28%–40% of adult NPSLE manifestations develop before or around the time of the diagnosis of SLE and 63% occur within the first year after diagnosis.

References: Levenson JL (2004). *The American Psychiatric Publishing Textbook of Psychosomatic Medicine*. Arlington, VA: American Psychiatric Publishing, p. 544; Popescu A, Kao AH (2011). Neuropsychiatric systemic lupus erythematosus. *Curr Neuropharmacol*, 9(3): 449–457.

Question 22 Answer: b, Clifton assessment procedures for the elderly
Explanation: This is a scale that can predict survival, placement and decline in elderly subjects. The Kew cognitive map assesses parietal lobe function and language functions in the patient with dementia. The Clifton assessment procedures for the elderly (CAPE) helps to assess the level of disability and thus allows for the prediction of need for support service. The National Adult Reading Test (NART) is used to determine the premorbid intelligence quotient (IQ) and thus help in the initial assessment of apparent cognitive impairment. Premorbid functioning is compared with the current functioning using the Wechsler Adult Intelligence Scale (WAIS).

Reference: Puri BK, Hall AD, Ho RC (2014). *Revision Notes in Psychiatry*. Boca Raton, FL: CRC Press, p. 691.

Question 23 Answer: d, Bupropion
Explanation: Selective serotonin re-uptake inhibitors (SSRIs) are suitable for patients with human immunodeficiency virus (HIV) because SSRIs do not affect the CD4 counts. Most of them are equally effective. They tend to have around 70%–90% response rate. With regard to (d), it is advised to be avoided in patients with advanced HIV, epilepsy and acquired immune deficiency syndrome (AIDS)-related dementia. Given his recent episode of delirium, the usage is contraindicated as well.

Reference: Puri BK, Hall AD, Ho RC (2014). *Revision Notes in Psychiatry*. Boca Raton, FL: CRC Press, p. 486.

Question 24 Answer: c, 5-Hydroxytryptamine (5-HT)2A antagonist
Explanation: The action of the antipsychotic on the D2 receptor would lead to improved negative and positive symptoms. It might also result in extrapyramidal side effects as well as prolactin changes. The action of the antipsychotic on the 5-HT2A receptor would result in sexual dysfunction.

References: Miyamoto S et al. (2005). Treatments for schizophrenia: A critical review of pharmacology and mechanisms of action of antipsychotic drugs. *Mol Psychiatry*, 10(1): 79–104; Shapiro DA et al. (2003). Aripiprazole, a novel atypical antipsychotic drug with a unique and robust pharmacology. *Neuropsychopharmacology*, 28(8): 1400–1411.

Question 25 Answer: c, Restricted, stereotyped and repetitive behaviour
Explanation: Studies have shown that most children with autism do show improvement in social relation and communication. The only area in which they do not show improvement is with regard to their rituals and repetitive behaviour. For some children, inappropriate sexual behaviours may emerge in adolescence and early adulthood. Childhood autism usually causes lifelong disability, in which 10% of people with autism ultimately lose their language skills and have intellectual deterioration.

Reference: Puri BK, Hall AD, Ho RC (2014). *Revision Notes in Psychiatry*. Boca Raton, FL: CRC Press, p. 628.

Question 26 Answer: d, Tall stature
Explanation: Nocturnal enuresis is associated more commonly with short stature. Seventy percent have a first-degree relative with late attainment of continence. Stressful life events might result in a doubling of the frequency. Delayed toilet training might result in a delay as well. Developmental delay is twice as common in enuretic children as in controls. Enuretic children are more likely than non-enuretics to have a different shape of bladder base plate and also to have a reduced functional bladder volume.

Reference: Puri B, Treasaden I (eds) (2010). *Psychiatry: An Evidence-Based Text*. London: Hodder Arnold, pp. 482–483, 1067.

Question 27 Answer: e, On average, girls are more distressed than boys by divorce
Explanation: On average, boys are more distressed than girls by divorce, while girls are more distressed than boys if their mothers remarry. Previous studies have shown that there is a raise in conduct problems, anxiety and depression for a year or two following the divorce. Eventually, most of the children become well-functioning individuals, but the divorce may leave a lasting concern on their intimate relationship that may result in failure of the child's future marriage.

Reference: Goodman R, Scoot S (2005). *Child Psychiatry* (2nd edition). Oxford, UK: Blackwell Publishing.

Question 28 Answer: c, In the United States, 17%–20% of elementary school children are estimated to suffer from reading disabilities
Explanation: It should be 2%–8%. For E, it was supported by Stevenson's study, which showed that the prevalence of reading disorders is similar in United States, Taiwan and Japan.

Reference: Stevenson HW et al. (1982). Reading disabilities: The case of Chinese, Japanese, and English. *Child Develop,* 53: 1164–1181.

Question 29 Answer: a, Neuroticism
Explanation: On the Minnesota Multiphasic Personality Inventory (MMPI), bulimics tend to have elevated scores for the psychopathic deviance. On the Eysenck Personality Inventory, they tend to score higher for psychoticism as well as neuroticism.

Reference: Puri BK, Hall AD, Ho RC (2014). *Revision Notes in Psychiatry*. Boca Raton, FL: CRC Press, p. 584.

Question 30 Answer: b, Shoplifting
Explanation: The typical symptoms include deliberately destroying properties, set-ting fire and breaking into someone's house. The early symptoms include stealing objects of value within the home or outside.

Further Reading: Puri BK, Treasaden I (eds) (2010). *Psychiatry: An Evidence-Based Text.* London: Hodder Arnold, p. 1059.

Question 31 Answer: e, Most elderly individuals who have committed suicide tend not to have sought consultation prior to their act
Explanation: This is incorrect. Previous studies have highlighted that 80% of those completing suicide had seen their general practitioner (GP) before their death. In addition, the incidence of physical illnesses in completed elderly suicide is higher than expected. Chronic pain is often a contributory factor. Living alone, a widowed or separated status and alcohol abuse are also risk factors.

Reference: Puri BK, Hall AD, Ho RC (2014). *Revision Notes in Psychiatry*. Boca Raton, FL: CRC Press, p. 715.

Question 32 Answer: c, Retrieval of information in the elderly is impaired, and in particular, cued recall is affected
Explanation: This is incorrect as it is the un-cued recall that shows an age-related decline.

Reference: Puri BK, Hall AD, Ho RC (2014). *Revision Notes in Psychiatry*. Boca Raton, FL: CRC Press, p. 679.

Question 33 Answer: d, 45%
Explanation: In terms of psychopathology, an estimated 46% of individuals with late-onset psychosis have at least one first-rank symptom. The most common hallucinatory experience is auditory, but visual, somatic and olfactory hallucinations also occur.

Reference: Puri BK, Hall AD, Ho RC (2014). *Revision Notes in Psychiatry*. Boca Raton, FL: CRC Press, p. 713.

Question 34 Answer: c, Repeated purposeless movements
Explanation: Tics are sudden, rapid and involuntary movements of circumscribed muscle groups without serving any purpose.

Reference: Puri BK, Treasaden I (eds) (2010). *Psychiatry: An Evidence-Based Text*. London: Hodder Arnold, p. 550.

Question 35 Answer: c, Personality Assessment Inventory (PAI)
Explanation: Objective personality measures involve the scoring of individual responses, by an observer based on a user manual and instructions. This includes Million Behavioural Health Inventory (MBHI), Million Clinical Multiaxial Inventory (MCMI), PAI and MMPI. Projective personality measures involve the eliciting of responses that allow psychodiagnostic interference and detect disorders of reality testing and thought processes; this includes Rorschach Inkblot Test (RIT) and the thematic apperception test (TAT).

Reference: Levenson JL (2004). *The American Psychiatric Publishing Textbook of Psychosomatic Medicine*. Arlington, VA: American Psychiatric Publishing, p. 22.

Question 36 Answer: e, Verbal abilities
Explanation: The Halstead–Reitan Neuropsychological Test Battery (HRNTB) is the most frequently used neuropsychological battery. It consists of five types of measures: (1) input measures; (2) test of verbal abilities; (3) measures of spatial, sequential, and manipulatory abilities; (4) test of abstraction, reasoning, logical analysis and concept formation; and (5) output measures. The popularity of the HRNTB stems from its ability to discriminate between brain-damaged and non-brain-damaged people and to identify the lateralization of damage. These measures have been found to be influenced by age, sex, and education and, to a lesser extent, race or ethnicity.

References: Levenson JL (2004). *The American Psychiatric Publishing Textbook of Psychosomatic Medicine*. Arlington, VA: American Psychiatric Publishing, pp. 16–17; Yantza CL Gavett BE, Lynch JK, McCaffrey RJ (2006 Dec). Potential for interpretation disparities of Halstead–Reitan neuropsychological battery performances in a litigating sample. *Arch Clin Neuropsychol*, 21(8): 809–817. Epub 2006 Oct 4.

Question 37 Answer: c, Acetylcholine
Explanation: Serotonin, dopamine and the catecholamines (adrenaline and noradrenaline) are neurotransmitters involved in the modulation of aggression. Dopamine and serotonin levels in the prefrontal cortex have been found to change in the opposite direction, with a sustained decrease in serotonin to 80% of baseline levels during and after the confrontation and an increase in dopamine to 120% after the confrontation. The temporal pattern of monoamine changes, which followed rather than preceded the confrontation, points to a significant role of cortical dopamine and 5-HT in the consequences as opposed to the triggering of aggressive acts.

References: Levenson JL (2004). *The American Psychiatric Publishing Textbook of Psychosomatic Medicine*. Arlington, VA: American Psychiatric Publishing, p. 176; van Erp AM, Miczek KA (2000). Aggressive behavior, increased accumbal dopamine, and decreased cortical serotonin in rats. *J Neurosci*, 15;20(24): 9320–9325.

Question 38 Answer: e, If a child presents with both enuresis and encopresis, enuresis should be treated first
Explanation: The encopresis should be treated first. Aggressive encopresis is associated with a poor prognosis. Diurnal enuresis is more common in females, owing to a higher prevalence of urinary tract infections.

Reference: Puri BK, Treasaden I (eds) (2010). *Psychiatry: An Evidence-Based Text*. London: Hodder Arnold, p. 1068.

Question 39 Answer: c, In patients with nephrogenic diabetes insipidus, the urine concentrates normally in response to desmopressin
Explanation: This refers to cranial diabetes insipidus. There is failure to concentrate urine in response to desmopressin in nephrogenic diabetes insipidus.

Reference: Puri BK, Hall AD, Ho RC (2014). *Revision Notes in Psychiatry*. Boca Raton, FL: CRC Press, p. 478.

Question 40 Answer: a, Analysis of variance (ANOVA)
Explanation: It is a statistical test to demonstrate statistically significant differences between the means of several groups. It allows the comparison of more than two means. It also assumes the variable to be normally distributed, that is, it is a parametric test. By partitioning the total variance of a set of observations into parts due to particular factors (e.g. sex, treatment group), differences in the mean values of the dependent variable can be assessed. The model underlying ANOVA is essentially the same as that involved in multiple linear regression, with the explanatory variables being dummy variables, coding factor levels and interactions between factors.

ANOVA may be a one-way or two-way (taking multiple relationships into account) analysis of variants. The chi square, Kruskal–Wallis and Mann–Whitney tests are all non-parametric tests that do not assume a normal distribution.

Reference: Everitt BS (2006). *Medical Statistics from A to Z* (2nd edition). Cambridge, UK: Cambridge University Press, p. 10.

Question 41 Answer: c, The probability of rejecting the null hypothesis when it is true

Explanation: Type one errors are generally considered to be more serious than type two errors. In a type one error, there is a false positive, and the null hypothesis has been wrongly rejected; thereby, the study shows an effect that in reality does not exist. A type two error, in contrast, is only an error in the sense that an opportunity to reject the null hypothesis was lost, that is, erroneously accepted and true differences not shown. There is a trade-off between type one and type two errors: the more the study restricts type one errors by setting a lower significance level of alpha (power of study to detect differences), the greater the chance that a type two error will occur.

Reference: Lewis GH, Sheringham J, Kalim K, Crayford TJ (2008). *Mastering Public Health: A Postgraduate Guide to Examination and Revalidation*. London: Royal Society of Medicine Press, p. 87.

Question 42 Answer: b, Chi-square

Explanation: Chi-squared tests are used to compare categorical data that are unpaired, forming a contingency table. In this case, nominal categorical data are collected. Chi-squared tests are used to calculate *p*-values that are then used to determine whether the two groups differed by chance or by some inherent differences. The test is based on the squared differences between the observed and expected frequencies. The test can be either paired or non-paired, so that, either within subject or between subject, comparisons can be studied.

Reference: Everitt BS (2006). *Medical Statistics from A to Z* (2nd edition). Cambridge, UK: Cambridge University Press, p. 42.

Question 43 Answer: c, Monetary incentives

Explanation: Research has shown that providing monetary incentives significantly improves rates compared with when no incentives are provided. Money is the only factor that has a significant independent effect on likelihood of response. Sending reminder postcards does not significantly increase response rates of mailed questionnaires. Informed consent must be obtained from all research participants.

Reference: Whiteman MK, Langenberg P, Kjerulff K et al. (2003). A randomized trial of incentives to improve response rates to a mailed women's health questionnaire. *J Womens Health (Larchmt)*, 12: 821–828.

Question 44 Answer: c, It blocks reuptake of dopamine

Explanation: Cocaine's primary pharmacodynamic action related to its behavioural effects is competitive blockage of dopamine reuptake by the dopamine transporter. This blockage increases the concentration of dopamine in the synaptic cleft and results in increased activation of both dopamine type 1 (D1) and type 2 (D2) receptors. It also blocks the reuptake of noradrenaline, but this is not its main mechanism of action.

Reference: Sadock BJ, Sadock VA (2003). *Kaplan and Sadock's Synopsis of Psychiatry* (9th edition). Philadelphia, PA: Lippincott, Williams & Wilkins, pp. 429–430.

Question 45 Answer: d, Disulfiram

Explanation: This is a commonly prescribed aversive agent, and the prescribing doctor should ensure that the person has not consumed any alcohol for at least 1 day before the commencement of the drug. It works via the inhibition of Aldehyde dehydrogenase 2 (ALDH2) and would lead to an acetaldehyde accumulation after drinking alcohol, thus resulting in unpleasant side effects.

Reference: Puri BK, Hall AD, Ho RC (2014). *Revision Notes in Psychiatry*. Boca Raton, FL: CRC Press, p. 524.

Question 46 Answer: c, Hyperthermia

Explanation: Use of 3,4-methylenedioxy-*N*-methylamphetamine (MDMA) drugs, such as ecstasy, can lead to the serious side effect of lethal hyperthermia, which is mediated by 5-HT. Other harmful effects include death occurring in those with pre-existing cardiac disease caused by cardiac arrhythmias, convulsions, hypertensive crises that may lead to strokes, neurotoxicity and even toxic hepatitis possibly related to impurities in the preparation.

References: Puri BK, Hall AD, Ho RC (2014). *Revision Notes in Psychiatry*. Boca Raton, FL: CRC Press, pp. 543–544; Brown PL, Klyatkin EA (2004). Brain hyperthermia induced by MDMA (ecstasy): Modulation by environmental conditions. *Eur J Neurosci*, 20(1): 51–58.

Question 47 Answer: c, Loss of appetite

Explanation: During cocaine withdrawal, appetite is usually increased rather than decreased. Other symptoms include fatigue, sleep disturbances (insomnia or hypersomnia), psychomotor agitation or retardation and nightmares. With mild-to-moderate cocaine use, these withdrawal symptoms end within 18 hours. With heavy use, withdrawal symptoms can last up to a week but usually peak in 2–4 days. Withdrawal symptoms can also be associated with suicidal ideation in affected persons.

Reference: Sadock BJ, Sadock VA (2003). *Kaplan and Sadock's Synopsis of Psychiatry* (9th edition). Philadelphia, PA: Lippincott, Williams & Wilkins, p. 433.

Question 48 Answer: b, 10
Explanation: About two-thirds of people convicted of homicide with an abnormal mental state at time of the offence are thought to be psychotic. Twenty-five percent of them were known to have refused drug treatment in the month before the homicide and 52% had missed their last appointment with services before the offence.

Reference: The University of Manchester. The National Confidential Inquiry into Homicide and Suicide by People with Mental Illness Annual Report, July 2012. http://www.bbmh.manchester.ac.uk/cmhr

Question 49 Answer: a, Antisocial
Explanation: Among those prisoners who had a clinical interview, the prevalence of any personality disorder was 78% for male remand, 64% for male sentenced and 50% for female prisoners. Antisocial personality disorder has been found to be the most common personality disorder in all prisoners, including females. Sixty-three percent of male remand prisoners, 49% of male sentenced prisoners and 31% of female prisoners were assessed as having antisocial personality disorder.

Reference: Department of Health (2001). *ONS Survey of Psychiatric Morbidity Among Prisoners in England and Wales, 1997.* Essex, UK: UK Data Service.

Question 50 Answer: d, It focuses on violence towards people and property
Explanation: The Historical, Clinical and Risk Management Questionnaire (HCR-20) is focused on violence towards people only and does not include violence to animals or property. The HCR-20 total score is a good predictor of both violent and other offences following discharge from medium secure units for male forensic psychiatric patients in the United Kingdom. Both the historical and risk sub-scales were able to predict offences, but the clinical sub-scale did not produce significant predictions. The predictive efficacy was highest for short periods (under 1 year) and showed a modest fall in efficacy over longer periods (5 years).

References: Douglas KS, Guy LS, Reeves KA (2008). *HCR-20 Violence Risk Assessment Scheme: Overview and Annotated Bibliography (Current up to November 24, 2008).* Tampa, FL: University of South Florida; Gray NS (2008). Predicting violent reconvictions using the HCR-20. *Brit J Psychiatr*, 192: 384–387.

Question 51 Answer: a, High levels of staff–patient interaction
Explanation: Other environmental risk factors include lack of structured activity, poorly defined staffing roles, unpredictable ward programmes and availability of weapons. The environment is very important, as it can be manipulated to reduce the risk of violence. Three groups of environmental factors seem particularly influential: the physical facilities provided for patients, visitors and staff; the experience, training, supervision and numbers of staff and the policies in place to manage the clinical environment.

Reference: Davison SE (2005). The management of violence in general psychiatry. *Adv Psychiatr Treat*, 11: 362–370.

Question 52 Answer: c, It is attributed to mutation on chromosome 22
Explanation: Cystathionine beta-synthase, together with vitamin B6, converts homocysteine to cystathionine. Deficiency of this enzyme causes accumulation of homocysteine and its precursor methionine. Homocystinuria leads primarily to vascular thrombotic events, particularly strokes in young and middle-aged adults, and mental retardation. The relationship between homocystinuria and strokes is so strong that an elevated serum homocysteine level is a risk factor for strokes. The other features of homocysteinuria that reflect malformation of multiple organs include dislocation of the ocular lens, pectus excavatum or carinatum and a tall, Marfan-like stature. There are also often behavioural disturbances, obsessive-compulsive symptoms and personality disorders.

Reference: Kaufman DM, Milstein MJ (2013). *Kaufman's Clinical Neurology for Psychiatrists* (7th edition). Philadelphia, PA: Saunders, p. 296.

Question 53 Answer: b, Fragile X syndrome
Explanation: The diagnosis is that of fragile X syndrome. It is the most common inherited cause of learning disability. It accounts for 10%–20% of mental retardation in men. It is an X-linked dominant genetic disorder with low penetrance. The clinical features include short stature, seizures (20% of patients), strabismus, mitral valve prolapse and single transverse palmer crease. Other associated comorbid psychiatric features include autism-like behaviour and speech and language delays.

Reference: Puri BK, Hall AD, Ho RC (2014). *Revision Notes in Psychiatry*. Boca Raton, FL: CRC Press, p. 666.

Question 54 Answer: d, Idiopathic or unknown
Explanation: There are multiple aetiologies contributing to mental retardation. In one-third of cases, no cause can be identified. Deprivation of nutrition, nurturance and social stimulation may contribute to the development of mental retardation. Current knowledge suggests that genetic, environmental, biological and psychosocial factors work additively in mental retardation. The more severe the mental retardation, the more likely it is that the cause is evident.

Reference: Sadock BJ, Sadock VA (2003). *Kaplan and Sadock's Synopsis of Psychiatry* (9th edition). Philadelphia, PA: Lippincott, Williams & Wilkins, pp. 1164–1165.

Question 55 Answer: c, Stimulants can relieve the stereotyped behaviours
Explanation: Stimulants reduce hyperactivity but not stereotyped behaviour.

Reference: Puri BK, Treasaden I (eds) (2010). *Psychiatry: An Evidence-Based Text*. London: Hodder Arnold, pp. 109, 1066–1067, 1088–1090.

Question 56 Answer: b, Interpersonal psychotherapy
Explanation: Both CBT and IPT are useful in the management of bulimia nervosa.

Reference: Puri BK, Treasaden I (eds) (2010). *Psychiatry: An Evidence-Based Text*. London: Hodder Arnold, pp. 687–703, 1063.

Question 57 Answer: b, Three times
Explanation: Approximately, 10% of patients with schizophrenia commit suicide, and for most individuals, it tends to happen earlier in the course of their illness. Paranoid schizophrenics are three times more likely compared with non-paranoid individuals to commit suicide.

Reference: Puri BK, Hall AD, Ho RC (2014). *Revision Notes in Psychiatry*. Boca Raton, FL: CRC Press, p. 370.

Question 58 Answer: e, Bupropion
Explanation: Based on previous research, it has been demonstrated that bupropion is associated with seizures if given to eating-disordered patients at doses of 600–800 mg per day. All the other options are appropriate choices in this case.

Reference: Bacaltuchuk J et al. (2001). Antidepressants versus placebo for people with bulimia nervosa. *Cochrane Database Syst Rev*, 4: CD003391.

Question 59 Answer: b, Pseudobulbar palsy
Explanation: The description above is classical for that of Binswanger's disease. The age of onset is usually between 50 and 65, and there is a gradual accumulation of neurological signs, which include those of disturbances of motor functioning as well as pseudobulbar palsy. There is often a history of severe hypertension, systemic vascular disease and stroke.

Reference: Puri BK, Hall AD, Ho RC (2014). *Revision Notes in Psychiatry*. Boca Raton, FL: CRC Press, p. 699.

Question 60 Answer: b, Resolution therapy
Explanation: This is a form of therapy that is a companion to reality orientation and looks for meaning in the "here and now" in the behaviour and confused talk of the patient. Reality orientation involves consistent use of orientation devices and other memory aids to remind the patients and environment. Reminiscent therapy involves reliving the past experience. Validation therapy empathizes with the feelings and meanings hidden behind their confused speech and behaviour. Snoezlen involves the utilization of a specially designed room with a soothing and stimulating environment.

Reference: Puri BK, Hall AD, Ho RC (2014). *Revision Notes in Psychiatry*. Boca Raton, FL: CRC Press, p. 698.

Question 61 Answer: c, Increased serotonin in the cortex
Explanation: The main neurotransmitter abnormality is that of the loss of the cholinergic neurons in the basal forebrain and associated low cortical cholinergic

activity and reduced choline acetyl-transferase, especially in the temporal cortex. This has been proposed to be due to the degeneration of the neurons in the nucleus basalis of Meynert, which provides the cortex with its cholinergic projection. Other neurochemical changes include decreased dopamine beta-hydroxylase and decreased dopamine, decreased noradrenaline and serotonin in the cortex.

Reference: Puri BK, Hall AD, Ho RC (2014). *Revision Notes in Psychiatry*. Boca Raton, FL: CRC Press, p. 694.

Question 62 Answer: d, Presence of coronary artery disease
Explanation: According to a meta-analysis done by Huffman and Pollack (2003), five variables that correlate with higher rates of panic disorder among people seeking treatment for chest pain in emergency rooms have been found. These are quality of atypical chest pain, the absence of coronary artery disease, female gender, younger age and a high level of self-reported anxiety.

Reference: Huffman JC, Pollack MH (2003). Predicting panic disorder among patients with chest pain: An analysis of the literature. *Psychosomatics*, 44: 222–236.

Question 63 Answer: d, The presence of comorbid medical illness is a poor prognostic factor
Explanation: The onset of hypochondriasis is between 20 and 30 years of age. It is associated with lower economic status and a history of medical illnesses. Good prognostic factors include the presence of a comorbid medical illness, acute onset, brief duration, mild symptoms, absence of secondary gain and absence of psychiatric comorbidity. Those with hypochondriasis have high rates of psychiatric comorbidity, and somatization disorder is commonly seen with it. Antidepressants such as SSRIs and psychotherapy are useful treatment options.

Reference: Puri BK, Hall AD, Ho RC (2014). *Revision Notes in Psychiatry*. Boca Raton, FL: CRC Press, pp. 470–471.

Question 64 Answer: c, Patients typically have experienced an actual infestation or exposure to organisms in the past
Explanation: This patient is suffering from delusional parasitosis, which is a delusional disorder in which she firmly believes that she is infested with living organisms. Most patients are not keen to receive psychiatric treatment, as they believe that their infestations are real. Patients commonly may have experienced an actual infestation or exposure to organisms in the past, and there is usually a specific precipitating event. Antipsychotics are useful to reduce the delusions.

Reference: Levenson JL (2004). *The American Psychiatric Publishing Textbook of Psychosomatic Medicine*. Arlington, VA: American Psychiatric Publishing, p. 35.

Question 65 Answer: b, Dependent personality disorder
Explanation: Trichotillomania is the compulsion to pull out one's hair. The peak age at onset is 12–13 years, and the disorder is often chronic and difficult to treat.

Trichotillomania is typically confined to one or two sites. It most frequently affects the scalp but can also involve the eyelashes, eyebrows, pubic hair, body hair, and facial hair. Patients tend to be highly secretive about the condition and to regard their behaviour as shameful. Many hair pullers also exhibit additional stereotypic movements, such as nail biting, knuckle cracking, touching or playing with pulled hair and hair eating (trichophagia). The common comorbid psychiatric disorders in trichotillomania include mood and anxiety disorder, substance and eating disorders. No particular personality disorder is characteristic of those with trichotillomania.

References: Levenson JL (2004). *The American Psychiatric Publishing Textbook of Psychosomatic Medicine*. Arlington, VA: American Psychiatric Publishing, p. 637; Chamberlain SR, Menzies L, Sahakian BJ, Fineberg NA (2007 Apr). Lifting the veil on trichotillomania. *Am J Psychiatry*, 164(4): 568–574.

Question 66 Answer: d, Topiramate
Explanation: Topiramate has the highest risk of cognitive side effects, followed by carbamazepine, valproate, lamotrigine and gabapentin. Its main cognitive impairments include reduction in verbal fluency and reaction time, resulting in high discontinuation rates. Topiramate is best tolerated when doses are titrated slowly, and lowest doses possible are used. The negative cognitive effects induced by topiramate often are temporary and resolve after discontinuation of medication.

References: Levenson JL (2004). *The American Psychiatric Publishing Textbook of Psychosomatic Medicine*. Arlington, VA: American Psychiatric Publishing, p. 885; Sommer BR, Mitchell EL, Wroolie TE (2013). Topiramate: Effects on cognition in patients with epilepsy, migraine headache and obesity. *Ther Adv Neurol Disord*, 6(4): 211–227.

Question 67 Answer: b, Cost-effectiveness analysis
Explanation: Table 3.1 illustrates cost-effectiveness analysis, which measures the total cost of providing a service to depressed patients with different levels of severity based on mean depression scores over 1 year. It also includes other outcome measures such as health-related quality of life (HRQOL) over 1 year. In this study, the direct and indirect costs incurred by each group were calculated in monetary values (i.e. US dollars). This study is not a cost–benefit analysis because it does not assess willingness to pay to treat a condition and trade-off measures (e.g. how much a patient is willing to pay in exchange for permanent cure). This study is not a cost-minimization analysis because it does not compare the cost of different interventions by assuming equal health benefits of each intervention. This study is not a cost-utility analysis because it does not report quality-adjusted life year (QALY). There is no such analysis known as cost–performance analysis.

Question 68 Answer: d, Cost of sick leave related to depressive disorder
Explanation: Cost of sick leave is an indirect cost. Monetary valuing of direct costs refers to the multiplication of unit cost by the number of health services or products consumed in a defined period. In this study, direct costs represent all the health resources utilization delivered to the patients because of depressive disorder

in 12 months, including direct healthcare resources as well as non-healthcare resources. Direct healthcare resources related to depressive disorder comprise visits to healthcare providers, which include GPs, specialists, psychologists and other healthcare providers; investigations including blood tests, urine tests, imaging tests such as conventional radiographical investigations (e.g. computed tomography (CT) scans and magnetic resonance imaging (MRI)); prescribed medication; emergency room visits; costs of inpatient care (including rehabilitation hospitalization); patients' out-of-pocket expenses for health products, non-traditional therapies and private hospital facilities. Indirect costs represent the productivity loss resulting from depressive disorder for the society in terms of lost earnings. In this study, the loss of productivity for those who were employed was the product of annual sick leave days and the salary reported by each patient. As for unemployment secondary to depressive disorder, lost wages based on the mean monthly salary of the previous job are calculated as productivity loss.

Reference: Ho RC, Mak KK, Chua AN, Ho CS, Mak A (2013). The effect of severity of depressive disorder on economic burden in a university hospital in Singapore. *Expert Rev Pharmacoecon Outcomes Res*, 13(4): 549–559.

Question 69 Answer: d, Mean Hamilton depression rating scale (HAMD) score over 1 year
Explanation: The candidate should refer to multivariate analysis under indirect cost (not direct cost). The mean HAMD score over 1 year remains significantly associated with indirect cost ($p = 0.004$) after adjustment for other variables. The other variables are not significantly associated with indirect cost, age ($p = 0.098$), gender ($p = 0.089$), education level ($p = 0.061$) and number of suicide attempts in 1 year ($p = 0.747$).

Question 70 Answer: a, The higher scores on the Dermatitis Family Impact Scale (DFIQ) correlate with poorer HRQOL in the children, and the correlation is significant
Explanation: Table 3.3 demonstrates the correlation between two variables. The higher scores on the DFIQ correlate with better (not poorer) HRQOL in the children, and the correlation is significant. The correlation between DFIQ and HRQOL is positive. It means that high score of the DFIQ correlates with high scores of the HRQOL or better HRQOL. This finding is hard to explain clinically, but this is the finding based on the correlational analysis.

Question 71 Answer: e, An inhalant
Explanation: Substance-induced dementia can be caused by alcohol, sedative-hypnotics or inhalants. Inhalant-inducing persisting dementia may be due to the neurotoxic effects of the inhalants themselves, the neurotoxic effects of the metals (e.g. lead) commonly used in inhalants or the effects of frequent and prolonged periods of hypoxia. Dementia caused by inhalants is likely to be irreversible in all but the mildest cases.

Reference: Sadock BJ, Sadock VA (2003). *Kaplan and Sadock's Synopsis of Psychiatry* (9th edition). Philadelphia, PA: Lippincott, Williams & Wilkins, p. 442.

Question 72 Answer: c, Four times

Explanation: There is good evidence that heavy drinking runs in families. The relatives of alcoholics have higher rates of alcoholism than relatives of controls. Twin studies indicate that monozygotic twins have a higher concordance rate than dizygotic twins. In normal twins, approximately one-third of the variance in drinking habits has been estimated to be genetic in origin. Adoption studies support the hypothesis of genetic transmission of alcoholism. The sons of alcoholic parents are three or four times more likely to become alcoholic than the sons of non-alcoholics, irrespective of the home environment.

References: Puri BK, Hall AD, Ho RC (2014). *Revision Notes in Psychiatry*. Boca Raton, FL: CRC Press, p. 516; Goodwin et al. (1973). Alcohol problems in adoptees raised apart from alcoholic biological parents. *Arch Gen Psychiatr*, 28: 238–243.

Question 73 Answer: a, Cardiac arrest

Explanation: Acute intoxication can lead to fatal accidents, particularly through falling or drowning. However, the greatest risk of death is during an episode of sniffing. They might also cause burns to the throat and the lung, in turn, causing cardiac arrest through vagal nerve stimulation. There have been reports of long-term damage to the central nervous system (CNS), heart, liver and kidneys. Chronic use may cause a persistent cerebellar syndrome and peripheral neuropathy.

Reference: Puri BK, Hall AD, Ho RC (2014). *Revision Notes in Psychiatry*. Boca Raton, FL: CRC Press, p. 546.

Question 74 Answer: e, Ketamine

Explanation: Ketamine is a shorter-acting derivative of phencyclidine (PCP). Ketamine is in the form of tablets, and it is snorted or injected. The action of ketamine is mediated by competitive inhibition from the *N*-methyl-*D*-aspartate (NMDA) receptor complex. It leads to cramps, fatigue, depression and irritability. It may lead to violent reactions (may harm other people) and flashbacks. Severe intoxication produces a state of virtual helplessness and lack of coordination. Ketamine is associated with moderate-to-severe lower urinary tract symptoms. These urinary symptoms include frequency, urgency, dysuria, urge incontinence and occasionally painful haematuria.

References: Puri BK, Hall AD, Ho RC (2014). *Revision Notes in Psychiatry*. Boca Raton, FL: CRC Press, p. 543; Chu PS, Ma WK, Wong SC et al. (2008). The destruction of the lower urinary tract by ketamine abuse: A new syndrome? *BJU Int*, 102(11): 1616–1622.

Question 75 Answer: e, MDMA

Explanation: MDMA causes potent release and reuptake inhibition of serotonin and associated with serotoninergic neurotoxicity in humans. MDMA could cause a feeling of closeness to other people, altered sensual and emotional overtones, increased in empathy and extroversion. The acute effects include sweating, tachycardia, dry mouth, jaw clenching, muscle aches, bruxism, jaw clenching and gait dependence.

Reference: Puri BK, Hall AD, Ho RC (2014). *Revision Notes in Psychiatry*. Boca Raton, FL: CRC Press, p. 543.

Question 76 Answer: a, 5%
Explanation: The National Confidential Inquiry into Suicide and Homicide by People with Mental Illness was conducted in England and Wales during the years 1996–1999. Of the 1594 convicted of homicide, 34% had a mental disorder, 5% had schizophrenia (lifetime) and 10% had symptoms of mental illness at the time of the offence; 9% received a diminished responsibility verdict and 7% a hospital disposal – both were associated with severe mental illness and symptoms of psychosis.

References: Puri BK, Treasaden I (eds) (2010). *Psychiatry: An Evidence-Based Text*. London: Hodder Arnold, pp. 1162–1163, 1173, 1176–1177; Shaw J, Hunt IM, Flynn S et al. (2006). Rates of mental disorder in people convicted of homicide. National clinical survey. *Br J Psychiatry*, 188: 143–147.

Question 77 Answer: e, 35%
Explanation: The conversion rate from first-episode psychosis to schizophrenia has been estimated to be 35%. Approximately, 70% of those diagnosed would achieve full remission within 3–4 months. Another 80% of individuals would achieve stable remission within 1 year.

Reference: Puri BK, Hall AD, Ho RC (2014). *Revision Notes in Psychiatry*. Boca Raton, FL: CRC Press, p. 371.

Question 78 Answer: e, Young age of first sexual offence conviction
Explanation: A history of sexual offending has been found to be among the strongest predictors of sexual recidivism. Predictors are classified into two categories: static and dynamic factors. Static factors refer to historical characteristics that cannot be altered. Dynamic factors are characteristics, circumstances and attitude that can change throughout one's life. Examples of dynamic characteristics include drug or alcohol use, poor attitude, deviant sexual preferences, negative peer influence and poor self-regulation and intimacy problems.

Reference: Hanson RK, Harris A (1998). *Dynamic Predictors of Sexual Recidivism*. Ottawa, Ontario: Solicitor General of Canada.

Question 79 Answer: c, Sporadic
Explanation: Klinefelter syndrome usually occurs as sporadic events in a family. About 50% is due to maternal non-dysjunction and 50% due to parental non-dysjunction. Eighty percent of men with Klinefelter syndrome have a 47 XXY karyotype with an additional X chromosome being derived equally from meiotic errors in each parent. Other karyotypes include 47 XXY or 46 XY mosaicism and severe X chromosome aneuploidy such as 48 XXXY and 49 XXXXY. These karyotypes usually occur as sporadic events in a family. Fertility can be achieved using haploid spermatocytes obtained by testicular biopsy.

Reference: Puri BK, Hall AD, Ho RC (2014). *Revision Notes in Psychiatry*. Boca Raton, FL: CRC Press, pp. 667–668.

Question 80 Answer: e, Vascular dementia
Explanation: Down syndrome is associated with increased risk of Alzheimer's disease (50–59 years old = 36%–40%; 60–69 years old = 55%) instead of vascular dementia. Over the age of 40 years, there is high incidence of neurofibrillary tangles and plaques with increase in P300 latency. Hearing loss, hypothyroidism, leukaemia and obstructive sleep apnoea are comorbidities of Down syndrome.

Reference: Moore DP, Puri BK (2012). *Textbook of Clinical Neuropsychiatry and Behavioral Neuroscience* (3rd edition). London: Hodder Arnold, p. 459.

Question 81 Answer: d, Moderate mental retardation
Explanation: Approximately 85% are due to a de novo deletion, whereas 10%–15% of cases are familial in nature. More than 90% are a result of parental transloca-tion. The characteristic features include round face with microcephaly, broad flat nose, low set ears, cardiac abnormality, gastrointestinal abnormalities, severe men-tal retardation, infantile cat-like cry, severe psychomotor retardation, hyperactivity and stereotypies. The rate of survival is expected to be low.

Reference: Puri BK, Hall AD, Ho RC (2014). *Revision Notes in Psychiatry*. Boca Raton, FL: CRC Press, p. 673.

Question 82 Answer: c, It occurs in expansion of CGG trinucleotide repeats of over 200 triplets
Explanation: An expansion of the sequence of CGG trinucleotide repeating to over 200 triplets constitutes full mutation, while expansion of 55–200 repeats is known as permutation. Those with full mutations develop fragile X syndrome but not permutation. Those with permutation, however, are at increased risk for develop-ing fragile X–associated tremor/ataxia syndrome (FXTAS) in middle or later years. Females tend to have much milder cases. It occurs secondary to mutations in the fragile mental retardation (FMR)1 gene. MRI studies reveal abnormalities that include hypertrophy of caudate nucleus, hypertrophy of the hippocampus and atrophy of the superior temporal gyrus and cerebellar vermis.

Reference: Moore DP, Puri BK (2012). *Textbook of Clinical Neuropsychiatry and Behavioural Neuroscience* (3rd edition). London: Hodder Arnold, pp. 461–462.

Question 83 Answer: b, Somnambulism is classified as insane automatism
Explanation: This individual cannot use voluntary intoxication with alcohol as a defence as voluntary intoxication does not constitute a defence by itself. Legal automatism results in decreased punishment or even acquittal, but there is no fixed maximum punishment. Automatism refers to unconscious, involuntary, non-purposeful acts where the mind is not conscious of what the body is doing. There is a separation between the mind and the act. Sane automatism is a once-only event,

resulting from external causes. Insane automatisms are caused by diseases of the mind such as mental illness or brain diseases.

Reference: Puri BK, Hall AD, Ho RC (2014). *Revision Notes in Psychiatry*. Boca Raton, FL: CRC Press, p. 731.

Question 84 Answer: b, A prolonged-release formulation of melatonin is licensed for the short-term treatment of insomnia in children in the United Kingdom

Explanation: A prolonged-release formulation was licensed in the United Kingdom as a short-term treatment of insomnia in patients aged over 55 years.

A is correct as melatonin is a hormone from the pineal gland and is secreted in a circadian manner with a nocturnal rise in level. This natural chemical does not cause much drug interaction, and it is metabolized by the liver. It has not been evaluated in children and adolescents. The dose of melatonin varies from 500 µg (physiological dose) to 5 mg.

Reference: Taylor D, Paton C, Kapur S (2009). *The Maudsley Prescribing Guidelines* (10th edition). London: Informa Healthcare.

Question 85 Answer: d, Psychiatric Research Interview for Substance and Mental Disorders (PRISM)

Explanation: PRISM is used for assessment of substance abuse and psychiatric comorbidity. It is a structured diagnostic interview and emphasizes that the assessment of alcohol and substance misuse be performed before the appointment of psychiatric disorders, so that the history of substance misuse can be linked to the development of psychiatric illnesses.

Reference: Goldberg D, Hilier VP (1979). A scaled version of the General Health Questionnaire (GHQ-28). *Psychol Med*, 9: 139–145.

Question 86 Answer: c, It focuses on functioning over the past 2 weeks

Explanation: The General Health Questionnaire (GHQ) focuses on functioning over the past month and is intended to screen for general non-psychotic psychiatric morbidity. The four versions are GHQ-60 Complete Version, GHQ-30 Measure of Physical Illness, GHQ-28 Measure of Somatic, Neurotic and Affective Symptoms and their Impact on Social Function, and GHQ-12 Short Research Version. The 28-item version is used most widely. This is not only because of time considerations but also because the GHQ-28 has been used most widely in other working populations, allowing for more valid comparisons.

References: Goldberg D, Hilier VP (1979). A scaled version of the General Health Questionnaire (GHQ-28). *Psychol Med*, 9: 139–145; Goldberg D (1972). *The Detection of Psychiatric Illness by Questionnaire: A Technique for the Identification and Assessment of Non-psychotic Psychiatric Illness*. Maudsley Monographs No 21. Oxford, UK: Oxford University Press.

Question 87 Answer: c, It is useful for people with concurrent physical illness as it places less emphasis on somatic symptoms
Explanation: The Montgomery and Asberg Depression Rating Scale (MADRS) is a clinician-rated 10-item scale for patients with major depressive disorder. It can be used for assessing patients who are likely to experience side effects from medication. Suggested cut-offs are 0–6 recovered, 7–19 mild depression, 20–34 moderate depression and 35–60 severe depression.

Reference: Montgomery SA, Asberg M (1979). A new depression scale designed to be sensitive to change. *Br J Psych*, 134: 382–389.

Question 88 Answer: e, One of its strengths is that behavioural symptoms, and somatic complaints are preferred over self-reported distress
Explanation: There are a number of criticisms about HAMD. These include poor reliability in some items, a heterogeneous and unstable factor analytic structure, no general factor and behavioural symptoms, and somatic complaints are preferred over self-reported distress.

Reference: Hamilton M (1960). A rating scale for depression. *J Neurol Neurosurg Psychiatry*, 23: 56–62.

Question 89 Answer: d, Sample size for parametric data is preferably >30, but for non-parametric, it is best for <50 data cases.
Explanation: The assumption for parametric tests is that data follows a known distribution (e.g. normal or Poisson), while non-parametric tests make no assumptions about the underlying distribution. The confidence interval (CI) calculation for parametric tests is straightforward, but that of non-parametric tests is more difficult. Examples of parametric tests include student's *t*-test, paired *t*-test, ANOVA, multivariate analysis of variance (MANOVA), correlation and regression (all types). Examples of non-parametric tests include Mann–Whitney *U*, Wilcoxon signed-rank, the Kruskal–Wallis test and chi-squared test.

Reference: Lewis GH, Sheringham J, Kalim K, Crayford TJB (2008). *Mastering Public Health: A Postgraduate Guide to Examination and Revalidation*. London: Royal Society of Medicine Press, pp. 88–96.

Question 90 Answer: b, Chi-square
Explanation: The chi-square test is a non-parametric test that can be used to compare independent qualitative and discrete quantitative variables presented in the form of contingency tables containing the data frequencies. Ethnicity is a categorical data. The chi-square test is used to measure differences in more than two independent groups.

Reference: Puri BK, Hall AD, Ho RC (2014). *Revision Notes in Psychiatry*. Boca Raton, FL: CRC Press, p. 307.

Question 91 Answer: d, Spearman correlation
Explanation: Spearman correlation is a measure of the relationship between two variables that uses only the ranks of the observations on each. Pearson correla-

tion is used for correlation analysis in continuous interval and ratio data, while kappa correlation is used in categorical data. The remaining options are not used for correlation analysis. The McNemar test is used for comparing proportions in data involving paired samples. The Wilcoxon signed-rank test is a distribution-free method for testing the difference between two populations using matched samples.

Reference: Everitt BS (2006). *Medical Statistics from A to Z* (2nd edition). Cambridge, UK: Cambridge University Press, pp. 148, 220, 246.

Question 92 Answer: e, Width of the CI is dependent on sample size: a larger sample generates wider CI
Explanation: CI is a range of values calculated from the sample observations that is believed, with a particular probability, to contain the true parameter value. A 95% CI, for example, would imply that if the estimation process was repeated again and again, 95% of the calculated intervals would be expected to contain the true parameter value. The width of the CI is dependent on sample size: larger samples produce narrower CIs.

Reference: Everitt BS (2006). *Medical Statistics from A to Z* (2nd edition). Cambridge, UK: Cambridge University Press, p. 56.

Question 93 Answer: b, It shows an autosomal-dominant inheritance pattern
Explanation: Hoarding is most commonly found in people with OCD. About 18%–42% of people with OCD report hoarding and saving compulsions. Hoarding symptoms show autosomal recessive inheritance patterns and have been associated with genetic markers on chromosomes 4, 5 and 17. Psychiatric comorbidities include schizophrenia, learning disability, neurodegenerative disorders (especially from frontal lobe dysfunction), autism-spectrum disorders, eating disorder and impulse control disorder.

Reference: Puri BK, Hall AD, Ho RC (2014). *Revision Notes in Psychiatry*. Boca Raton, FL: CRC Press, pp. 425–426.

Question 94 Answer: c, There are decreased levels of interleukin (IL)-6 and IL-1-beta
Explanation: Studies of the cerebrospinal fluid (CSF) of depressed patients showed increased levels of IL-6 and soluble IL-6 receptor and increased levels of IL-1-beta. In the peripheral blood, there is decreased lymphocyte number, increased neutrophil number and decreased natural killer (NK) cell activity. There is also increased level of acute-phase proteins in depressed patients. Patients with depression showed increased levels of tumour necrosis factor (TNF)-alpha compared with healthy controls. Studies have shown that higher somatoform symptoms during the last 2 years significantly predicted an increase in TNF-alpha in women with major depression but not in men. A syndrome of 'sickness behaviour' that resembles major depression can occur with the administration of cytokine therapies such as interferon (IFN)-alpha and IL-2.

Reference: Liu Y, Ho RC, Mak A (2011). Interleukin (IL)-6, tumour necrosis factor alpha (TNF-<alpha>) and soluble interleukin-2 receptors (sIL-2R) are elevated in patients with major depressive disorder: A meta-analysis and meta-regression. *J Affect Disorder*, 139(3): 230–239.

Question 95 Answer: c, 15

Explanation: Sensory gating refers to the pre-attentional habituation of responses to repeated exposure to the same sensory stimulus. The inhibition of responsiveness to repetitive stimulation provides humans with the ability to negotiate a sensory-laden environment by blocking out irrelevant, meaningless or redundant stimuli. P50 is an electroencephalogram (EEG) event-related potential waveform used to assess sensory gating. A large percentage of patients with schizophrenia are characterized by an abnormality in P50 sensory gating. This abnormality has been shown to be genetically linked to the α-7 nicotinic receptor and is transiently reversed by acute nicotine administration. Chromosome 15 has been linked to the failure to inhibit the P50 auditory-evoked response to repeated stimuli in schizophrenia.

References: Yudofsky SC, Hales RE (2002). *The American Psychiatric Publishing Textbook of Neuropsychiatry and Clinical Neurosciences* (4th edition). Arlington, VA: American Psychiatric Publishing, p. 383; Potter D, Summerfelt A, Gold J, Buchanan RW (2006). Review of clinical correlates of P50 sensory gating abnormalities in patients with schizophrenia. *Schizophr Bull*, 32(4): 692–700.

Question 96 Answer: d, 72%

Explanation: Based on a previous review article, neuroimaging studies have identified that approximately 65%–78% receptor blockade would help individuals to achieve the best benefits from the medications, while experiencing the least amount of side effects. However, it should be noted that clozapine does not conform to the typical therapeutic window.

Approximately, 72% affinity of the antipsychotic to the dopamine receptor would result in an elevated prolactin level.

Reference: Ginovart N, Kapur S (2012). Role of dopamine D(2) receptors for antipsychotic activity. *Handb Exp Pharmacol*, 212: 27–52.

Question 97 Answer: e, Acetylcholine dysregulation

Explanation: Common biological abnormalities shared by schizophrenia and schizotypal disorder include dopamine dysregulation, raised CSF homovanillic acid (HVA) concentrations, reduction in temporal lobe volumes, impaired smooth pursuit eye movements and impaired tests of executive functioning. Almost all studies of the families of schizophrenic probands have found an excess of both schizophrenia and schizotypal personality disorder among relatives (22% in the biological relatives of schizophrenics vs. 2% of adoptive relatives and controls). Schizotypal disorder has a relatively stable course, with only about 10% of people going on to develop schizophrenia.

Reference: Puri BK, Hall AD, Ho RC (2014). *Revision Notes in Psychiatry*. Boca Raton, FL: CRC Press, pp. 440–442.

Question 98 Answer: e, Masked depression
Explanation: In masked depression, depressed mood is not always the main concern but rather somatic symptoms. It tends to be more common in the undeveloped world and also in those who are unable to articulate their emotions. The presence of biological symptoms would be helpful in making the diagnosis. Diurnal variation in abnormal behaviour could mirror the diurnal variation in mood.

Reference: Puri BK, Hall AD, Ho RC (2014). *Revision Notes in Psychiatry*. Boca Raton, FL: CRC Press, p. 380.

Question 99 Answer: e, Analysis of communication
Explanation: Dialectical thinking involves a process in which the client has been advised not to think linearly. Dialectical behavior therapy (DBT) also includes behavioural therapy with homework assignment; mindfulness 'how' skills as well as mindfulness 'what' skills. It also includes life-skill training and the use of metaphors. The usage of metaphors would help to enhance effectiveness of communication, allowing for the discovery of one's own wisdom and strengthening the therapeutic alliance.

Reference: Puri BK, Hall AD, Ho RC (2014). *Revision Notes in Psychiatry*. Boca Raton, FL: CRC Press, p. 339.

Question 100 Answer: e, Tower of London Test
Explanation: The Cambridge Cognition Examination is a neuropsychological screening instrument used in the United Kingdom. It is actually a part of the Cambridge Mental Disorders of the Elderly Questionnaire (CAMDEX) and incorporates the Mini Mental State Examination (MMSE), Blessed dementia rating scale and the Hachinski ischaemic score, NART, Kendrick object learning test for memory and the Wisconsin card sorting test for executive function. The Tower of London Test is not part of the assessment battery.

Reference: Puri BK, Hall AD, Ho RC (2014). *Revision Notes in Psychiatry*. Boca Raton, FL: CRC Press, p. 688.

Question 101 Answer: d, Visual hallucinations
Explanation: Visual hallucinations are quite common with prolonged usage of dopamine agonists. The hallucinations are typically complex in nature, involving scenes, animals or people and may last from minutes to hours or even days. Auditory hallucinations and olfactory hallucinations might occur, but these are usually less common.

Reference: Puri BK, Treasaden I (eds) (2010). *Psychiatry: An Evidence-Based Text*. London: Hodder Arnold, p. 542.

Question 102 Answer: b, Being unmarried
Explanation: There are multiple good prognostic factors mentioned in the vignette. These include having good premorbid social adjustment, abrupt onset of his illness, lack of negative symptoms and cognitive impairment and having paranoid symptoms. Being married is a positive prognostic factor.

Reference: Puri BK, Hall AD, Ho RC (2014). *Revision Notes in Psychiatry*. Boca Raton, FL: CRC Press, p. 370.

Question 103 Answer: d, Motivating interviewing
Explanation: In motivational interviewing, the therapist uses a non-judgmental, non-confrontational and supportive approach to explore the patient's ambivalence about change. The main techniques include expressing empathy and establishing understanding from the patient's perspectives; developing discrepancy in the behaviour and patient's personal goals/values; identifying the advantages and disadvantages of change; rolling with patient's resistance by understanding his or her hesitancy to change; supporting self-efficacy to reach personal goals; and allowing the patient to realize optimism about change and providing a menu of options for change.

Reference: Puri BK, Hall AD, Ho RC (2014). *Revision Notes in Psychiatry*. Boca Raton, FL: CRC Press, p. 348.

Question 104 Answer: a, The incidence of sudden and unexpected death is usually around 5%
Explanation: The incidence of sudden and unexpected death is around 2%. The condition is a predominantly female disorder, but men with clinical features similar to Rett syndrome have been described. It is due to a mutation of the transcription regulatory gene methyl CpG binding protein 2 (MECP2) at chromosome Xq28. The developmental decline usually begins from the age of 7–24 months. Anticonvulsant treatment is helpful in the prevention of seizures. Behaviour therapy is helpful with prevention of self-injurious behaviour.

Reference: Puri BK, Hall AD, Ho RC (2014). *Revision Notes in Psychiatry*. Boca Raton, FL: CRC Press, p. 630.

Question 105 Answer: b, 2 years
Explanation: The prevalence of the disorder is 1.7 per 1,000. The average age of onset is between 3 and 4 years of age. There is a male predominance. There is normal development for at least 2 years after birth. However, there is a progressive loss of previously acquired skills before the age of 10 years, especially so in the following areas: language, social skills, bowel and bladder control, motor skills and play. There are qualitative impairments in social interactions involving non-verbal behaviour and communication using spoken language. Stereotypic behaviour is also present.

Reference: Puri BK, Hall AD, Ho RC (2014). *Revision Notes in Psychiatry*. Boca Raton, FL: CRC Press, p. 630.

Question 106 Answer: a, Motor tics
Explanation: Motor tics are usually the first to appear. Simple motor tics include blinking, brow wrinkling, grimacing and shoulder shrugging. Complex motor tics may include touching, smelling, hopping, throwing, clapping and bending over.

Reference: Puri BK, Treasaden I (eds) (2010). *Psychiatry: An Evidence-Based Text*. London: Hodder Arnold, p. 550.

Question 107 Answer: d, Depression
Explanation: The Connors' rating scale is a diagnostic scale for ADHD using the *Diagnostic and Statistical Manual of Mental Disorders, 4th Edition* (DSM-IV) criteria. This scale includes measures of behaviour described by parents and teachers. The behaviour scale includes the following: (1) ADHD symptoms, (2) anxiety, (3) cognitive problems, (4) oppositional behaviour, (5) perfectionism and (6) social problems.

Reference: Puri BK, Hall AD, Ho RC (2014). *Revision Notes in Psychiatry*. Boca Raton, FL: CRC Press, p. 632.

Question 108 Answer: e, One in six
Explanation: If undetected and/or untreated, postnatal depression can last up to 2 years with serious consequences for the marital relationship as well as for the development of the child. There is good evidence for a link between depressive disorder in mothers and emotional disturbance in their children. The relapse rate for subsequent non-psychotic depression is one in six.

Reference: Puri BK, Hall AD, Ho RC (2014). *Revision Notes in Psychiatry*. Boca Raton, FL: CRC Press, p. 568.

Question 109 Answer: b, One in three
Explanation: The initial prognosis of postpartum psychosis is quite good. Cases often settle within 6 weeks and most have fully recovered by 6 months. After an episode of post-partum psychosis, the risk of a further episode in each subsequent pregnancy has been estimated to be around one in three and one in five. For those with a previous psychiatric history or a family history, the risk is higher.

Reference: Puri BK, Hall AD, Ho RC (2014). *Revision Notes in Psychiatry*. Boca Raton, FC: CRC Press, p. 570.

Question 110 Answer: b, For bipolar disorder, lithium, at low doses, can be used and is safe for neonates
Explanation: For bipolar disorder, valproate can be used, but the mother has to be advised to ensure adequate contraception to avoid pregnancy. Lithium's concentration in the breast milk is 50% of the serum concentration. If the patient is taking lithium during pregnancy, it will be necessary to augment with an antipsychotic during the postpartum period because the risk of a relapse is high. For depressive disorder, the recommended medications are paroxetine and sertraline as well as tricyclic antidepressants. Methadone is compatible with breastfeeding, but the dose should be kept as low as possible.

Reference: Puri BK, Hall AD, Ho RC (2014). *Revision Notes in Psychiatry*. Boca Raton, FL: CRC Press, p. 570.

Extended Match Items

Theme: Psychotherapy

Question 111 Answer: b, Denial
Explanation: Denial is the avoidance of awareness of an external reality that is difficult to face. In this case, the issue of amputation is difficult for the patient to face, and he decides to avoid it by saying that everything is fine.

Question 112 Answer: e, Projection
Explanation: In projection, unacceptable qualities, feelings, thoughts or wishes are projected onto another person or thing. This is often seen in paranoid patients. In this case, the patient gets defensive and blames the psychiatrist for probing too much about his situation and deliberately making his mood worse.

Question 113 Answer: c, Displacement
Explanation: In displacement, emotions, ideas or wishes are transferred from their original object to a more acceptable substitute. In this case, the patient vents his frustration only on his wife instead of his colleagues, as it is safer and more acceptable for the patient.

Question 114 Answer: h, Sublimation
Explanation: Sublimation refers to channelling socially objectionable or internally unacceptable motives into socially acceptable ones. In this case, the patient copes by devoting his energy into doing volunteering work, which is socially acceptable; this helps his mood get better.

Reference: Puri BK, Hall AD, Ho RC (2014). *Revision Notes in Psychiatry*. Boca Raton, FL: CRC Press, pp. 136–137.

Theme: Psychotherapy

Question 115 Answer: a, Acting out
Explanation: Acting out is enacting an unconscious wish or fantasy impulsively as a way of avoiding painful affect. In this case, the patient expresses her unconscious emotional conflicts and feelings regarding her father and the physical abuse directly through hitting the nurse, without being consciously aware of the meaning.

Question 116 Answer: i, Suppression
Explanation: Suppression refers to the conscious effort not to attend to certain feelings or impulses, while repression refers to the blockage or expulsion of unacceptable ideas or impulses in the inner states to stop them from entering consciousness. In this case, the patient consciously makes an attempt to block her memories of the past so as not to affect her mood.

Question 117 Answer: g, Rationalization
Explanation: Rationalization refers to the justification of unacceptable attitudes, beliefs or behaviours, making them tolerable to oneself. In this case, the patient tries to justify and explain her rationale for self-cutting, which she perceives as an acceptable way of coping with her emotions.

Question 118 Answer: d, Intellectualization

Explanation: Intellectualization refers to the excessive use of abstract ideation to avoid difficult feelings or conflicts. In this case, the patient uses abstract thinking to explain her situation, and this in turn prevents her from facing her inner conflicts and feelings.

Question 119 Answer: b, Idealization

Explanation: Idealization refers to attributing perfect or near-perfect qualities onto others as a way of avoiding negative feelings. In this case, the patient idealizes the doctor despite having only seen him once, and she has strong positive feelings towards him.

Question 120 Answer: h, Regression

Explanation: In regression, there is transition, at times of stress and threat, to moods of expression and functioning that are on a lower level of complexity so that one returns to an earlier level of maturational functioning. In this case, the patient acts in a childlike manner when the stress becomes overwhelming.

Question 121 Answer: e, Isolation of affect

Explanation: Isolation of affect refers to the separation of an idea from its associated affect to avoid emotional pain. By doing this, the patient's link with the unhappy thoughts and memories is broken.

Question 122 Answer: c, Identification

Explanation: Identification refers to internalization of the qualities of another person by behaving like that person. In this case, the patient takes on the qualities of her aunt by behaving like her.

Reference: Puri BK, Hall AD, Ho RC (2014). *Revision Notes in Psychiatry*. Boca Raton, FL: CRC Press, pp. 136–137.

Theme: Research Methodology

Question 123 Answer: a, Kruskal – Wallis

Explanation: The Kruskal–Wallis test is a distribution-free method that is the analogue of the ANOVA of a one-way design, used to test whether a series of populations have the same median.

Question 124 Answer: c, One-way ANOVA

Explanation: ANOVA is the acronym for analysis of variance. It is the separation of variation attributable to one factor from that attributed to others. By partitioning the total variance of a set of observations into parts due to particular factors, differences in the mean values of the dependent variable can be assessed. The simplest analysis of this type involves a one-way design: a sample of individuals from a number of different populations compared with respect to some outcome measure of interest. The total variance in the observations is partitioned into a part due to differences between the group means and a part due to differences between subjects in the same group.

Question 125 Answer: g, Two-way ANOVA

Explanation: The two-way ANOVA test is an extension of the one-way ANOVA test, which examines the influence of different categorical independent variables on one dependent variable. While the one-way ANOVA measures the significant effect of one independent variable, the two-way ANOVA is used when there is more than one independent variable and multiple observations for each independent variable. The two-way ANOVA not only is able to determine the main effect of contributions of each independent variable but also identifies if there is a significant interaction effect between the independent variables.

References: Everitt BS (2006). *Medical Statistics from A to Z* (2nd edition). Cambridge, UK: Cambridge University Press, p. 130; Lewis GH, Sheringham J, Kalim K, Crayford TJB (2008). *Mastering Public Health: A Postgraduate Guide to Examination and Revalidation*. London: Royal Society of Medicine Press, pp. 93–94.

Theme: Research Methodology

Question 126 Answer: i, Level 4

Question 127 Answer: f, Level 2C

Question 128 Answer: j, Level 5

Explanation: The Centre for Evidence-Based Medicine (CEBM) has ranked the different types of research evidence based on how likely they are to be true. The strongest evidence comes from a systematic review that demonstrates consistent findings from several high-quality RCTs. This is termed as level 1 evidence, and recommendations based on level 1 results are called grade A. Further down the hierarchy come more heterogeneous findings and evidence from less robust sources.

Reference: Lewis GH, Sheringham J, Kalim K, Crayford TJ (2008). *Mastering Public Health*. London: Royal Society of Medicine Press, p. 62.

Theme: Learning Disability

Question 129 Answer: d, 60

Explanation: According to *International Classification of Diseases* (ICD)-10 criteria for mental retardation, for mild mental retardation, the IQ range is 50–69, with mental age of 9–12 years. About 85% of those with learning disability have mild mental retardation.

Question 130 Answer: c, 40

Explanation: According to ICD-10 criteria for mental retardation, for moderate mental retardation, the IQ range is 35–49, with mental age of 6–9 years. It accounts for about 10% of those with learning disability.

Question 131 Answer: b, 30

Explanation: According to ICD-10 criteria for mental retardation, for severe mental retardation, the IQ range is 20–34, with mental age of 3–6 years. This accounts for 3% of those with learning disability.

Question 132 Answer: a, 15
Explanation: According to ICD-10 criteria for mental retardation, for profound mental retardation, the IQ range is difficult to measure but is <20. This accounts for 2% of those with learning disability.

Reference: Puri BK, Hall AD, Ho RC (2014). *Revision Notes in Psychiatry*. Boca Raton, FL: CRC Press, p. 663.

Theme: Old-Age Psychiatry

Question 133 Answer: a, MMSE, b, Addenbrooke's cognitive assessment revised, c, Montreal cognitive assessment, d, Clinical dementia rating scale
Explanation: NICE guidelines recommend that clinical cognitive assessment should include examination on attention, concentration, orientation, short- and long-term memory, praxis, language and executive function. Standardized instruments for formal cognitive testing include all of the above. In addition, other instruments include the General Practitioner Assessment of Cognition and 6-item Cognitive Impairment Test and 7-minute screen.

Question 134 Answer: e, Dementia questionnaire for the mentally retarded, f, Dementia scale for Down syndrome
Explanation: Patients with learning disability require different tests, such as the dementia questionnaire for mentally retarded persons or dementia scale for Down syndrome.

Question 135 Answer: a, MMSE, h, Blessed dementia rating scale, i, Hachinski ischaemic score, j, NART, k, Kendrick object learning test for memory, l, Wisconsin card sorting test
Explanation: The Cambridge cognition examination is a neuropsychological screening instrument used in the United Kingdom. It is part of the CAMDEX, which incorporates the MMSE, Blessed dementia rating scale and the Hachinski ischaemic score, NART, Kendrick object learning test for memory and also the Wisconsin card sorting test.

Reference: Puri BK, Hall AD, Ho RC (2014). *Revision Notes in Psychiatry*. Boca Raton, FL: CRC Press, p. 688.

Theme: Neuroimaging in the Elderly

Question 136 Answer: f, Gross atrophy in fronto-temporal regions
Explanation: The EEG is always abnormal in Creutzfeldt–Jakob disease (CJD), showing an increase in slow-wave activity and a reduction in a rhythm; as the disease progresses, bilateral slow spike wave discharges may accompany myoclonic jerks. Gross atrophy is usually seen in the fronto-temporal regions (knife-blade atrophy) in Pick disease, but the diagnosis cannot be made on this evidence alone.

Question 137 Answer: e, Anterior hypo-perfusion on functional imaging
Explanation: Dementia of frontal lobe type and Pick disease affect the frontal and anterior temporal areas of the brain. Structural imaging may not show characteristic lesion in the early stage, and functional imaging shows anterior hypo-perfusion. EEG is usually normal in this particular form of dementia.

Question 138 Answer: c, Subcortical vascular encephalopathy, d Small, well-localized subcortical infarcts
Explanation: Binswanger disease is a progressive subcortical vascular encephalopathy with CT scan revealing markedly enlarged ventricles secondary to infection in hemispheric white matter. Infarcts are observed to affect periventricular and central white matter. In multiple lacunar states, there are CT scan appearances of small well-localized subcortical infarcts. It is usually associated with dementia characterized by dysarthria, incontinence and explosive laughing, secondary to frontal lobe disturbances.

Question 139 Answer: a, Cortical atrophy and ventricular enlargement, b Atrophy of the hippocampus
Explanation: CT scans of the brain do not reliably differentiate normal from those with Alzheimer's dementia, with approximately 20% overlap between these groups. Generally, cortical atrophy and ventricular enlargement are greater than in controls with increasing cognitive dysfunction correlating with increasing cerebral atrophy, but more so with increasing ventricular size. An increase in ventricular size over a span of 1 year is suggestive of Alzheimer's dementia. MRI scan may reveal atrophy of the hippocampus. MRI is the preferred modality to assist with early diagnosis or detect subcortical vascular changes.

Reference: Puri BK, Hall AD, Ho RC (2014). *Revision Notes in Psychiatry*. Boca Raton, FL: CRC Press, pp. 696–705.

Theme: General Adult
Question 140 Answer: a, Conversion disorder
Explanation: This person is suffering from conversion disorder. There is no evidence of a physical disorder that could explain the symptoms. Conversion disorder is associated with psychological conflict or need, traumatic events, insoluble problems and/or disturbed relationships. The unpleasant effect associated with these conflicts is displaced and converted unconsciously into symptoms, the primary gain being relief from intolerable intrapsychic conflict.

Question 141 Answer: c, Factitious disorder
Explanation: This person is suffering from a factitious disorder, Munchhausen syndrome (hospital addiction syndrome), in which physical or psychological symptoms are voluntarily and intentionally produced, the motivation is largely

unconscious but directed towards achieving the sick role. Common presenting symptoms and signs include bleeding, diarrhoea, hypoglycaemia, infection, rashes and seizures. When the nature of feigned or intentionally produced symptoms and/or signs come to light, such individuals may discharge themselves or abscond from hospital, travel to another hospital (peregrination) and present with the same clinical scenario. Depression should be excluded. The prognosis is poor. Psychological treatment is the treatment of choice, but the patient will often refuse this.

Question 142 Answer: e, Hypochondriasis
Explanation: This person is suffering from hypochondriasis (hyperchondriacal or severe health anxiety disorder). There is an intense persistent fear of disease. Disease conviction occurs despite repeated negative investigations and medical reassurance. Hypochondriacal symptoms are most frequently secondary to depressive illness.

Question 143 Answer: f, Malingering
This person is malingering. In this condition, the person intentionally produces physical or psychological symptoms. Motivation is conscious and for external gain.

Reference: Puri BK, Hall AD, Ho RC (2014). *Revision Notes in Psychiatry*. Boca Raton, FL: CRC Press, pp. 470–471.

Theme: Forensic Psychiatry

Question 144 Answer: i, 45%
Explanation: While violence in people with schizophrenia is uncommon, they have a higher risk than the general population. The prevalence of recent aggressive behaviour among outpatients with schizophrenia is around 5%. Among the types of aggression, verbal aggression is the commonest at around 45%, followed by physical violence towards objects (29%), violence towards others (19%) and self-directed violence (8%). Recent episodes of aggression of any severity are more likely among patients with a history of violence and also if there have been relapses within the previous year and with low treatment satisfaction.

Question 145 Answer: e, 30%
Explanation: Among the types of aggression, verbal aggression is the commonest at around 45%, followed by physical violence towards objects (29%), violence towards others (19%) and self-directed violence (8%).

Question 146 Answer: d, 20%
Explanation: Among the types of aggression, verbal aggression is the commonest at around 45%, followed by physical violence towards objects (29%), violence towards others (19%) and self-directed violence (8%).

Question 147 Answer: b, 10%
Explanation: Among the types of aggression, verbal aggression is the commonest at around 45%, followed by physical violence towards objects (29%), violence towards others (19%) and self-directed violence (8%).

Question 148 Answer: j, 50%

Explanation: In chronically ill and disabled patients with schizophrenia, acts of violence are often less severe but are particularly directed towards family members, friends, caregivers and healthcare providers. In treatment settings, aggression and violence frequently occur when providers attempt to modify patients' behaviour. Family members are victims in 50% of the assaults. Strangers are attacked in 20% of cases.

Question 149 Answer: d, 20%

Explanation: In chronically ill and disabled patients with schizophrenia, acts of violence are often less severe but are particularly directed towards family members, friends, caregivers and healthcare providers. In treatment settings, aggression and violence frequently occurs when providers attempt to modify patients' behaviour. Family members are victims in 50% of the assaults. Strangers are attacked in 20% of cases.

References: Sadock BJ, Sadock VA, Ruiz P (2009). *Kaplan and Sadock's Comprehensive Textbook of Psychiatry* (9th edition). Philadelphia, PA: Lippincott, Williams & Wilkins, p. 1449; Bobes J, Fillat O, Arango C (2009). Violence among schizophrenia out-patients compliant with medication: Prevalence and associated factors. *Acta Psychiatr Scand*, 119(3): 218–225.

Theme: Hospital Liaison Psychiatry

Question 150 Answer: g, Emotionalism

Explanation: Emotionalism is characterized by an increase in episodes of laughing or crying that are sudden or unheralded and not all under normal social control. Post-stroke, there is a prevalence rate of 15% of patients at 1 month, 21% at 6 months and 11% at 12 months. Lesions in the left frontal and temporal regions are associated with emotionalism.

Question 151 Answer: d, Catastrophic reaction

Explanation: A catastrophic reaction is a rare affective disorder characterized by a disruptive emotional outburst involving anxiety, agitation and aggressive behaviour. It is associated with non-fluent aphasias and left opercular lesions. Catastrophic reactions appear to be a specific consequence of the intense frustration and perceived loss associated with an expressive aphasia.

Question 152 Answer: j, Vascular dementia

Explanation: Vascular dementia occurs as a result of an impairment of the vascular supply to the brain. This impairment can have many causes, but atherosclerotic changes are the most common. Neurological signs include haemiparesis, sensory change, dysphasia or visual disturbances. Mood disturbances, including mood lability, depression and anxiety, are more common than in Alzheimers disease and may predate cognitive impairment.

Question 153 Answer: e, Depression

Explanation: Depression is common following a stroke. Some 30%–40% of patients who survive intracerebral haemorrhage develop depression, which can impair rehabilitation. Treatment with antidepressants is effective and leads to faster rehabilitation. There is particularly good evidence for the efficacy of fluoxetine, citalopram and nortriptyline.

References: House A, Dennis M et al. (1989). Emotionalism after stroke. *BMJ*. 298: 991–994; Puri BK, Treasaden I (eds) (2010). *Psychiatry: An Evidence-Based Text.* London: Hodder Arnold, pp. 438, 613, 621; Teasell R (1993). Catastrophic reaction after stroke: A case study. *Am J Phys Med Rehabil*, 72: 151–153.

Theme: Psychotropic Medications in Breastfeeding

Question 154 Answer: a, Lithium
Explanation: Lithium should not be used. Instead valproate could be used. The concentration of lithium in the breast milk is approximately 50% of the serum concentration. If the patient is taking lithium during pregnancy, it is necessary to augment with an antipsychotic during the postpartum period if the risk of relapse is considered to be high.

Question 155 Answer: c, Paroxetine, d Sertraline
Explanation: Paroxetine and sertraline could be used to help treat postnatal depression and are not contraindicated if the mother wishes to breastfeed her child. They are present in the breast milk in relatively low levels. Citalopram and fluoxetine should not be used, as they are present in the breast milk at relatively high levels.

Question 156 Answer: j, Clozapine
Explanation: For schizophrenia, only sulpiride and olanzapine is indicated. Clozapine is not indicated for patients with psychosis who are breastfeeding.

Question 157 Answer: k, Methadone
Explanation: Methadone is compatible with breastfeeding, but the dose has to be kept to a minimum.

Reference: Puri BK, Hall AD, Ho RC (2014). *Revision Notes in Psychiatry*. Boca Raton, FL: CRC Press, p. 570.

Theme: Cardiovascular Disease and Psychotropics

Question 158 Answer: a, Clozapine, b Olanzapine
Explanation: Clozapine, olanzapine and paliperidone are not indicated in patients with atrial fibrillation. Only aripiprazole is indicated.

Question 159 Answer: d, Mirtazapine
Explanation: Mirtazapine is often used for patients with atrial fibrillation and who are on non-steroidal anti-inflammatory drugs (NSAIDs) and warfarin. Tricyclic antidepressants are not recommended in patients with atrial fibrillation.

Question 160 Answer: f, Lithium g, Valproate
Explanation: Lithium and valproate are the mood stabilizers that can be used in patients with atrial fibrillation.

Question 161 Answer: i, Rivastigmine
Explanation: Rivastigmine seems to be the safest medication for use for patients with atrial fibrillation. Other acetyl-cholinesterase inhibitors should be avoided.

Reference: Puri BK, Hall AD, Ho RC (2014). *Revision Notes in Psychiatry*. Boca Raton, FL: CRC Press, p. 473.

Theme: Research Methodology

Question 162 Answer: d, Incremental validity
Explanation: Incremental validity is the extent to which the test provides a significant improvement in addition to the use of another approach. A test has incremental validity if it helps more than if it were not used.

Question 163 Answer: b, Content validity
Explanation: Content validity is the extent to which the test measures variables that are related to the parameter that should be measured by the test.

Question 164 Answer: a, Concurrent validity
Explanation: Concurrent validity is the extent to which the test correlates with a measure that has been previously validated.

References: Puri BK, Hall AD, Ho RC (2014). *Revision Notes in Psychiatry*. Boca Raton, FL: CRC Press, p. 318; Gosall N, Gosall G (2012). *The Doctor's Guide to Critical Appraisal*. Cheshire: PasTest, pp. 72–73.

Theme: Research Methodology

Question 165 Answer: f, Snowball
Explanation: Snowball sampling is a method of survey sample selection that is often used to locate rare or difficult-to-find populations. The procedure usually involves two stages: (1) identification of a sample of respondents with a particular characteristic and (2) asking initial sample members to provide names of other potential sample members. This is very cost efficient, but there is volunteer bias and the sampling error cannot be calculated.

Question 166 Answer: a, Convenience
Explanation: Convenience sampling is done as convenient, often allowing the subject to choose whether or not he or she is sampled. This type of sampling is the easiest and potentially the most dangerous. This is useful for preliminary research, as it is extremely efficient. However, there is volunteer bias, and the sampling error cannot be calculated.

Question 167 Answer: g, Stratified
Explanation: In stratified sampling, different populations of people are recruited from particular subgroups or strata in the target population. This is achieved by dividing the target population into two or more strata based on one or more characteristics and sampling each stratum (usually randomly). This improves accuracy of the estimation and allows calculation of the sampling error, but it requires accurate information about the population, and choice of relevant stratification variable can be difficult.

References: Lewis GH, Sheringham J, Kalim K, Crayford TJ (2008). *Mastering Public Health*. London: Royal Society of Medicine Press, pp. 46–47; Gosall N, Gosall G (2012). *The Doctor's Guide to Critical Appraisal*. Cheshire, UK: PasTest, pp. 42–43.

Theme: Psychotherapy

Question 168 Answer: g, Melanie Klein

Explanation: Melanie Klein evolved a theory of internal object relations that was intimately linked to drives. She postulated that the ego undergoes a splitting process to deal with the terror of annihilation. She viewed projection and introjection as the primary defensive operations in the first months of life. Infants project derivatives of the death instinct into the mother and then fear attack from the 'bad mother', a phenomenon that Klein referred to as 'persecutory anxiety'. This anxiety is intimately associated with the paranoid–schizoid position, in which the infants' mode of organising experience is to split all aspects of infant and mother into good and bad elements.

Question 169 Answer: c, Carl Jung

Explanation: Carl Jung expanded in his work, which he termed analytical psychology on Freud's concept of the unconscious, by describing the collective unconscious as consisting of all humankind's common, shared mythological and symbolic past. The collective unconscious includes archetypes – representational images and configurations with universal symbolic meanings. Archetypal figures exist for the mother, father, child and hero, among others. Archetypes contribute to complexes, feeling-toned ideas that develop as a result of personal experience interacting with archetypal imagery.

Question 170 Answer: a, Balint

Explanation: Balint believed that the urge for a primary love object underlies virtually all psychological phenomena. Infants wish to be loved totally and unconditionally, and when a mother is not forthcoming with appropriate nurturance, a child devotes his or her life to a search for the love missed in childhood. He coined the terms 'ocnophilia' and 'philobatism' to specify what he saw as two basic defensive modes of object relations. In the ocnophilic mode, denial of basic-fault separateness is promoted essentially by a clinging to the object and an avoiding of 'horrid' intervening space. For the philobat, the lost continuity of primary love is illusorily recreated by developing skilful mobility through which objects (here seen as obstacles) may be navigated around, while inhabiting the intervening 'friendly' spaces.

Question 171 Answer: f, Margaret Mahler

Explanation: Margaret Mahler proposed a theory of separation-individuation to describe how young children acquire a sense of identity separate from their mothers'. Her theory was based on observations of the interactions of children and their mothers. It consists of normal autism (from birth to 2 months), symbiosis (2–5 months), differentiation (5–10 months), practicing (10–18 months), rapprochement (18–24 months) and object constancy (2–5 years).

Question 172 Answer: h, Wilfred Bion

Explanation: Wilfried Bion expanded Melanie Klein's concept of projective identification to include an interpersonal process in which a therapist feels coerced by a patient into playing a particular role in the patient's internal world. He also developed the notion that the therapist must contain what the patient has projected so that it is processed and returned to the patient in modified form.

Question 173 Answer: d, Fairburn

Explanation: Ronald Fairbairn replaced the Freudian structural ideas of superego, ego and id with the notion of dynamic structures (object relations theory, developed originally by Winnicott, Guntrip and others). When an infant encounters frustration, a portion of the ego is defensively split off in the course of development and functions as an entity in relation to internal objects and to other subdivisions of the ego. He also stressed that not only an object but also an object relationship is internalized during development, so that a self is always in relationship to an object and the two are connected with an affect.

Question 174 Answer: i, Winnicott

Explanation: Donald W. Winnicott's theory of multiple self-organizations included a true self, which develops in the context of a responsive holding environment provided by a good-enough mother. When infants experience a traumatic disruption of their developing sense of self, however, a false self emerges and monitors and adapts to the conscious and unconscious needs of the mother; it thus provides a protected exterior behind which the true self is afforded a privacy that it requires to maintain its integrity.

Question 175 Answer: b, Bowlby

Explanation: John Bowlby formulated the theory that normal attachment in infancy is crucial to a person's healthy development, with maternal deprivation resulting in separation anxiety. Attachment develops gradually; it results in an infant wanting to be with a preferred person, who is perceived as stronger, wiser and able to reduce anxiety or distress. Attachment thus gives infants feelings of security. The process is facilitated by interaction between mother and infant; the amount of time together is less important than the amount of activity between the two.

Question 176 Answer: e, Heinz Kohut

Explanation: Heinz Kohut is best known for his writings on narcissism and the development of self psychology. He viewed the development and maintenance of self-esteem and self-cohesion as more important than sexuality or aggression. He conceived two separate lines of development, one moving in the direction of object relatedness and the other in the direction of greater enhancement of the self.

Reference: Sadock BJ, Sadock VA (2003). *Kaplan and Sadock's Synopsis of Psychiatry* (9th edition). Philadelphia, PA: Lippincott, Williams & Wilkins, pp. 29, 140, 218, 220, 222–223.

Theme: Addictions and Mechanism of Actions

Question 177 Answer: e, Phencyclidine

Explanation: PCP is a dissociative agent as the person remains conscious. PCP blocks NMDA glutamate receptors. It leads to emotional withdrawal, concrete thinking, catatonic or bizarre posturing, assaultive behaviour and prolonged psychotic reaction.

Question 178 Answer: f, MDMA
Explanation: MDMA is a designer drug and serotonin neurotoxin.

Question 179 Answer: c, Cannabis
Explanation: There are two subtypes of the cannabinoid receptor, CB1 and CB2. CB1 receptors are highly expressed in the hippocampus, cortex, basal ganglia and cerebellum and spinal cord. Both CB1 and CB2 are coupled to inhibitory G-proteins. Activation of the cannabinoid receptors causes inhibition of adenylate cyclase and a subsequent decrease in the concentration of cAMP in the cells.

Question 180 Answer: b, Opioid
Explanation: This is the correct mechanism of action for opioid. The increased activation of dopaminergic neurons in the nucleus accumbens and the ventral tegmental areas that are part of the brain's reward pathway and the release of dopamine into the synaptic results in sustained activation of the post-synaptic membrane.

Reference: Puri BK, Hall AD, Ho RC (2014). *Revision Notes in Psychiatry*. Boca Raton, FL: CRC Press, pp. 519–545.

Theme: Learning Disability and Clinical Phenotypes

Question 181 Answer: a, Primary prevention
Explanation: This is true with regard to primary prevention. It usually also involves population screening, carrier detection and prenatal diagnosis by utlilization of molecular genetics. It is also important to prevent exposure to ionizing radiation and teratogenic drugs. It also involves smoking cessation and avoiding alcohol misuse during pregnancy.

Question 182 Answer: c, Tertiary prevention
Explanation: At the community level, active resettlement programmes with expansion of support network, such as special education services, training placements, day and residential services can prevent long-term hospital care.

Question 183 Answer: b, Secondary prevention
Explanation: This involves prentatal diagnosis, maternal serum alpha foetoprotein and triple tests. It also involves neonatal screening to detect endocrine diseases such as congenital hypothyroidism and metabolic diseases.

Reference: Puri BK, Hall AD, Ho RC (2014). *Revision Notes in Psychiatry*. Boca Raton, FL: CRC Press, p. 614.

Theme: Child Psychiatry

Question 184 Answer: b, 3%

Question 185 Answer: e, 10%
Explanation: The heritability is over 90%. The recurrence rate in siblings is roughly 3% for narrowly defined autism but is about 10%–20% for milder variants. There is an association between autism and learning disabilities.

Seventy percent of children with autism do have mental retardation, mild-to-moderate mental retardation (30%) and severe-to-profound mental retardation (50%). Commonly, it is also associated with academic learning problems in literacy or numeracy. It is associated with ADHD (50%). 10% of individuals with autism do have OCD. Tics and Tourette's syndrome have been associated as well.

Reference: Puri BK, Hall AD, Ho RC (2014). *Revision Notes in Psychiatry*. Boca Raton, FL: CRC Press, p. 627.

Theme: Old-Age Psychiatry

Question 186 Answer: h, Vascular dementia
Explanation: Vascular dementia is characterized by a stepwise deteriorating course with a patchy distribution of neurological and neuropsychological deficits. There is evidence of vascular diseases on physical examination.

Question 187 Answer: g, Pseudodementia
Explanation: In pseudodementia, there is the presence of family or personal history of mood disorder. In addition, the onset is acute in nature. There is lack of motivation in the individual, and he or she usually answers with 'don't know' for most of the questions. Memory deficits are usually reported by patients. Mood is typically low and irritable at times. Individuals cannot enjoy things in life and are preoccupied with somatic complaints. There is the absent of aphasia, and there is the presence of mood-congruent hallucinations.

Question 188 Answer: e, Lewy body dementia
Explanation: The common cognitive symptoms include enduring and progressive cognitive impairment with impairments in consciousness, alertness and also attention. It is associated with apathy, depression and hallucinations (complex visual hallucinations: 80% and auditory hallucinations: 20%). It is also associated with extrapyramidal signs and parkinsonism. There might be neuroleptic sensitivity, falls, syncope as well as spontaneous loss of consciousness.

Question 189 Answer: c, Cerebral autosomal-dominant arteriopathy with sub-cortical infarcts and leukoencephalopathy (CADSIL)
Explanation: CADSIL is a genetic disease with Notch 3 mutations in chromosome 19 and results in recurrent subcortical cerebrovascular accidents (CVAs) (80%), cognitive deterioration (50%), mood changes (30%), epilepsy (10%) and gait abnormalities.

Question 190 Answer: f, Psychogenic fugue

Explanation: In dissociative fugue, there are all the features of dissociative amnesia plus an apparently purposeful journey away from home. A new identity may be assumed.

Question 191 Answer: d, Frontal lobe dementia

Explanation: Patients with frontotemporal lobe dementia have younger age of onset, more severe apathy, disinhibition, reduction in speech output, loss of insight, and coarsening of social behaviour but less spatial disorientation compared with patients with Alzheimer's dementia.

Question 192 Answer: b, Binswanger's disease

Explanation: This is a progressive subcortical vascular encephalopathy with CT scan revealing markedly enlarged ventricles secondary to infarction in hemispheric white matter. Infarcts are observed to affect periventricular and central white matter. The age of onset is 50–65 years, with a gradual accumulation of neurological signs, dementia and disturbances in motor function including pseudobulbar palsy. There is often a history of severe hypertension, systemic vascular disease and stroke.

Question 193 Answer: i, Vitamin B1 deficiency

Explanation: Wernicke's encephalopathy is caused by severe deficiency of thiamine (vitamin B1), which is usually caused by alcohol abuse in Western countries. Other causes do include hyperemesis as well as starvation. The important clinical features include ophthalmoplegia, nystagmus, ataxia and clouding of consciousness.

Reference: Puri BK, Hall AD, Ho RC (2014). *Revision Notes in Psychiatry*. Boca Raton, FL: CRC Press, pp. 517, 681–723.

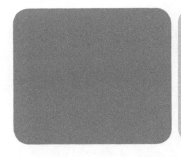

MRCPYSCH PAPER B MOCK EXAMINATION 3: QUESTIONS

GET THROUGH MRCPSYCH PAPER B MOCK EXAMINATION

Total number of questions: 188 (109 MCQs, 79 EMIs)
Total time provided: 180 minutes

Question 1
Which of the following is not a typical symptom of classic chronic Lyme encephalopathy?
  a. Amnesia
  b. Daytime hypersomnolence
  c. Depression
  d. Hypophosphataemia
  e. Peripheral neuropathy

Question 2
What is the estimated incidence of developing Ebstein anomaly if the mother is exposed to lithium in the first trimester?
  a. 0.01%
  b. 0.02%
  c. 0.05%
  d. 0.2%
  e. 0.4%

Question 3
If a mother with bipolar disorder is maintained on sodium valproate throughout pregnancy, what is the estimated incidence of neural tube defects?
  a. 1 in 10
  b. 1 in 50
  c. 1 in 80
  d. 1 in 100
  e. 1 in 200

Question 4
Which particular chromosomal loci have been implicated with autistic disorder?
a. Chromosomal 1q
b. Chromosomal 2q
c. Chromosomal 6q
d. Chromosomal 10q
e. Chromosomal 22q

Question 5
An 18-year-old female has been referred by her school counsellor, as he was concerned that she might have depression. In adolescent-onset bipolar disorder, which of the following symptoms is less likely to occur compared with adult-onset depression?
a. Persistent low mood
b. Loss of interest
c. Significant weight loss
d. Feelings of worthlessness
e. Psychomotor retardation

Question 6
Psychotherapy is one of the core modalities for the treatment of individuals with borderline personality disorder. Which of the following therapies targets mainly the distorted perceptions of significant others?
a. Supportive psychotherapy
b. Cognitive behavioural therapy (CBT)
c. Schema-focused therapy
d. Transference-focused therapy
e. Family therapy

Question 7
A 32-year-woman has always had difficulties with trusting others. She also does not feel that her spouse has been faithful towards her. She has been referred and seen by the outpatient psychiatry team, who has diagnosed her with paranoid personality disorder. Which of the following treatments is least likely to be suitable for her?
a. Supportive psychotherapy
b. Problem-based therapy
c. Cognitive behavioural therapy
d. Group-based therapy
e. Antidepressant treatment

Question 8
A 50-year-old man with a history of cardiac arrhythmia and a pacemaker implant has been admitted to the National Health Service (NHS) service following a severe

bout of depression with strong suicidal ideations. All the following are relative contraindications against electroconvulsive therapy (ECT) with the exception of

a. Cerebral aneurysm
b. Recent cerebrovascular accident
c. Presence of a pacemaker
d. Sick-cell disease
e. Intra-cerebral haemorrhage

Question 9
Which of the following statements is false about the findings from the Multimodal Treatment Study (MTA) on attention-deficit hyperactivity disorder (ADHD)?

a. There is a small but detectible reduction in overall growth in height for children who remain on stimulants.
b. Loss of growth is maximal in the first year of treatment.
c. 35% showed a moderate and gradual improvement, and 50% showed significant improvement over the 3-year study period.
d. 15% initially responded well but deteriorated over 3 years.
e. Drug treatment was associated with a reduction in the rate of delinquency and substance abuse in children with ADHD, compared to the rate found in normal controls.

Question 10
The male-to-female ratio is hypothyroidism is

a. 1:2
b. 1:8
c. 1:16
d. 1:32
e. 1:64

Question 11
A 65-year-old woman has been having difficulties with her sleep. Which of the following are not characteristic sleep changes that take place in aging?

a. Decreased duration of slow-wave sleep
b. Decreased sleep efficiency
c. Decreased total sleep time
d. Decreased episodes of rapid eye movement (REM) sleep
e. Increased sleep latency

Question 12
Which of the following is a feature of non-REM sleep?

a. Decreased parasympathetic activity
b. Increased cerebral blood flow
c. Increased tendon reflexes
d. Decreased complexity of dreams
e. Increased respiratory rate

Question 13

Which of the following statements is false?

a. Hypomagnesaemia is associated with hyperparathyroidism.
b. After treatment of hyperthyroidism, psychiatric symptoms usually resolve.
c. Hypothyroidism causes hirsutism.
d. One-third of patients with hyperthyroidism meet the criteria for major depressive disorder.
e. Delusions and hallucinations are equally common in hypothyroidism.

Question 14

Which of the following is not considered to be subcortical dementia?

a. Human immunodeficiency virus (HIV)-related dementia
b. Huntington chorea
c. Parkinson disease
d. Frontal temporal dementia
e. Vascular dementia

Question 15

Which of the following neuroanatomical areas shows decreased blood flow during the Wisconsin card sorting test (WCST) in patients with schizophrenia?

a. Dorsolateral temporal cortex
b. Parietal cortex
c. Parahippocampal gyrus
d. Prefrontal cortex
e. Occipital cortex

Question 16

Which of the following statements regarding the standard error of the mean (SEM) is false?

a. It decreases as the sample size increases.
b. It increases as the standard deviation increases.
c. It is a measure of the variability of the observations.
d. It measures the variability of the sample statistic in relation to the true but unknown population characteristic.
e. None of the above.

Question 17

Twenty depressed patients were given escitalopram and matched with another 20 depressed patients, who were given agomelatine. The Montgomery–Asberg Depression Rating Scale was used to assess these patients' response to the medication. Which of the following tests below can be used to compare treatment effect?

a. Independent sample t-test
b. Mann–Whitney U test

c. McNemar test
d. Paired *t*-test
e. Sign test

Question 18

Referring to Figure 5.1, intention to treat analysis was used. How many participants should be included?
  a. 12 participants
  b. 14 participants
  c. 26 participants
  d. 32 participants
  e. 58 participants

Question 19

Based on Table 5.1, calculate the rate of depressed subjects with intervention.
  a. 0.27
  b. 0.37
  c. 0.47
  d. 0.57
  e. 0.67

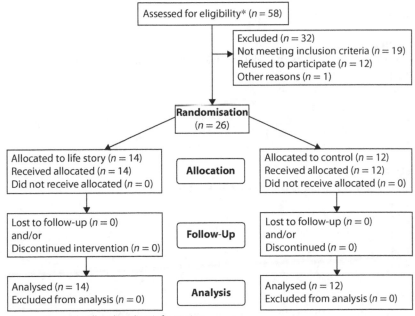

Figure 5.1 CONSORT diagram: participant recruitment, intervention and assessment. (From Chan MF, Ng SE, Tien A, Ho RC, Thayala J (2013). A randomised controlled study to explore the effect of life story review on depression in older Chinese in Singapore. *Health Soc Care Commun*, 21(5): 545–553.)

Table 5.1 Comparison of outcome between intervention and control groups

	Depressed subjects	Not depressed subjects	Total number of subjects
Intervention group	28	31	59
Control group	36	21	57

Question 20
Based on Table 5.1, calculate the rate of rate of depressed subjects with the control group?
  a. 0.33
  b. 0.43
  c. 0.53
  d. 0.63
  e. 0.73

Question 21
Based on Table 5.1, what is the absolute benefit increase?
  a. 0.16
  b. 0.26
  c. 0.36
  d. 0.46
  e. 0.56

Question 22
Based on Table 5.1, what is the relative risk of remaining depressed?
  a. 0.34
  b. 1.34
  c. 2.34
  d. 3.34
  e. 4.34

Question 23
Based on Table 5.1, what is the relative benefit increase?
  a. 0.34
  b. 1.34
  c. 2.34
  d. 3.34
  e. 4.34

Question 24
Based on Table 5.1, what is the number needed to treat (NNT)?
  a. 6 patients
  b. 16 patients
  c. 26 patients
  d. 36 patients
  e. 46 patients

Question 25
If the confidence interval (CI) of absolute risk reduction (ARR) is 0.16 (95% CI: 0.04–0.35), what is the CI of NNT?
 a. 0.86–10
 b. 1.86–15
 c. 2.86–25
 d. 3.86–30
 e. 4.86–35

Question 26
Which of the following is not a sign of inhalant intoxication?
 a. Diplopia
 b. Euphoria
 c. Hyper-reflexia
 d. Nystagmus
 e. Slurred speech

Question 27
A 64-year-old man with Parkinson disease is noted by the family to persistently gamble in the casino, despite having lost huge sums of money and being in debt. Premorbidly, he only gambled small amounts sparingly. Which one of the following drugs that he was taking could potentially cause pathological gambling?
 a. Bromocriptine
 b. Galantamine
 c. L-Dopa
 d. Pramipexole
 e. Selegiline

Question 28
Which of the following offences or misconduct are not more predominantly committed by male offenders?
 a. Murder and manslaughter
 b. Robbery with violence
 c. Sexual aggression
 d. Homosexual offences
 e. Threat and fraud

Question 29
A 37-year-old male sex offender is being assessed for risk of recidivism. Which of the following is the best predictor of sexual reoffending?
 a. Antisocial orientation
 b. Denial of sex crime
 c. Lack of victim empathy
 d. Low motivation for treatment
 e. Psychological distress

Question 30

Which of the following statements is false regarding tuberous sclerosis?
a. Approximately two-thirds of all cases are spontaneous mutations, while one-third are inherited on an autosomal dominant basis.
b. It is associated with mental retardation in approximately half of patients.
c. It is associated with seizures.
d. It is associated with cardiac rhabdolipomas and pulmonary cysts.
e. Progression of adult-onset cases tends to be much faster than childhood-onset cases.

Question 31

Which of the following statements is false regarding foetal alcohol syndrome?
a. Binge alcohol drinking in pregnant mothers may be as dangerous as daily drinking in this syndrome.
b. It is associated with mental retardation, which, in most cases, is of mild severity.
c. It is associated with behavioural problems similar to those of ADHD, but hyperactivity is more prominent than distractibility and inattentiveness.
d. It is caused by in utero exposure to alcohol.
e. There is often some resolution of the dysmorphic features by adulthood.

Question 32

A morbidly obese 13-year-old boy has difficulty controlling his overeating. He often goes to extreme length to satisfy his hunger. He also tends to prick his skin and gets irritable easily. He attends a special school because of a diagnosis of mild learning disability when he was younger. On physical examination, he is short in stature and has micropenis with cryptorchidism. Which one of the following diagnoses is most likely?
a. Bardet–Biedl syndrome
b. Fragile X syndrome
c. Lesch–Nyhan syndrome
d. Phenylketonuria
e. Prader–Willi syndrome

Question 33

Which of the following is a risk factor for suicide in patients with schizophrenia?
a. Regaining insight
b. Discharge from inpatient care 3 months and beyond
c. Just recently employed
d. Female gender
e. Having low educational attainment before onset of the illness

Question 34

Risk of future antisocial personality disorder in a 14-year-old child with conduct disorder is
a. 10%
b. 20%
c. 30%

d. 40%
e. 50%

Question 35
Which of the following disorders is recognized to cause schizophrenia-like psychosis in a 40-year-old man?
a. Cerebral autosomal-dominant arteriopathy with subcortical infarcts and leukoencephalopathy (CASDIL)
b. Mitochondrial encephalomyopathy, lactic acidosis and stroke-like episodes (MELAS) syndrome
c. Huntington disease
d. Kennedy disease
e. Polyneuropathy, organomegaly, endocrinopathy, monoclonal gammopathy and skin changes (POEM) syndrome

Question 36
A 22-year-old university student suffers from first episode psychosis and has great difficulty with her studies. She was diagnosed to have schizophrenia. Which of the following neurocognitive functions is most impaired?
a. Language functions
b. Immediate verbal memory
c. Visuospatial skills
d. Working memory
e. Vigilance

Question 37
Nicotine causes addiction through its action as which of the following?
a. Acetylcholine agonist
b. Acetylcholine antagonist
c. Dopamine agonist
d. Dopamine antagonist
e. Stimulating nicotine receptors

Question 38
Which of the following is not a general principle behind motivational interviewing?
a. Develop discrepancy
b. Express empathy
c. Psychoeducation
d. Roll with resistance
e. Support self-efficacy

Question 39
A 49-year-old male offender with a history of schizophrenia is released from a medium-secure unit. What is the probability that he will reoffend within 2 years?
a. 2%
b. 10%

c. 20%
d. 22%
e. 30%

Question 40
What percentage of perpetrators of homicide have symptoms of mental illness at the time of the offence?
a. 1%
b. 5%
c. 7%
d. 10%
e. 15%

Question 41
A newborn child with Down syndrome is found on genetic testing to have an unbalanced Robertsonian translocation, and you are asked to counsel the parents. Which one of the following pieces of advice is incorrect?
a. Both parents should be offered chromosome analysis, as one may carry the translocation in a balanced form.
b. If the mother is found to be a carrier, the recurrence risk is 50%.
c. Ultrasound monitoring of nasal bone formation will be useful in future antenatal screening for Down syndrome.
d. If parents are carriers of translocation, they have 46 chromosomes.
e. In translocation, patients with Down syndrome have 46 chromosomes

Question 42
Hachinski score is indicated for which particular form of dementia?
a. Alzheimer's dementia
b. Frontal temporal dementia
c. Vascular dementia
d. HIV-related dementia
e. Mixed dementia

Question 43
Based on your understanding of Lewy body dementia (LBD), how common is the presence of visual hallucinations?
a. 10%
b. 20%
c. 40%
d. 60%
e. 80%

Question 44
In Figure 5.2, cluster 1 has more cases of depressive disorder, adjustment, stress, panic attack, first suicide attempt and no admissions. Cluster 2 has more cases of borderline personality disorder, hallucination, insomnia, headache, multiple

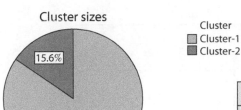

Size of smallest cluster	65 (15.6%)
Size of largest cluster	353 (84.4%)
Ratio of sizes: Largest cluster to Smallest cluster	5.43

Figure 5.2 Summary of two-step clustering. (From Choo C, Diederich J, Song I, Ho RC (2014). Cluster analysis reveals risk factors for repeated suicide attempts in a multi-ethnic Asian population. *Asian J Psychiatr*, 8: 38–51.)

attempts and multiple admissions. Which of the clustering algorithms was used to generate Figure 5.2?
  a. Centroid-based clustering
  b. Connectivity-based clustering
  c. Density-based clustering
  d. Distribution-based clustering
  e. Regression-based clustering.

Question 45
Referring to Figure 5.3, which of the following should be the *x*-axis?
  a. Sensitivity
  b. Specificity
  c. Sensitivity/specificity
  d. 1 sensitivity
  e. 1 – specificity

Question 46
The cut-off score of an anxiety inventory is 40. If the sensitivity and specificity of this inventory of diagnosing anxiety are 0.42 and 0.95, respectively, what is the likelihood ratio for positive test result (LR+)?
  a. 2.4
  b. 4.4
  c. 6.4
  d. 8.4
  e. 10.4

Question 47
Which of the following is false about type II error?
  a. The null hypothesis is wrongly rejected.
  b. The study does not detect an effect that existed in reality.
  c. Type II errors are considered to be less serious than type I error.
  d. Type II errors occur when the sample size of a study is too small.
  e. Type II errors represents false negatives.

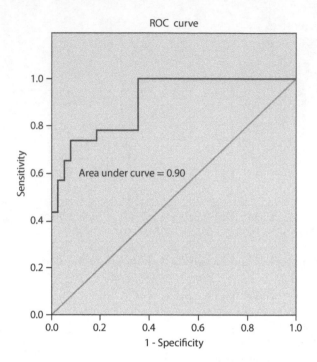

ROC curve

Figure 5.3 Result of receiver operating characteristic (ROC) analysis of the logistic regression model. (From Mak A, Tang CS, Chan MF, Cheak AA, Ho RC (2011). Damage accrual, cumulative glucocorticoid dose and depression predict anxiety in patients with systemic lupus erythematosus. *Clin Rheumatol*, 30(6): 795–803.)

Question 48

A 25-year-old man has been using cannabis for a year. He experiences withdrawal effects if he misses his regular dose. He is now keen to quit his habit. Which of the following medications would be helpful in treating his cannabis dependence syndrome?
a. Fluoxetine
b. Sodium valproate
c. Lithium
d. Diazepam
e. Busprione

Question 49

A 15-year-old boy is convicted of rape and undergoes treatment for sexual offenders. Which one of the following statements is most accurate about his recidivism rate compared with that of a 30-year-old man?
a. A 15-year-old has a higher rate of recidivism for sexual offence compared with a 30-year-old.
b. A 15-year-old has a lower rate of recidivism for sexual offence compared with a 30-year-old.
c. A 15-year-old has a higher rate of recidivism for non-sexual offence compared with the 30-year-old.

d. A 15-year-old has a lower rate of recidivism for non-sexual offence compared with a 30-year-old.
e. Their risk of recidivism for sexual offences is similar.

Question 50
Which of the following antibiotics can cause euphoria, delusions, depersonalization and illusions?
a. Cephalosporin
b. Clarithromycin
c. Gentamicin
d. Quinolone
e. Trimethoprim-sulfamethoxazole

Question 51
Which of the following statements about cannabis and schizophrenia is not true?
a. Cannabis has been known to lead to a twofold increase in the risk of schizophrenia.
b. Cannabis has been known to lead to a fourfold increase in the risk of psychosis.
c. Not all cannabis users develop schizophrenia, and this is dependent on the catechol-O-methyltransferase (COMT) genotype.
d. Patients who have homozygous VAL/VAL alleles in the COMT genotype have relatively higher risk.
e. Patients who are homozygous for MET/MET alleles in the COMT genotype have a twofold higher risk.

Question 52
Which of the following is not a good prognostic factor for patients with schizophrenia?
a. Being male
b. Being female
c. Good premorbid social adjustment
d. Family history of mood disorder
e. Abrupt or late onset of the illness

Question 53
The STAR*D trial main purpose is to determine the effectiveness of different treatments for people who have been diagnosed with major depressive disorder and have not responded to an initial antidepressant. In Level 2 of the treatment, which one of the following is not one of the treatment strategies considered and used in the trial?
a. Switching to other antidepressants from the selective serotonin re-uptake inhibitor (SSRI) class (sertraline)
b. Medication and psychotherapy augmentation
c. Antidepressant-only switch
d. Psychotherapy-only switch
e. Augmentation with physical therapies

Question 54

A 28-year-old man comes to the fertility clinic with his wife, citing inability to conceive after 2 years of marriage. On examination, he is noted to have tall stature, small penis and small testes. He also has low libido and erectile dysfunction, and his hormonal profile shows a low testosterone level and elevated follicle-stimulating hormone level. There is no family history of similar problems. Which one of the following is his most likely diagnosis?

a. Bardet–Biedl syndrome
b. Edward syndrome
c. Klinefelter syndrome
d. Phenylketonuria
e. Tay–Sachs disease

Question 55

In the United Kingdom, which of the following occupations is associated with the highest rate of suicide?

a. Elementary professionals
b. Working-age population
c. Machine operators
d. Deck crew
e. Agricultural workers

Question 56

Generally, the outcome for patients diagnosed with bulimia improves with time and has been noted to be better than that of anorexia nervosa. In terms of long-term outcomes, which of the following psychiatric conditions is highly associated with bulimia nervosa?

a. Depressive disorder
b. Generalized anxiety disorder
c. Panic disorder
d. Alcohol abuse
e. Opiate abuse

Question 57

Which of the following statements is false regarding the correlation coefficient?

a. The correlation coefficient can be strong but statistically non-significant because of sample size.
b. Spearman's and Kendall's rank correlation coefficients are non-parametric alternatives to Pearson's correlation coefficient.
c. The value of a correlation coefficient can range from –1 to +1.
d. A value of 0.5–0.8 signifies strong correlation.
e. None of the above.

Question 58

Which one of the following statements is true regarding type II error?

a. It can lead to false negatives.
b. The null hypothesis was wrongly rejected.
c. Study shows an effect that in reality does not exist.

d. The more the study restricts type I errors by setting a low level of alpha, the less the chance that a type II error will occur.

e. Type II errors are generally considered to be more serious than type I errors.

Question 59
Which of the following statements about type I error is false?
a. Bonferroni correction can be used to keep type II errors at a low level.
b. The null hypothesis is wrongly rejected.
c. The study shows an effect that does not exist.
d. The more the study restricts type I errors by setting a low level of alpha, the greater the chance that a type II error will occur.
e. Type I errors are more serious than type II errors.

Question 60
Approximately, what percentage of patients with schizophrenia are non-concordant with their medications?
a. 10%
b. 20%
c. 30%
d. 40%
e. 80%

Question 61
Which of the following is true about exhibitionism?
a. Exhibitionism is commonly associated with homosexual behaviour.
b. Exhibitionism is commonly associated with exposure of the genitalia to an unsuspecting stranger of the opposite gender.
c. Exhibitionism is commonly associated with sexual assault.
d. Exhibitionism is commonly associated with voyeurism.
e. Exhibitionism is commonly associated with young men.

Question 62
Which of the following medications is likely to be helpful for patients with agoraphobia as well as social phobia?
a. Fluoxetine
b. Sertraline
c. Bupropion
d. Mirtazapine
e. Monoamine oxidase inhibitor (MAOI)

Question 63
A 20-year-old man has been diagnosed with kleptomania. All the following are possible comorbid psychiatric disorders that a psychiatrist should assess for, with the exception of which of the following?
a. Depression
b. Bulimia nervosa
c. Sexual dysfunction

d. Fetishistic disorder

e. Somatoform disorder

Question 64

Which of the following biases could be minimized by blinding in a randomized controlled trial?

a. Berkson's bias

b. Measurement bias

c. Misclassification bias

d. Neyman bias

e. Volunteer bias

Question 65

A researcher wants to compare the responses (graded as mild, moderate and high responses) of a group of depressed patients on bupropion, with that of a control group on amitriptyline. Which of the following tests would be most appropriate?

a. Mann–Whitney U test

b. McNemar test

c. Sign test

d. Spearman's correlation test

e. Wilcoxon signed-rank test

Question 66

Which of the following statements is not true for confounders?

a. It can be adjusted for at the analysis stage.

b. It can be adjusted for at the study design stage.

c. It may be an intermediate step along the causal chain.

d. It must be associated with the disease and be independently associated with the exposure under study.

e. It must predict disease independently of the exposure under study.

Question 67

Which of the following statements regarding meta-analysis is incorrect?

a. Patricia Forest published the first Forest plot in 1958.

b. Meta-analysis allows combination of effect sizes from different studies.

c. Meta-analysis allows comparison of results from studies from different categories.

d. Meta-analysis is best complemented by meta-regression.

e. The pooled effect-size is dependent on the variability of source data.

Question 68

A 23-year-old man, Samuel, has been recently diagnosed with first-episode psychosis and has been started on a dose of olanzapine. He is having muscular rigidity and fever at the moment. The core trainee is suspecting that he might have neuroleptic malignant syndrome (NMS). All the following should be suspected as possible differentials with the exception of which one?

a. Central nervous system (CNS) infection
b. Sepsis
c. Malignant hyperthermia
d. Thyroid storm
e. Heavy metal (lead) poisoning

Question 69

Which of the following regarding hyperparathyroidism is false?

a. It leads to an increase in serum Mg^{2+}.
b. Affective disturbance and personality change occur when the serum Ca^{2+} is 3–4 mmol/L.
c. Delirium, impaired cognition and psychosis occur when the serum Ca^{2+} is 4–4.75 mmol/L.
d. Somnolence and coma occur when the serum Ca^{2+} is higher than 4–4.75 mmol/L.
e. One-third of patients with hyperparathyroidism have severe psychiatric problems.

Question 70

The purposes for conducting meta-regression include all the following except which of the following?

a. To evaluate the evidence obtained from multiple studies involving cost–benefit analysis studies of a health policy across multiple studies.
b. To examine the impact of different variables on study effect size.
c. To explain heterogeneity.
d. To identify potential bias.
e. To identify which independent variables are predictors of a dependent variable after adjustment of confounding factors.

Question 71

Which of the following is not a predictor for the persistence of hyperkinetic symptoms into adulthood?

a. Comorbid conduct disorder
b. Comorbid depressive disorder
c. Comorbid anxiety disorder
d. Comorbid language disorders
e. Psychosocial adversity

Question 72

Which of the following common psychiatric disorders has been known to be associated with the highest heritability?

a. Autistic disorder
b. Attention-deficit hyperkinetic disorder
c. Conduct disorder

d. Depressive disorder
e. Bipolar disorder

Question 73
An 8-year-old boy demonstrates only speak selectively in certain situations. His mother is very concerned about his condition and wants to know the long-term prognosis of his condition. Based on current evidence, poor prognosis is associated with duration of the condition being longer than?
a. 2 months
b. 5 months
c. 10 months
d. 12 months
e. 24 months

Question 74
All the following are implicated in the pathophysiology of tic disorder, with the exception of
a. Increase in D2 receptor sensitivity
b. Increase in serotonin 5Ht3 receptor sensitivity
c. Reduction in the levels of noradrenaline
d. Reduction in choline in the left putamen
e. Presence of abnormalities in the caudate nucleus

Question 75
Pica refers to the persistent eating of non-nutritive substances for at least twice per week for a total minimum duration of 1 month. It usually affects children above the age of
a. 2 years
b. 3 years
c. 4 years
d. 5 years
e. 10 years

Question 76
Which of the following is not a feature of melancholia?
a. Anhedonia
b. Excessive guilt
c. Loss of appetite
d. Mood reactivity
e. Psychomotor agitation

Question 77
A 32-year-old woman has just given birth to her newborn son 3 days ago. Her husband has noted that she has been very tearful, with significant irritability as well as anxiety. Which of the following is a recommended treatment of choice based on the National Institute for Health and Care Excellence (NICE) guidelines?
a. Supportive reassurance
b. Commencement of benzodiazepines

c. Commencement of mood stabilizers
d. Immediate admission to the inpatient psychiatry unit
e. Psychological therapies

Question 78
Which of the following is not a risk factor for tardive dyskinesia?
a. Being elderly
b. Diffuse brain damage
c. Duration of antipsychotic treatment
d. Affective psychosis
e. Male gender

Question 79
A researcher wants to find out which groups of depressed patients will benefit from taking a new antidepressant recently released on the market. The variables include age, gender, socio-economic status, number of depressive episodes and changes in Hamilton depression scale. Which one of the following analyses is this researcher doing?
a. Cluster analysis
b. Factor analysis
c. Individual analysis
d. Path analysis
e. Principal component analysis

Question 80
A psychiatrist works in an academic institution with no substance abuse unit. Based on patients with consecutive schizophrenia admitted having no substance abuse, he concludes that there is no real association between schizophrenia and substance abuse. Which bias has this psychiatrist made?
a. Ascertainment bias
b. Berkson's bias
c. Misclassification bias
d. Recall bias
e. Selection bias

Question 81
A researcher wants to study the prevalence of cannabis-induced psychosis in the community. He recruits patients who are on follow-up in the psychosis clinic. Which type of bias is he experiencing?
a. Ascertainment bias
b. Berkson's bias
c. Neyman bias
d. Selection bias
e. Volunteer bias

Question 82
A 20-year-old woman suffers from anorexia nervosa, and she is 30 weeks pregnant. The obstetrician consults you on the potential problems that may occur during the delivery. The use of which of the following obstetric procedures is known to be increased in pregnant women with anorexia nervosa?
a. Caesarean section
b. Episiotomy
c. Forceps delivery
d. Induction of labour
e. Vacuum delivery

Question 83
In separation anxiety disorder, the child has anticipatory anxiety of separation. The onset is usually before which one of the following ages?
a. 2 years
b. 3 years
c. 4 years
d. 5 years
e. 6 years

Question 84
Which of the following statements regarding treatment of ADHD is true?
a. Very low birth weight and perinatal insult are risk factors for ADHD.
b. The half-life of atomoxetine is 15 hours.
c. Atomoxetine can be given only as second-line agent under all circumstances.
d. There is evidence to support the use of second-generation antipsychotics to treat hyperactivity in ADHD.
e. Hyperactivity and epilepsy are mutually exclusive.

Question 85
In which of the following conditions would an electroencephalogram (EEG) demonstrate an increase in slow-wave activity and a reduction in rhythm?
a. Alzheimer's dementia
b. Frontal-temporal dementia
c. Creutzfeldt–Jakob disease (CJD)
d. Dementia due to Parkinson disease
e. Mixed dementia

Question 86
Which of the following about the prognosis of Huntington disease is correct?
a. 2 years
b. 5 years
c. 8 years
d. 10 years
e. 12 years

Question 87

A 40-year-old man presents with memory loss and ataxia. The radiologist gives you a call as he has discovered pulvinar signal in his magnetic resonance imaging (MRI). This MRI finding is associated with which of the following conditions?

a. CJD
b. Kuru
c. Gerstmann–Straussler–Scheinker syndrome
d. Familiar fatal insomnia
e. New variant CJD

Question 88

A male adolescent suffers from depression as he has difficulty in coping with changes associated with puberty. He wants to know the average duration of puberty in boys. Your answer is

a. 1–2 years
b. 3–4 years
c. 5–6 years
d. 7–8 years
e. 9–10 years

Question 89

Which of the following statements is incorrect?

a. Postpartum blues are common and usually have an onset between the third and the fifth days after pregnancy.
b. The incidence of depression in women in spontaneous abortion and ectopic pregnancy is much higher than that of the general population.
c. Postpartum psychosis should be regarded as a psychiatric emergency and warrants inpatient hospitalization.
d. There needs to be careful selection of psychotropic medications as these medications could have potential adverse effects on the infant.
e. Delusional disorders tend to be worsened in pregnancy.

Question 90

A 45-year-old man presents to the emergency department with clouding of consciousness, hallucinations and marked tremors. The core trainee who examined him noted that he has nystagmus and ophthalmoplegia on examination as well. He went into sustained ventricular fibrillation, which was not responsive to pharmacological management and demised shortly after. If a brain autopsy was performed for him, it is expected that there will be the presence of which of the following changes?

a. Temporal lobe sclerosis
b. Frontal lobe atrophy
c. Petechial haemorrhages in the periaqueductal gray matter
d. Enlarged lateral ventricles
e. Tau accumulation in the basal ganglia

Question 91

Which of the following statements regarding confounder and bias is incorrect?
a. Both confounder and bias can be adjusted for at the analysis stage.
b. Both confounder and bias can be prevented by having proper study design.
c. Confounder is a variable that is associated with exposure and outcome, while bias is a systematic error.
d. Confounder does not lead to false association between exposure and outcome, but bias does.
e. Confounder is introduced by a third factor independently related to the exposure and outcome, while bias is introduced by the researcher.

Question 92

A new drug, created by a drug company, is being administered to a small group of subjects in an inpatient clinic where they are being monitored constantly. Which phase of the clinical trial is this?
a. O
b. I
c. II
d. III
e. IV

Question 93

A new drug, created by a drug company, is being compared with the current standard treatment for a particular condition. Which phase of the clinical trial is this?
a. O
b. I
c. II
d. III
e. IV

Question 94

A 28-year-old man has been referred by his general practitioner (GP) for help in your mental health service. You understand from the referring memo by the GP that the referred gentleman has been having obsessions involving non-living objects and is not be able to control his sexual desire and, at times, engages in masturbation. Which of the following statements about his behaviour and diagnosis is incorrect?
a. This condition is usually more prevalent in males.
b. Approximately, 50% of men are considered to be homosexuals.
c. The behaviour is caused by classical conditioning.
d. This behaviour may be associated with temporal lobe dysfunction.
e. Treatment usually involves behavioural therapy focusing masturbatory reconditioning and response prevention.

Question 95

Chronic abuse of which of the following substances might result in the development of Goodpasture syndrome?

a. Khat
b. Steroid
c. Solvents
d. Nicotine
e. Ketamine

Question 96

A 55-year-old woman suffered from a heart attack and was resuscitated by the doctors in the emergency department. She has recovered from the episode. She then consults her GP and complains of recurrent nightmares and hypervigilance. She worries that she may suffer from nervous shock, and her GP has referred her for a psychiatric assessment. During the interview, she mentions that she did not have a heart attack. She thinks she developed an anaphylactic shock after an injection and wants to sue the hospital for compensation as she is incapable of working owing to the nervous shock. Which of the following statements is most likely to be correct?
a. There is a high chance that she will be able to return to work after settlement of this case.
b. She meets the criteria for nervous shock but not post-traumatic stress disorder (PTSD).
c. You should refer her to see a forensic psychiatrist for a formal and proper medico-legal assessment.
d. After you write the medical report, she is likely to be unhappy with the fact that you did not support her claim of having nervous shock and will lodge a formal complaint to the chief executive through her lawyer.
e. She should be referred to see an expert in PTSD for trauma-focused CBT.

Question 97

A 20-year-old woman suffers from anorexia nervosa. Her parents are concerned about her outcome. Which of the following factors indicates a poor prognosis based on the medical literature?
a. Early age of onset
b. Family history of anorexia nervosa
c. Female gender
d. Family history of bulimia nervosa
e. Later age of onset

Question 98

You are a forensic psychiatrist assessing a 33-year-old man convicted of child sexual abuse for his risk of recidivism. What is the likelihood of him being reconvicted of the same crime?
a. 10%
b. 15%
c. 20%
d. 25%
e. 30%

Question 99

Which of the following is not a way of reducing bias?
a. Blinding
b. Blinding of intervention group but not the observer who collects the measurements
c. Intention to treat analysis
d. Random allocation
e. True concealment

Question 100

Which of the following is not a risk factor for development of PTSD?
a. Female gender
b. Low intelligence quotient (IQ)
c. Low socioeconomic status
d. Pre-existing psychiatric disorder
e. Psychopathic traits

Question 101

Which of the following is not a feature of Ganser syndrome?
a. Amnesia
b. Confusion
c. Frank hallucinations
d. Somatic conversion
e. Vorbeireden

Question 102

A 70-year-old man was admitted to a general hospital as he felt pain when passing urine. Three days later, he began complaining to his relatives that the ward staff were not treating him well and were poisoning his food. He also saw insects crawling on the wall. The likely diagnosis is
a. Delirium
b. Delusional disorder
c. Late-onset schizophrenia
d. Lewy body dementia
e. Psychotic depression

Question 103

Which of the following is not usually found in Addison's disease?
a. Low sodium
b. Low potassium
c. High urea
d. Low glucose
e. Hypercalcaemia

Question 104

What percentage of patients with anorexia nervosa eventually develop symptoms of bulimia?

a. 10%
b. 20%
c. 30%
d. 50%
e. 70%

Question 105
Which of the following classes of drug has been known to be associated with a high incidence of pulmonary hypertension in the newborn?
a. Tricyclic antidepressant
b. Selective serotonin reuptake inhibitor (SSRI)
c. Noradrenergic and specific serotonergic antidepressants (NASSA)
d. Monoamine oxidase inhibitor (MAOI)
e. Antipsychotics

Question 106
Which of the following is not a risk factor for suicide in multiple sclerosis?
a. Male gender
b. Old age at onset of illness
c. Previous history of depression
d. Social isolation
e. Substance abuse

Question 107
A 55-year-old man presents with coronary artery disease (CAD). His wife asks you what the percentage of patients with CAD who develop depression is. Your answer is
a. 3%
b. 10%
c. 20%
d. 40%
e. 60%

Question 108
A 65-year-old bus driver suffers from post-cerebrovascular accident (CVA) cognitive impairment, and he is referred for assessment of pre-morbid intelligence. A junior psychologist consults you on which test to use. Which of the following would you recommend?
a. Hayling and Briston test
b. National adult reading test
c. Luria–Nebraska neuropsychological battery
d. Mini Mental State Examination (MMSE)
e. Verbal fluency test

Question 109
The mortality by suicide in Huntington disease is increased by
a. 5 times
b. 10 times
c. 15 times

d. 25 times

e. 30 times

Extended Match Items

Theme: Learning Disability
Options:
  a. 5
  b. 10
  c. 15
  d. 20
  e. 30
  f. 40
  g. 60
  h. 70
  i. 80

Lead in: Match one number to each of the following. Each option may be used once, more than once or not at all.

What is the percentage of patients with Turner syndrome:

Question 110
Suffering from renal malformations. (Choose one option.)

Question 111
Suffering hypothyroidism. (Choose one option.)

Question 112
Suffering coarctation of aorta. (Choose one option.)

Question 113
With a meiotic error that occurred in a paternal meiotic division. (Choose one option.)

Theme: Research Methodology
Options:
  a. Cox regression
  b. Linear regression
  c. Kaplan–Meier estimates
  d. Multiple linear regression
  e. Multiple logistic regression

Lead in: Match one correct statistical technique with each of the following descriptions of use. Each option may be used once, more than once or none at all.

Question 114
Analysis of the effect of several variables upon the time it takes for a specified event to happen. (Choose one option.)

Question 115
Describes the relationship between two numerical variables. (Choose one option.)

Question 116
Analysis of several explanatory variables with one outcome variable. (Choose one option.)

Theme: Research Methodology

Options:
- a. Cluster sampling
- b. Convenience sampling
- c. Event sampling
- d. Matched random sampling
- e. Panel sampling
- f. Progressive sampling
- g. Quota sampling
- h. Snowball sampling
- i. Systematic sampling
- j. Simple random sampling

Lead in: Select one appropriate sampling method to match each of the scenarios below. Each option may be used once, more than once or not at all.

Question 117
Subjects are first matched based on some demographic characteristics and then randomly assigned into groups. (Choose one option.)

Question 118
Subjects are selected based on an ordering scheme such as odd-numbered houses. (Choose one option.)

Question 119
Involves monitoring of ongoing experiences that vary across and within days in the ward environment. (Choose one option.)

Question 120
Subjects are first selected as a group through a random method, and the group will be given the same questionnaire three times in 1 year to seek their view on stigma in mental health. (Choose one option.)

Question 121
This is a non-probability sampling and subjects are drawn from the part of the population that is available in a clinical service. (Choose one option.)

Question 122
Subjects are first identified based on characteristics and are then required to provide names of other potential subjects. (Choose one option.)

Question 123
Subjects are arranged in areas such as inner-city, suburban and rural areas, and subjects from these areas are selected. (Choose one option.)

Theme: Neuroimaging in the Elderly

Options:
a. Alzheimer's dementia
b. Frontal-lobe dementia
c. HIV-related dementia
d. Huntington chorea
e. Parkinson disease dementia
f. CJD
g. Vascular dementia
h. LBD

Lead in: Match the classifications with the following questions. Each option may be used once or more than once or not at all.

Question 124
Name three examples of cortical dementia. (Choose three options.)

Question 125
Name three examples of subcortical dementia. (Choose three options.)

Question 126
Name two examples of mixed cortical and subcortical dementia. (Choose two options.)

Theme: Forensic Psychiatry

Options:
a. 1
b. 5
c. 10
d. 20
e. 30
f. 35
g. 45
h. 50
i. 60
j. 70
k. 80

Lead in: Match one number to each of the following statements. Each option may be used once, more than once or not at all.

Question 127
The percentage of prisoners with epilepsy. (Choose one option.)

Question 128
The percentage of arsonists who are male. (Choose one option.)

Question 129
The percentage of psychiatric patients released from medium secure units who re-offend. (Choose one option.)

Question 130
The percentage heritability of antisocial behaviour in prisoners. (Choose one option.)

Question 131
The percentage of prisoners who screen positive for adult ADHD. (Choose one option.)

Question 132
The percentage of female prisoners with antisocial personality disorder. (Choose one option.)

Theme: Dementia

Options:
 a. Behaviour Dimensions Scale (BDS)
 b. Cambridge Examination for Mental Disorders of the Elderly (CAMDEX)
 c. Cambridge Neuropsychological Test Automated Battery (CANTAB)
 d. Geriatric Mental State Schedule (GMS)
 e. Mini Mental State Examination (MMSE)
 f. Gresham Ward Questionnaire (GWQ)
 g. Manchester and Oxford Universities Scale for the Psychopathological Assessment of Dementia (MOUSEPAD)
 h. Present Behavioural Examination (PBE)
 i. Sandoz Clinical Assessment (SCAG)
 j. Performance Test of Activities of Daily Living (PADL)

Lead in: Match one test with each of the following questions. Each option may be used once, more than once or not at all.

Question 133
A rating scale used to screen for dementia. (Choose one option.)

Question 134
An automated computerized battery used for cognitive assessment of dementia. (Choose one option.)

Question 135
An assessment schedule consisting of a structured clinical interview, a range of objective tests and a structured interview with a relative of the patient with dementia. (Choose one option.)

Theme: Management of PTSD

Options:
  a. Cognitive behavioral therapy
  b. Eye movement desensitization reprocessing
  c. Interpersonal therapy
  d. Psychodynamic therapy
  e. Fluoxetine
  f. Paroxetine
  g. Sertraline
  h. Venlafaxine
  i. Carbamazepine
  j. Clonidine
  k. Buspirone

Lead in: Match the management options with each of the following questions. Each option may be used once, more than once or not at all.

Question 136
Based on NICE guidelines, which modality of therapy has been recommended to be offered to individuals with severe PTSD within 3 months of the trauma? (Choose one option.)

Question 137
Which of the above modalities of therapy help to stop the symptoms of PTSD? (Choose two options.)

Question 138
Based on NICE guidelines, which medications are likely to be beneficial for PTSD and should be used first? (Choose four options.)

Question 139
Which medications can help to reduce the hyperarousal and intrusive symptoms? (Choose two options.)

Question 140
Which medications can help to reduce and lessen the fear-induced startle response? (Choose one option.)

Theme: Learning Disability

Options:
  a. 1
  b. 2
  c. 5
  d. 10
  e. 30
  f. 40
  g. 50

h. 55
i. 66
j. 70
k. 80

Lead in: Choose one number to match each of the following statements. Each option may be used once, more than once or not at all.

Regarding patients with Down syndrome:

Question 141
What is the approximate highest prevalence of epilepsy commonly reported in studies? (Choose one option.)

Question 142
What is the prevalence of Alzheimer's disease at the age of 50–59 years? (Choose one option.)

Question 143
What is the prevalence of Alzheimer's disease at the age of 60–69 years? (Choose one option.)

Question 144
What is the percentage resulting from translocation of chromosome 21? (Choose one option.)

Question 145
What is the average life expectancy? (Choose one option.)

Question 146
What is the percentage with leukaemia? (Choose one option.)

Question 147
What is the percentage with hearing loss? (Choose one option.)

Question 148
What is the percentage with obsessive-compulsive disorder (OCD)? (Choose one option.)

Theme: Research Methods and Statistics
Options:
a. Correlation coefficient estimated by confirmatory factor analysis
b. Endogenous (latent) variable
c. Error variance
d. Exogenous (observed) variable

Lead in: Match one variable with Roman numerals in Figure 5.4 for each of the following statements. Each option may be used once, more than once or not at all.

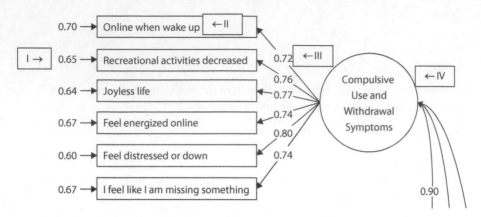

Figure 5.4 Standardized parameter estimates for the first-order four-factor confirmatory factor analysis of the Revised Chen Internet Addiction Scale (CIAS-R). (From Mak KK, Lai CM, Ko CH, Chou C, Kim DI, Watanabe H, Ho RC (2014). Psychometric properties of the Revised Chen Internet Addiction Scale (CIAS-R) in Chinese adolescents. *J Abnorm Child Psychol.*, 42(7): 1237–1245.)

Question 149
The name of variable indicated by I. (Choose one option.)

Question 150
The name of variable indicated by II. (Choose one option.)

Question 151
The name of variable indicated by III. (Choose one option.)

Question 152
The name of variable indicated by IV. (Choose one option.)

Theme: Psychiatry and Endocrine Disorders

Options:
  a. Hyperthyroidism
  b. Hypothyroidism
  c. Cushing syndrome
  d. Addison disease
  e. Syndrome of inappropriate antidiuretic hormone hyper-secretion
  f. Diabetes mellitus
  g. Diabetes insipidus
  h. Hyperparathyroidism
  i. Hypoparathyroidism

Lead in: Match one condition to each of the following statements. Each option may be used once, more than once or not at all.

Question 153
A 45-year-old woman is no longer able to meet the demands of her job and has been complaining of excessive tiredness, lethargy and constipation. She does not

have any medical history. Which one of the endocrine disorders might account for her symptoms? (Choose one option.)

Question 154
A 30-year-old woman is referred to your clinic. She has been complaining that she has been feeling quite anxious lately. She has frequent facial flushing and tachycardia. She has lost a significant amount of weight despite her having good appetite. Which one of the endocrine disorders might account for her symptoms? (Choose one option.)

Question 155
A 25-year-old woman has a long-standing history of irregular menses, along with weight gain. She has acne on her face, and she has been feeling depressed. At times, she has passive ideations of suicide. Which endocrine disorder might account for her symptoms? (Choose one option.)

Question 156
A 30-year-old woman presents to the emergency department with weakness, dizziness, anorexia, weight loss and gastrointestinal disturbances. On physical examination, generalized hyperpigmentation of the skin and the mucous membrane is noted. She also has postural hypotension and loss of pubic hair. Her family members have been reporting her having difficulties with her memory. Which endocrine disorder might account for her symptoms? (Choose one option.)

Question 157
A 60-year old woman has informed the psychiatrist that she has been feeling increasingly thirsty and needing to pass urine very often. She has been noted to have low urine osmolality and high plasma osmolality. Which endocrine disorder could she be having? (Choose one option.)

Theme: Learning Disability

Options:
a. 7
b. 10
c. 20
d. 35
e. 40
f. 70
g. 80
h. 90

Lead in: Choose one number to match each of the following statements. Each option may be used once, more than once or not at all.

What is the approximate percentage of the following?

Question 158
Children and young people with learning disability who have an additional diagnosable psychiatric disorder. (Choose one option.)

Question 159
Patients with learning disability developing dementia at the age of 65 years. (Choose one option.)

Question 160
Patients with epilepsy who have mild learning disability. (Choose one option.)

Question 161
Children with autism who have learning disability. (Choose one option.)

Theme: Side Effects of Anti-Dementia Medications

Options:
   a. Donepezil
   b. Rivastigmine
   c. Galantamine
   d. Memantine

Lead in: Match the medication with each of the following questions. Each option may be used once, more than once or not at all.

Question 162
Anti-dementia drugs can help with the stabilization of cognitive decline, improvement of ADL and the reduction of behavioural problems. In the event that the patient has asthma, which one of the anti-dementia drugs is contraindicated? (Choose one option.)

Question 163
The following side effects, as listed, are common for which of the above medications? Side effects include nausea, diarrhoea, dizziness, urinary incontinence, parasympathetic stimulation and a reduction in heart rate. (Choose three options.)

Theme: Sleep Disorders

Options:
   a. Insomnia
   b. Narcolepsy
   c. Obstructive sleep apnoea
   d. Central sleep apnoea
   e. Restless leg syndrome
   f. Somnambulism
   g. Sleep terrors

Lead in: Match one condition to each of the following statements. Each option may be used once, more than once or not at all.

Question 164
In this condition, the first symptom is always daytime sleepiness, and this usually occurs during adolescence. There is hypersomnia, sleep attacks and sleep paralysis. (Choose one option.)

Question 165
This is considered to be the most common breathing-related sleep disorder. (Choose one option.)

Question 166
This is a common sleep condition that is associated with autoimmune thyroid disorders, iron deficiency and diabetes mellitus. (Choose one option.)

Question 167
This is a sleep condition that is common in children and occurs on a frequent basis in 1%–4%. (Choose one option.)

Theme: Genetic Risk of Schizophrenia

a. 0%–4%
b. 5%–9%
c. 10%–14%
d. 15%–19%
e. 20%–24%
f. 25–29%
g. 30%–34%
h. 35%–50%
i. 60%–65%
j. 70%–75%
k. 80%–85%

Lead in: A 30-year-old man has suffered from schizophrenia for the past 5 years. He has recently gotten married. He and his wife are planning to have children. He is here for a consultation, as he is concerned about the genetic risks of schizophrenia.

Question 168
The risk of schizophrenia in his child if his wife also suffers from schizophrenia.

Question 169
The risk of schizophrenia in his child if his wife does not suffer from schizophrenia.

Question 170
The risk of schizophrenia if he adopted a child with DiGeorge syndrome.

Question 171
The risk of schizophrenia in his half-siblings.

Question 172
The risk of schizophrenia in his younger cousin.

Question 173
The risk of schizophrenia in his nephew or nieces.

Question 174

The risk of schizophrenia in his biological uncles or aunties.

Question 175

The percentage of people with schizophrenia who do not continue with antipsychotic after 1 year.

Question 176

The percentage of people with schizophrenia who smoke.

Theme: Statistical Tests

a. One-way analysis of variance (ANOVA)
b. Two-way ANOVA
c. Chi-squared test
d. Kruskal–Wallis
e. Mann–Whitney U test
f. McNemar test
g. Paired *t*-test
h. Wilcoxon rank sum test
i. Median and range

Lead in: Select the above statistical tests to the following scenarios. Each option might be used once, more than once or not at all.

Question 177

A study was conducted to analyse the effects of antidepressants on immunological functions. 30 female depressed patients were treated with SSRI and placebo for 6 weeks using a crossover design and a washout period in between. Cytokine levels were measured during treatment with SSRI and placebo according to the protocol. (Choose one option.)

Question 178

Five years ago, a group of 60-year-old patients who were diagnosed to suffer from mild cognitive impairment (MCI) were recruited into a longitudinal study. Their homocysteine levels were measured at baseline and were found to be skewed. Now, this sample is assessed for the presence or absence of dementia. The homocysteine levels are measured again and compared with levels 5 years ago. Which tests will be useful to test the hypothesis of changes in homocysteine levels in the presence or absence of dementia? (Choose one option.)

Question 179

Five years ago, a group of 60-year-old patients who were diagnosed to suffer from MCI and a group of age-matched controls without MCI were recruited into a longitudinal study. Their homocysteine levels were measured at baseline and were classified as low, medium and high levels. Now, this sample is assessed for the presence or absence of dementia. Which tests will be useful to test the hypothesis of (1) the baseline status MCI or normal controls and (2) the effect of baseline homocysteine levels on the presence or absence of dementia? (Choose two options.)

Question 180
A researcher wants to find out which types of antidepressants, tricyclicantidepressants (TCAs), SSRIs and serotonin–norepinephrine reuptake inhibitors (SNRIs), lead to a better quality of life in depressed patients. The health-related quality of life is measured by Short Form Health Survey 36 (SF-36), and the scores of three groups are compared. It was assumed that SF-36 follows normal distribution. (Choose one option.)

Question 181
In a postgraduate psychiatric clinical examination, which follows the close marking system (i.e. candidates usually score the marks between 4 and 7, 4 = fail, 5 = pass and 7 = distinction); the chief examiner wants to compare the median examination score among local, immigrant and refugee doctors. (Choose one option.)

Question 182
A study was conducted to test for a difference in income for patients with schizophrenia and aged-matched normal controls. The researchers also need to decide the best way to summarize income in the two groups. (Choose two options.)

Theme: Substance Misuse in Forensics
  a. 10%
  b. 20%
  c. 25%
  d. 40%
  e. 50%
  f. 60%

Lead in: Select the appropriate option for each of the following questions.

Question 183
The lifetime prevalence of substance misuse of dependence in people with schizophrenia.

Question 184
The lifetime prevalence of substance misuse or dependence in people with bipolar affective disorder.

Question 185
The lifetime prevalence of substance misuse or dependence in people with bipolar affective disorder.

Question 186
The percentage of male prisoners on remand who have moderate drug dependence.

Question 187
The percentage of male prisoners on remand who have severe drug dependence.

Question 188
The percentage of psychiatric patients who have committed homicide with a history of substance misuse.

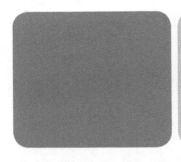

MRCPYSCH PAPER B MOCK EXAMINATION 3: ANSWERS

GET THROUGH MRCPSYCH PAPER B MOCK EXAMINATION

Question 1 Answer: d, Hypophosphataemia
Explanation: Lyme disease is caused by spirochaete *Borrelia burgdorferi* that is transmitted by *Ixodes* ticks. It has three stages: stage 1, rash; stage 2, early neurological signs, including lymphocytic meningitis, radicular pains, facial palsy, transverse myelitis and cranial and peripheral neuropathies; stage 3 (occurs 7 years after the initial diagnosis), late neurological signs, including Bell's palsy, dementia, encephalomyelitis, hemianopsia, hemiplegia, radiculo-neuropathy and seizures. Other typical symptoms of chronic Lyme encephalopathy include poor memory and concentration, fatigue, daytime hypersomnolence, irritability and depression.

References: Levenson JL (2004). *The American Psychiatric Publishing Textbook of Psychosomatic Medicine*. Arlington, VA: American Psychiatric Publishing, p. 583; Puri BK, Hall AD, Ho RC (2014). *Revision Notes in Psychiatry*. Boca Raton, FL: CRC Press, pp. 502–503.

Question 2 Answer: c, 0.05%
Explanation: The incidence has been estimated to be between 0.05% and 0.1% after maternal exposure to lithium the first trimester.

Reference: Puri BK, Hall AD, Ho RC (2014). *Revision Notes in Psychiatry*. Boca Raton, FL: CRC Press, p. 561.

Question 3 Answer: e, 1 in 200
Explanation: The incidence of foetal birth defect (mainly neural tube defect) has been estimated to be around 1 in 100.

Reference: Puri BK, Hall AD, Ho RC (2014). *Revision Notes in Psychiatry*. Boca Raton, FL: CRC Press, p. 561.

Question 4 Answer: b, Chromosomal 2q
Explanation: The heritability of the disorder has been found to be over 90%. The recurrence rate in siblings is roughly 3% for narrowly defined autism but is around

10%–20% for milder variants. The loci may involve chromosomes 2q and 7q. Family history of schizophrenia-like psychosis or affective disorder has been implicated as well.

Reference: Puri BK, Hall AD, Ho RC (2014). *Revision Notes in Psychiatry*. Boca Raton, FL: CRC Press, p. 623.

Question 5 Answer: e, Psychomotor retardation
Explanation: The mean duration of a depressive episode in children is around 7–9 months. The symptoms are similar to that of adults with a minimum of 2 weeks period of sadness, irritability, loss of interest and loss of pleasure. There is usually also impairment in social and role functions. Anxiety symptoms and conduct disorders are commonly associated disorders. It should be noted that children tend to have lesser psychomotor retardation in comparison with adults.

Reference: Puri BK, Hall AD, Ho RC (2014). *Revision Notes in Psychiatry*. Boca Raton, FL: CRC Press, p. 648.

Question 6 Answer: d, Transference-focused therapy
Explanation: In transference-focused therapy, it aims at correcting distorted perceptions of significant others and decreasing symptoms and self-destructive behaviours.

Reference: Puri BK, Hall AD, Ho RC (2014). *Revision Notes in Psychiatry*. Boca Raton, FL: CRC Press, p. 446.

Question 7 Answer: d, Group-based therapy
Explanation: Supportive therapy and problem-solving therapy are indicated for her. Cognitive-behavioural therapy (CBT) is also helpful for her condition. Cognitive therapy would help to target at the core beliefs, such as how others are malicious and deceptive. In behaviour therapy, the patient is involved in role play to handle hostility and personal attacks in their daily life. A course of antidepressant is likely also to be helpful for her.

Reference: Puri BK, Hall AD, Ho RC (2014). *Revision Notes in Psychiatry*. Boca Raton, FL: CRC Press, p. 443.

Question 8 Answer: b, Presence of a pacemaker
Explanation: Studies have demonstrated that, with proper pre-electroconvulsive therapy (ECT) cardiac and pacemaker/defibrillator assessment, ECT can be safely and effectively administered to patients with an implanted cardiac device.

Reference: Dolenc TJ et al. (2004). Electroconvulsive therapy in patients with cardiac pacemakers and implantable cardioverter defibrillators. *Pacing Clin Electrophysiol*, 27(9): 1257–1263.

Question 9 Answer: e, Drug treatment was associated with a reduction in the rate of delinquency and substance abuse in children with attention-deficit hyperactivity disorder (ADHD) to the rate found in normal controls
Explanation: The Multimodal Treatment Study (MTA) study shows that children with ADHD continue to show higher than normal rates of delinquency (four times) and substance use (two times). In the MTA study, 485 children took part in the 3-year follow-up study. Their mean age was 12 years. The primary outcome measures were ADHD and oppositional defiant disorder symptoms, reading scores, social skills, level of impairment and diagnosis. At the end of the first year, the research protocol was dropped, allowing for more naturalistic and personalized treatment.

Reference: Bates G (2009). Drug treatments for attention-deficit hyperactivity disorder in young people. *Adv Psych Treat*, 15: 162–171.

Question 10 Answer: b, 1:8
Explanation: This is a condition that affects 2%–5% of all women, mostly between the age of 20 and 45 years, with a female-to-male ratio of 5:1.

Reference: Puri BK, Treasaden I (eds) (2010). *Psychiatry: An Evidence-Based Text*. London: Hodder Arnold, pp. 576–577, 1081.

Question 11 Answer: d, Decreased episodes of rapid eye movement (REM) sleep
Explanation: Sleep parameters that increase amongst old people include sleep latency, frequency of awakenings at night, episodes and fragmentation of REM sleep. Sleep parameters that decrease amongst old people include duration of slow-wave sleep, sleep efficiency and total sleep time.

Reference: Puri BK, Hall AD, Ho RC (2014). *Revision Notes in Psychiatry*. Boca Raton, FL: CRC Press, p. 679.

Question 12 Answer: d, Decreased complexity of dreams
Explanation: Non-REM sleep occurs when there is reduced neuronal activity. Features of non-REM sleep include decreased complexity of dreams, increased parasympathetic activity, abolition of tendon reflexes, decreased heart rate, decreased systolic blood pressure, decreased respiratory rate, decreased cerebral blood flow and, usually, no penile erection. The following stages normally occur: stage 0, quiet wakefulness and shut eyes (electroencephalogram (EEG: alpha activity); stage 1, falling asleep (EEG: low amplitude, decreased alpha activity, low-voltage theta activity); stage 2, light sleep (EEG: 2–7 Hz, occasional sleep spindles and K complexes); stage 3, deep sleep (EEG: increased delta activity in 20%–50%) and stage 4, deep sleep (EEG: further increase in delta activity at more than 50%).

Reference: Puri BK, Hall AD, Ho RC (2014). *Revision Notes in Psychiatry*. Boca Raton, FL: CRC Press, p. 216.

Question 13 Answer: c, Hypothyroidism causes hirsutism
Explanation: Hypothyroidism is associated with hair loss.

Further Reading: Puri BK, Treasaden I (eds) (2010). *Psychiatry: An Evidence-Based Text*. London: Hodder Arnold, pp. 576–577, 1081.

Question 14 Answer: d, Frontal temporal dementia
Explanation: The typical examples of cortical dementia include Alzheimer dementia, frontal-lobe dementia and Creutzfeldt–Jakob disease (CJD). The typical examples of subcortical dementia include human immunodeficiency virus (HIV)–related dementia, Huntington chorea and Parkinson disease. Examples of mixed cortical and subcortical dementia include vascular dementia, dementia with Lewy bodies and neuropsychiatric conditions following carbon monoxide poisoning.

Reference: Puri BK, Hall AD, Ho RC (2014). *Revision Notes in Psychiatry*. Boca Raton, FL: CRC Press, p. 693.

Question 15 Answer: d, Prefrontal cortex
Explanation: People with schizophrenia performing the Wisconsin Card Sorting Test (WCST, which normally activates the frontal lobe) have been shown to have decreased blood flow in the frontal cortex during the WCST. Hypofrontality is associated with the presence of negative symptoms of schizophrenia. Cognitive impairment is common amongst patients with schizophrenia. Cognitive deficits include reduction in learning potential, poor semantic memory, impaired spatial delayed response, impaired visually oriented working memory, impaired source monitoring, executive dysfunction, social deficits, poor selective and sustained memory and reduced pre-pulse inhibition. Lesions in the dorsolateral frontal cortex lead to difficulties in delayed response requiring memory for spatial location.

Reference: Puri BK, Hall AD, Ho RC (2014). *Revision Notes in Psychiatry*. Boca Raton, FL: CRC Press, p. 363.

Question 16 Answer: c, It is a measure of the variability of the observations
Explanation: The standard error of the mean (SEM) is the standard deviation (SD) of the sample mean's estimate of a population mean. It describes the uncertainty of how the sample mean represents the population mean. The SD, however, describes the variability between individuals in a sample. As the SEM is always less than the SD, it misleads the reader into underestimating the variability between individuals within the study sample.

Reference: Nagele P (2003). Misuse of standard error of the mean (SEM) when reporting variability of a sample. A critical evaluation of four anaesthesia journals. *Br J Anaesth*, 90(4): 514–516.

Question 17 Answer: a, Independent sample *t*-test
Explanation: The independent sample *t*-test is used to test two groups using matched samples. It assumes that the differences between pairs are normally distributed.

The null hypothesis is that there is no difference between paired observations. It is commonly used in case–control trials and matched-pair randomized controlled trials.

Reference: Everitt BS (2006). *Medical Statistics from A to Z* (2nd edition). Cambridge, UK: Cambridge University Press, pp. 225–226.

Question 18 Answer: c, 26 participants

Explanation: In this trial, there are patients who lost to follow-up or discontinued from the trial. Intention to treat (ITT) analysis includes all the patients who were involved in the initial randomisation during the final analysis. Those who were lost to follow-up or discontinued from the trial are either considered as treatment failures or as last observation carried forwards and being included in the final analysis. As a result, 26 participants who consented and randomized were included in the final analysis. If those who were lost to follow-up or discontinued were excluded from the analysis, the results may overestimate the effect of treatment.

Question 19 Answer: c, 0.47

Explanation:

	Depressed subjects	Not depressed subjects	Total number of subjects
Intervention group	28 (A)	31 (B)	59
Control group	36 (C)	21 (D)	57

The rate of depressed subjects with intervention = A/(A + B) = 28/59 = 0.47. This is also known as experimental event rate (EER).

Question 20 Answer: d, 0.63

Explanation:

	Depressed subjects	Not depressed subjects	Total number of subjects
Intervention group	28 (A)	31 (B)	59
Control group	36 (C)	21 (D)	57

The rate of depressed subjects with control = C/(C + D) = 36/57 = 0.63 This is known as control event rate (CER).

Question 21 Answer: a, 0.16

Explanation: Absolute benefit increase = EER – CER = 0.63 – 0.47 = 0.16.

Question 22 Answer: b, 1.34

Explanation: Relative risk of remaining depressed = EER/CER = 0.63/0.47 = 1.34.

Question 23 Answer: a, 0.34
Explanation: Relative benefit increase = (EER – CER)/CER = (0.63 – 0.47)/0.47 = 0.34.

Question 24 Answer: a, Six patients
Explanation: Number needed to treat (NNT) = 1/absolute risk reduction (ARR) = 1/|CER – EER| = 1/0.16 = 6.25 = 6 patients.

Question 25 Answer: c, 2.86–25
Explanation: Lower limit of the confidence interval (CI) of NNT = 1/higher limit of CI of ARR = 1/0.35 = 2.86.
   Upper limit of the CI of NNT = 1/lower limit of CI of ARR = 1/0.04 = 25.

Question 26 Answer: c, Hyper-reflexia
Explanation: Inhalant intoxication leads to depressed reflexes (hyporeflexia) instead of hyper-reflexia. This is due to the inhalants acting as central nervous system depressant. Other signs of intoxication include giddiness, poor coordination, unsteady gait, nystagmus, diplopia, lethargy, tremors, generalized muscle weakness, euphoria, psychomotor slowing and stupor or coma.
   A recent research studying the adverse consequences of acute inhalant intoxication amongst youths has reported that high-frequency inhalant users were significantly more likely than moderate and low frequency users to experience adverse consequences. Certain risky behaviours, such as engaging in unprotected sex or acts of physical violence while high on inhalants, were dramatically more common amongst high-frequency users compared with low-frequency users.

References: Sadock BJ, Sadock VA (2003). *Kaplan and Sadock's Synopsis of Psychiatry* (9th edition). Philadelphia, PA: Lippincott, Williams & Wilkins, pp. 441–442; Garland EL, Howard MO (2014). Adverse consequences of acute inhalant intoxication. *Exp Clin Psychopharmacol*, 19(2): 134–144.

Question 27 Answer: d, Pramipexole
Explanation: Pathological gambling has been found to be a rare potential complication related to the treatment of Parkinson disease. Based on a study by Dodd et al. (2005), it was found that dopamine agonist therapy was associated with potentially reversible pathological gambling. Pramipexole was predominantly the medication found to be implicated in this. This might be related to disproportionate stimulation of dopamine D3 receptors, which are mainly localized to the limbic system.

Reference: Dodd ML, Klos KJ, et al. (2005). Pathological gambling caused by drugs used to treat Parkinson disease. *Arch Neurol*, 62: 1377–1381.

Question 28 Answer: e, Threat and fraud
Explanation: The male-to-female ratio for recorded crime is 10:1, and the age distribution of female offenders is similar to that of males due to secondary peak of middle-aged shoplifters. Options A–D are predominantly male offences.

Predominantly male offences include breaking and entering, sex offenses of any kind, non-sexual aggression to person, grievous bodily harm, larceny and motoring offences. Women are responsible for over one-third of all homicides in which the offender has a psychiatric disorder. Women predominate amongst depressive homicides, and the commonest victim is their child. Child stealing is exclusively committed by females. There are three types: (1) Comforting offence is usually committed by a young woman who has a need to look after a young child. She is more likely to take a child whom she has already known and often has a history of personality disorder and delinquency. (2) Manipulative offence is usually committed by a woman to maintain a relationship by claiming the baby to replace the one lost by miscarriage. (3) Impulsive psychotic offence is usually committed by a woman during the acute relapse of a psychotic illness.

Reference: Chiswick, D, Cope R (1995). *Seminars in Forensic Psychiatry*. London: Gaskell.

Question 29 Answer: a, Antisocial orientation
Explanation: A meta-analysis of 82 recidivism studies identified antisocial orientation and deviant sexual preferences as the major predictors of sexual recidivism for sexual offenders. The other options listed have little or no relationship with sexual recidivism. Standardized measures of risk in sexual reoffending tend to concentrate on a small number of variables, such as psychopathy, non-sexual offending, victims unknown to the offender, paraphilias, male victims and inability to form stable relationships.

References: Hanson RK, Morton-Bourgon KE (2005). The characteristics of persistent sexual offenders: A meta-analysis of recidivism studies. *J Consult Clin Psychol*, 73: 1154–1163; Puri BK, Treasaden I (eds) (2010). *Psychiatry: An Evidence Based Text*. London: Hodder Arnold, pp. 767–9, 772, 773, 1242.

Question 30 Answer: e, Progression of adult-onset cases tends to be much faster than childhood-onset cases
Explanation: In adult-onset cases, the progression tends to be much slower than in childhood onset cases, and it may be compatible with a normal lifespan. Those with early-onset cases, especially those with severe epilepsy, rarely survive for more than 15 years, succumbing to status epilepticus or cardiac or renal complications.

Reference: Moore DP, Puri BK (2012). *Textbook of Clinical Neuropsychiatry and Behavioral Neuroscience* (3rd edition). London: Hodder Arnold, pp. 456–457.

Question 31 Answer: c, It is associated with behavioural problems similar to those of ADHD, but hyperactivity is more prominent than distractibility and inattentiveness
Explanation: Foetal alcohol syndrome is clearly related to maternal alcohol ingestion, but it is not clear whether it is the first or later trimesters that constitute the greatest period of risk. It is also unclear whether it is the total amount of alcohol consumed that is important or whether relative brief exposures to high levels are

more toxic. A profile similar to ADHD is common. However, distractibility and inattentiveness are more prominent than hyperactivity. There is often some resolution of the dysmorphic features by adulthood, but other symptoms tend to persist.

Reference: Moore DP, Puri BK (2012). *Textbook of Clinical Neuropsychiatry and Behavioral Neuroscience* (3rd edition). London: Hodder Arnold. p. 466.

Question 32 Answer: e, Prader–Willi syndrome
Explanation: Prader–Willi syndrome is characterized by extreme hyperphagia, obesity, mild mental retardation and various dysmorphic features. Patients may have behavioural problems that include skin pricking, ritualized behaviour and temper tantrums. Hypogonadism is present, presenting in males as micropenis and cryptorchidism.

Reference: Moore DP, Puri BK (2012). *Textbook of Clinical Neuropsychiatry and Behavioral Neuroscience* (3rd edition). London: Hodder Arnold, p. 465.

Question 33 Answer: a, Regaining insight
Explanation: About 10% of patients with schizophrenia commit suicide, and for most, it happens early in their illness. Risk factors for suicide are being male, young, unemployed; having chronic illness with relapses and remissions; having high educational attainment before onset of the illness; having akathisia; abruptly stopping medication and recent discharge from inpatient care.

Reference: Puri BK, Hall AD, Ho RC (2014). *Revision Notes in Psychiatry*. Boca Raton, FL: CRC Press, p. 371.

Question 34 Answer: d, 40%
Explanation: 40% of young people with conduct disorder develop dissocial personality disorder in adulthood. Borderline intelligence quotient (IQ), mental retardation and family history of dissocial personality disorder are predictive factors.

Reference: Puri BK, Hall AD, Ho RC (2014). *Revision Notes in Psychiatry*. Boca Raton, FL: CRC Press, p. 635.

Question 35 Answer: c, Huntington disease
Explanation: Huntington disease is a dominantly inherited, neurodegenerative disorder due to expansion of a polymorphic tri-nucleotide repeat in the short arm of chromosome 4. Clinical manifestations consist of a triad of choeric movements, cognitive decline and psychiatric syndromes starting in the fourth to the fifth decade. Psychiatric manifestations vary and may precede motor and cognitive changes. Personality changes and depression occur more commonly. Paranoid schizophrenia-like symptoms occur in 6%–25% of cases.

Reference: Correa BB et al. (2006). Association of Huntington's disease and schizophrenia-like psychosis in a Hungtinton's disease pedigree. *Clin Pract Epidemiol Ment Health*, 15(2): 1.

Question 36 Answer: b, Immediate verbal memory
Explanation: Meta-analysis has found that neurocognitive deficits are maximal in immediate verbal memory and processing speed in people suffering from the first episode of schizophrenia.

Reference: Mesholam-Gately RI, Giuliano AJ, Goff KP et al. (2009). Neurocognition in first-episode schizophrenia: A meta-analytic review. *Neuropsychology*, 23(3): 315–336.

Question 37 Answer: c, Dopamine agonist
Explanation: Nicotine is believed to produce its positive reinforcing and addictive effects by activating the dopaminergic pathway projecting from the ventral tegmental area to the cerebral cortex and the limbic system. In addition to activating this dopamine reward system, nicotine causes an increase in the concentration of circulating noradrenaline and adrenaline and an increase in the release of vasopressin, beta-endorphin, adrenocorticotropic hormone and cortisol. These hormones are thought to contribute to the basic stimulatory effects of nicotine on the central nervous system.

Reference: Sadock BJ, Sadock VA (2003). *Kaplan and Sadock's Synopsis of Psychiatry* (9th edition). Philadelphia, PA: Lippincott, Williams & Wilkins, p. 445.

Question 38 Answer: c, Psychoeducation
Explanation: Psychoeducation (refers to the education provided to patients and families with mental health problems regarding illness and treatment) is not a general principle of motivational interviewing. Express empathy involves seeing the world through the patient's eyes and sharing in his or her experiences. When patients feel that they are understood, they are able to be more open about their experiences and share them with others. To support self-efficacy, a patient's belief that change is possible is an important motivator in making a change. As patients are responsible for choosing and acting on their actions to change, supporting their sense of self-efficacy is important to help them stay motivated. In roll with resistance, the counsellor does not fight resistance of the patient but 'rolls with it' instead. The counsellor uses the patient's momentum and further explores the patient's views. Using this approach, resistance tends to be decreased. To develop discrepancy, the motivation to change occurs when people perceive the discrepancy between where they are and where they want to be. The counsellor aims to achieve this through helping patients examine the discrepancies between their current behaviour and future goals.

Reference: Miller WR, Zweben A, DiClemente CC, Rychtarik RG (1992). *Motivational Enhancement Therapy Manual: A Clinical Research Guide for Therapists Treating Individuals with Alcohol Abuse and Dependence*. Rockville, MD: National Institute on Alcohol Abuse and Alcoholism, pp. 13–35.

Question 39 Answer: b, 10%
Explanation: Medium-secure units were set up for people whose severely disruptive or dangerous behaviour required psychiatric treatment in conditions of medium

security. The majority of inmates have severe mental illness, mostly schizophrenia. A national cohort study conducted in England and Wales concluded that women were less likely than men to be reconvicted within 2 years of discharge with reoffending rates within 2 years at 9% and 16%, respectively. The Sainsbury Centre for Mental Health found that 7% reoffended within 2 years of discharge.

References: Maden A, Skapinakis P, Lweis G et al. (2006). Gender differences in reoffending after discharge from medium-secure units. National cohort study in England and Wales. *Br J Psychiatry*, 189: 168–172; Puri BK, Treasaden I (eds) (2010). *Psychiatry: An Evidence-Based Text*. London: Hodder Arnold, pp. 1154, 1157; Rutherford M, Duggan S (2008). Forensic mental health services: facts and figures on current provision. *Br J Forensic Pract*, 10: 4–10.

Question 40 Answer: d, 10%
Explanation: The National Confidential Inquiry into Suicide and Homicide by People with Mental Illness was conducted in England and Wales during the years 1996–1999. Of the 1594 convicted of homicide, 10% had symptoms of mental illness at the time of the offence, 34% had a mental illness (lifetime) and 5% had schizophrenia (lifetime); 9% received a diminished responsibility verdict and 7% received a hospital disposal – both were associated with severe mental illness and symptoms of psychosis.

References: Puri BK, Treasaden I (eds) (2010). *Psychiatry: An Evidence-Based Text*. London: Hodder Arnold, pp. 1162–1163, 1173, 1176–1177; Shaw J, Hunt IM, Flynn S et al. (2006). Rates of mental disorder in people convicted of homicide. National clinical survey. *Br J Psychiatry*, 188: 143–147.

Question 41 Answer: b, If the mother is found to be a carrier, the recurrence risk is 50%
Explanation: The recurrence risk is 10%–15%. With regard to Down syndrome, 94% of cases are caused by meiotic nondisjunction of trisomy 21 (47 chromosomes). Five percent of cases are caused by translocation that refers to a fusion between chromosomes 21 and 44 (46 chromosomes). One percent of cases are caused by mosaicism that refers to non-disjunction occurring after fertilisation in any cell division. Robertsonian translocations are caused by the fusion of chromosomes 14 and 21. The extra chromosome is usually of maternal origin (90%), and most maternal errors occur during the first meiotic division. The risk of recurrence of translocation is around 10%.

Reference: Puri BK, Hall AD, Ho RC (2014). *Revision Notes in Psychiatry*. Boca Raton, FL: CRC Press, p. 661.

Question 42 Answer: c, Vascular dementia
Explanation: The scoring is important as it helps to distinguish between vascular dementia and dementia of Alzheimer type. A score more than 7 is indicative of vascular dementia, whereas a score less than 4 is indicative of Alzheimer type. The

following aspects are being scored: course of the illness, symptoms, history and focal neurological symptoms and focal neurological signs.

Reference: Puri BK, Hall AD, Ho RC (2014). *Revision Notes in Psychiatry*. Boca Raton, FL: CRC Press, p. 700.

Question 43 Answer: e, 80%

Explanation: Lewy body dementia (LBD) is the third most common cause of late-onset dementia and less common cause of early onset dementia. It frequently occurs in combination with Alzheimer dementia. It more commonly affects men than women. Apart from the presence of cognitive symptoms, there is also the presence of non-cognitive symptoms. Common non-cognitive symptoms include apathy, depression and hallucinations (complex visual hallucinations are present in 80% of individuals and auditory hallucinations in 20%), and 65% of individuals also have delusions.

Reference: Puri BK, Hall AD, Ho RC (2014). *Revision Notes in Psychiatry*. Boca Raton, FL: CRC Press, p. 702.

Question 44 Answer: b, Connectivity-based clustering

Explanation: The above study explores the risk factors for single and repeated suicide attempters. Cluster 1 represents single suicide attempters, and cluster 2 represents repeated suicide attempters. The authors used the connectivity-based clustering algorithms to connect objects (e.g. borderline personality disorder, hallucination, multiple admissions) being more related to form a cluster. Centroid-based clustering is represented by a central vector, but no vector is mentioned in the analysis. This study does not report distribution and density of objects. As a result, density-based and distribution-based clustering are not relevant for this study.

Question 45 Answer: e, 1 – Specificity

Explanation: Figure 5.3 is a receiver operating characteristic (ROC) curve, which is a plot of sensitivity versus (1 – specificity). The name derives from its original use in radar technology. We found that higher damage accrual, higher cumulative glucocorticoid dose, more severe depression and fewer regular medications were predictive of the presence of anxiety in patients with lupus. By ROC analysis, this model was 90% accurate in predicting the presence of anxiety in patients with lupus, with the area under curve of sensitivity versus 1-sensitivity plot.

Reference: Mak A, Tang CS, Chan MF, Cheak AA, Ho RC (2011). Damage accrual, cumulative glucocorticoid dose and depression predict anxiety in patients with systemic lupus erythematosus. *Clin Rheumatol*, 30(6): 795–803.

Question 46 Answer: d, 8.4

Explanation: Positive likelihood ratio (LR+) = sensitivity/(1 – specificity) = 0.42/(1 – 0.95) = 0.42/0.05 = 8.4. LR+ indicates the odds of increasing the risk of having a disease when a test is positive. As the LR+ is far away from 1, there is strong evidence for the presence of disease if a participant scores higher than 40 points on this scale.

Question 47 Answer: a, The null hypothesis is wrongly rejected
Explanation: The null hypothesis is wrongly rejected in type I error. For type II error, the null hypothesis is not rejected when it should have been. Type II error is less serious than type I error because it represent false-negative but not false-positive results.

Question 48 Answer: e, Busprione
Explanation: Thus far, no medications have been shown broadly and consistently effective, and none have been approved thus far by any of the regulatory bodies. Medications that have been studied include those that help alleviate symptoms of cannabis withdrawal, those that directly affect endogenous cannabinoid receptor function and those that have shown efficacy in treatment of other psychiatric conditions. Busprione is the only medication to date that has shown efficacy for cannabis dependence in a controlled clinical trial.

Reference: AM Weinstein et al. (2011). Pharmacological treatment of cannabis dependence. *Curr Pharm Des*, 17(4): 1351–1358.

Question 49 Answer: b, A 15-year-old has a lower rate of recidivism for sexual offence compared with a 30-year-old
Explanation: A review of 79 sexual offender treatment outcome studies showed that the overall sexual recidivism rate for adolescent sex offenders who receive treatment is low compared with adults. Research has shown that adolescent sex offenders are more responsive to treatment than adult sex offenders and have low rates of recidivism in adulthood when provided with appropriate treatment. Adolescent sex offenders' rates of recidivism range from 5% to 14%.

References: National Centre on Sexual Behaviour of Youth (2003). NCSBY Fact Sheet: What research shows about adolescent sex offenders. ncsby.org/What%20 Research%20Shows%20About%20Adolescent%20Sex%20Offenders%20060404. pdf; Puri BK, Treasaden I (eds) (2010). *Psychiatry: An Evidence-Based Text*. London: Hodder Arnold, pp. 769, 774 1156, 1183, 1184, 1197.

Question 50 Answer: a, Cephalosporin
Explanation: Risk factors of neuropsychiatric side effects from antibiotics have included prior psychopathology, coexisting medical conditions, slow acetylator status, advanced age, concomitant medications and increased permeability of the blood–brain barrier, as well as high antibiotic dosage and intrathecal or intravenous administration. Psychiatric toxicity may result from various mechanisms of action, including antagonism of gamma-aminobutyric acid or pyridoxine, adverse interactions with alcohol, or inhibition of protein synthesis. The psychiatric side effects of cephalosporins include euphoria, delusions, depersonalization and illusions. The side effects of clarithromycin include delirium and mania, whereas the side effects of gentamicin and trimethoprim-sulfamethoxazole include delirium and psychosis. The side effects of quinolones include psychosis, paranoia, mania, agitation and Tourette-like syndrome.

References: Levenson JL. *The American Psychiatric Publishing Textbook of Psychosomatic Medicine*. Arlington, VA: American Psychiatric Publishing, p. 592; Sternbach H, State R (1997). Antibiotics: Neuropsychiatric effects and psychotropic interactions. *Harv Rev Psychiatry*, 5(4): 214–226.

Question 51 Answer: e, Patients who are homozygous for MET/MET alleles in the catechol-*O*-methyltransferase (COMT) genotype have a twofold higher risk
Explanation: Research studies have shown that individuals with VAL/VAL alleles in the COMT genotype have higher risk, but those individuals with MET/MET alleles in the COMT genotype have no increase in risk. Cannabis might lead to the following symptoms: amotivational syndrome, flashback phenomena, changes in affect, changes in heart rate, red eyes, motor incoordination and memory problems.

Reference: Puri BK, Hall AD, Ho RC (2014). *Revision Notes in Psychiatry*. Boca Raton, FL: CRC Press, p. 361.

Question 52 Answer: a, Being male
Explanation: Approximately 25% of cases of schizophrenia show good clinical and social recovery. Factors associated with good prognosis include being female, being married, good premorbid social adjustment, family history of affective disorder, short duration of illness prior to treatment, no ventricular enlargement, abrupt or late onset of the illness.

Reference: Puri BK, Hall AD, Ho RC (2014). *Revision Notes in Psychiatry*. Boca Raton, FL: CRC Press, p. 370.

Question 53 Answer: e, Augmentation with physical therapies
Explanation: Option (e) is not part of the STAR*D trial. The level 2 treatment strategies include (1) switching to other antidepressants (sertraline, venlafaxine, buproprion) and cognitive therapy, (2) medication and psychotherapy augmentation, (3) antidepressant only switch, (4) antidepressant only augmentation, (5) psychotherapy only switch and (6) psychotherapy only augmentation.

Reference: Puri BK, Hall AD, Ho RC (2014). *Revision Notes in Psychiatry*. Boca Raton, FL: CRC Press, p. 392.

Question 54 Answer: c, Klinefelter syndrome
Explanation: Klinefelter syndrome occurs secondary to the presence of one or more extra X chromosomes. It is characterized by tall stature, hypogonadism and infertility. Some patients may come to clinical attention only during a workup for infertility or erectile dysfunction.

Reference: Moore DP, Puri BK (2012). *Textbook of Clinical Neuropsychiatry and Behavioral Neuroscience* (3rd edition). London: Hodder Arnold, p. 460.

Question 55 Answer: a, Elementary professionals
Explanation: A recent meta-analysis looked at a total of 34 studies. Elementary professionals were at elevated risk compared with the working-age population. This was followed by machine operators and deck crew and then agricultural workers.

Reference: Allison Milner et al. (2013). Suicide by occupation: systematic review and meta-analysis. *BJP*, 203: 409–416.

Question 56 Answer: a, Depressive disorder
Explanation: It is true that the outcome for bulimia nervosa improves with time and is better than anorexia nervosa. The majority of patients make a full recovery or suffer only moderate abnormalities in eating attitudes after 10 years. There is comorbidity with depression, with prominent anorectic features increasing the likelihood of a poor response. Depression in itself is a negative prognostic factor for the outcome for bulimia nervosa.

Reference: Puri BK, Hall AD, Ho RC (2014). *Revision Notes in Psychiatry*. Boca Raton, FL: CRC Press, p. 587.

Question 57 Answer: d, A value of 0.5–0.8 signifies strong correlation
Explanation: The correlation coefficient is an index that quantifies the linear relationship between a pair of variables. Various correlation coefficients are available, all taking values between –1 and 1, with the extreme values indicating a perfect linear relationship and the sign indicating the direction of the relationship. *r* (degree of correlation): 0–0.2 (negligible), 0.2–0.5 (weak), 0.5–0.8 (moderate) and 0.8–1.0 (strong).

Reference: Everitt BS (2006). *Medical Statistics from A to Z* (2nd edition). Cambridge, UK: Cambridge University Press, p. 60.

Question 58 Answer: a, It can lead to false negatives
Explanation: For type II errors, the null hypothesis was not rejected when it should have been, and the study does not detect an effect that existed in reality. The more the study restricts type I errors by setting a low level of alpha, the higher the chance that a type II error will occur. Type II errors are generally considered to be less serious than type I errors as they are only errors in the sense that the opportunity to reject the null hypothesis is lost.

Reference: Lewis GH, Sheringham J, Kalim K, Crayford T JB (2008). *Mastering Public Health: A Postgraduate Guide to Examination and Revalidation*. London: Royal Society of Medicine Press, pp. 87–88.

Question 59 Answer: a, Bonferroni correction can be used to keep type II errors at a low level
Explanation: Type I error is the error that results when the null hypothesis is rejected falsely. Type II error is the error that results when the null hypothesis is

accepted falsely. There is a trade-off between type I and type II errors: the more the study restricts type I errors by setting a low level of alpha, the greater the chance that a type II error will occur. As more and more tests are performed on the data set, the likelihood of a type I error increases; that is, the chance of falsely concluding that an association is significant. To compensate for multiple comparisons, Bonferroni correction is used. It helps to keep type I error at a low level.

References: Everitt BS (2006). *Medical Statistics from A to Z* (2nd edition). Cambridge, UK: Cambridge University Press, p. 238; Lewis GH, Sheringham J, Kalim K, Crayford T JB (2008). *Mastering Public Health: A Postgraduate Guide to Examination and Revalidation*. London: Royal Society of Medicine Press, pp. 87–88.

Question 60 Answer: d, 40%
Explanation: Between 40% and 60% of patients with schizophrenia are non-concordant with oral medications. Possible reasons will include the following: limited insight, limited beneficial effect, unpleasant side effects, pressure from family and friends and poor therapeutic engagement with their medical team.

Reference: Puri BK, Hall AD, Ho RC (2014). *Revision Notes in Psychiatry*. Boca Raton, FL: CRC Press, p. 365.

Question 61 Answer: b, Exhibitionism is commonly associated with exposure of the genitalia to an unsuspecting stranger of the opposite gender
Explanation: Exhibitionism describes the continual or repetitive desire to expose one's genitals to strangers, usually of the opposite sex, without seeking or desiring any further contact.

Reference: Puri BK, Treasaden I (eds) (2010). *Psychiatry: An Evidence-Based Text*. London: Hodder Arnold, pp. 749, 762, 766–767.

Question 62 Answer: e, Monoamine oxidase inhibitor (MAOI)
Explanation: Selective serotonin re-uptake inhibitors (SSRIs) are usually the first-line treatments for phobic anxiety disorder. MAOIs are effective for patients with social phobia and agoraphobia. Of note, 80%–90% of pure social phobic are almost asymptomatic at week 16, based on a previous research.

Reference: Puri BK, Hall AD, Ho RC (2014). *Revision Notes in Psychiatry*. Boca Raton, FL: CRC Press, p. 407.

Question 63 Answer: e, Somatoform disorder
Explanation: Kleptomania is an impulse-control disorder characterized by repeated failure to resist the impulse to steal, in which tension is then relieved by stealing. The sex ratio of female to male is 4:1. Pure kleptomania is extremely rare. The treating psychiatrist should look out for other psychiatric disorders, such as depression, anxiety, bulimia nervosa, sexual dysfunction as well as fetishistic stealing.

Reference: Puri BK, Hall AD, Ho RC (2014). *Revision Notes in Psychiatry*. Boca Raton, FL: CRC Press, p. 724.

Question 64 Answer: b, Measurement bias
Explanation: Measurement bias results in errors that occur in instruments and inaccuracies or incompleteness of data collection, which affects the groups to differing degrees. There are three types of measurement bias: instrument bias, recall bias and observer bias. Blinding of participants avoids respondent bias, blinding of practitioners who are treating study participants avoids instrument bias and blinding of observer who collect measurements or analyse results avoids observer bias.

Reference: Lewis GH, Sheringham J, Kalim K, Crayford T JB (2008). *Mastering Public Health: A Postgraduate Guide to Examination and Revalidation*. London: Royal Society of Medicine Press, pp. 27–30.

Question 65 Answer: a, Mann–Whitney *U* test
Explanation: The data in this question are not paired data, so options C and E are incorrect as they are used for paired data. The Mann–Whitney *U* test is used for unpaired data from small samples taken from a non-normally distributed population, which is appropriate for this case. The McNemar test is used for matched analyses and only for actual numbers but not proportions or percentages. Spearman's correlation is a measure of the relationship between two variables that uses only the ranks of the observations on each.

Reference: Lewis GH, Sheringham J, Kalim K, Crayford T JB (2008). *Mastering Public Health: A Postgraduate Guide to Examination and Revalidation*. London: Royal Society of Medicine Press, pp. 88, 539.

Question 66 Answer: c, It may be an intermediate step along the causal chain
Explanation: Criteria for confounders are it must be associated with the disease and be independently associated with the exposure under study; it must predict disease independently of the exposure under study and it cannot simply be an intermediate step in the causal chain. It can be countered and controlled for at the design stage or it can be adjusted for at the analysis stage.

Reference: Lewis GH, Sheringham J, Kalim K, Crayford T JB (2008). *Mastering Public Health: A Postgraduate Guide to Examination and Revalidation*. London: Royal Society of Medicine Press, pp. 31–34.

Question 67 Answer: a, Patricia Forest published the first Forest plot in 1958
Explanation: There is a misunderstanding that Forest plot is named after a person. Lewis and Clark stated that the origin of Forest refers to the forest of lines produced in the Forest plot. Meta-analysis combines results or effect sizes from different studies and allows comparison of results from different categories by sensitivity analysis. The pooled effect size is dependent on the variability of source data, and such variability is known as heterogeneity. Researchers often perform meta-analysis alone without including meta-regression. It is best to be complemented by meta-regression to identify moderators that explain heterogeneity.

Reference: Lewis S, Clarke M (2001). Forest plots: Trying to see the wood and the trees. *BMJ*, 322(7300): 1479–1480.

Question 68 Answer: e, Heavy mental (lead) poisoning

Explanation: The core signs and symptoms of neuroleptic malignant syndrome (NMS) include muscle rigidity and fever, as well as altered consciousness, mutism, labile blood pressure, tachycardia, tremor, incontinence and leukocytosis. The differential diagnoses to be considered include central nervous system (CNS) infection, sepsis, serotonin syndrome, lethal catatonia, catatonia, myocardial infarction, heat stroke, malignant hyperthermia and thyroid storm. Heavy metals such as thallium and arsenic are possible differentials but not lead poisoning.

Reference: Hall RCW et al. (2006). Neuroleptic malignant syndrome in the elderly: Diagnostic criteria, incidence, risk factors, pathophysiology and treatment. *Clin Geriatrics*, 14: 39–46.

Question 69 Answer: a, It leads to an increase in serum Mg^{2+}

Explanation: It leads to reduction in Mg^{2+}. Some of the commonly associated neuropsychiatric symptoms include disturbance of mood and drive, delirium (caused by high calcium levels), cognitive impairment and psychosis (5%–20%). The correction of serum calcium usually results in a reversal of the psychiatric symptoms.

Reference: Puri BK, Hall AD, Ho RC (2014). *Revision Notes in Psychiatry*. Boca Raton, FL: CRC Press, p. 478.

Question 70 Question: e, To identify which independent variables are predictors of a dependent variable after adjustment of confounding factor

Explanation: In meta-analysis, meta-regression is mainly used to examine the impact of different variables on study effect size and to identify moderators that explain heterogeneity. Heterogeneity arises when combining results from different studies, and this can identify potential bias in selection of studies or research participants. Meta-regression is used in policy analysis by evaluating the evidence in cost–benefit analysis studies of a health policy across multiple studies. Option E refers to multivariate linear or logistic regression conducted in a single study. A lot of researchers and MRCPsych candidates believe that meta-regression serves the same purpose as multivariate linear or logistic regression, and this concept is incorrect.

Reference: Stanley TD, Jarrell SB (1989). Meta-regression analysis: A quantitative method of literature surveys. *J Econ Surv*, 19(3): 299–308.

Question 71 Answer: d, Comorbid language disorder

Explanation: ADHD symptoms still persist at the age of 30 years in one-quarter of ADHD children. Most of these patients with persistent ADHD symptoms do not require medication. As they age, the symptoms of hyperactivity usually improve. However, the inattention component is likely to persist. It should be noted that remission is usually considered to be unlikely before the age of 12 years. The predictors for the persistence of ADHD symptoms into adulthood include having a family history of ADHD, the presence of psychosocial adversity, the presence of comorbid conduct, depressive and/or anxiety disorder.

Reference: Puri BK, Hall AD, Ho RC (2014). *Revision Notes in Psychiatry*. Boca Raton, FL: CRC Press, p. 635.

Question 72 Answer: a, Autistic disorder
Explanation: The heritability of autistic disorder has been known to be over 90%. The recurrence rate in siblings is roughly 3% for narrowly defined autism but is about 10%–20% for milder variants. The loci usually involve chromosomes 2q and 7q.

Reference: Puri BK, Hall AD, Ho RC (2014). *Revision Notes in Psychiatry*. Boca Raton, FL: CRC Press, p. 623.

Question 73 Answer: d, 12 months
Explanation: In general, in the long term, the prognosis is good unless there are other disorders that are also present. Poor prognosis is associated with duration of the condition being longer than 12 months.

Reference: Puri BK, Hall AD, Ho RC (2014). *Revision Notes in Psychiatry*. Boca Raton, FL: CRC Press, p. 642.

Question 74 Answer: b, Increase in serotonin 5HT3 receptor sensitivity
Explanation: This is incorrect. All the above are related pathophysiology. Abnormalities in the basal ganglia and caudate nucleus have been implicated as well. The onset is usually before the age of 18 years. Tics are sudden, rapid and involuntary movements of circumscribed muscles without any purpose.

Reference: Puri BK, Hall AD, Ho RC (2014). *Revision Notes in Psychiatry*. Boca Raton, FL: CRC Press, p. 640.

Question 75 Answer: a, 2 years old
Explanation: Pica, based on the 10th revision of *International Classification of Diseases* (ICD-10) diagnostic criteria, refers to the persistent eating of non-nutritive substances at least twice per week for a total minimum duration of 1 month. The chronological and mental age of the child is usually above that of 2 years old. It is associated with other psychiatric disorders, such as learning disability, psychosis and social deprivation.

Reference: Puri BK, Hall AD, Ho RC (2014). *Revision Notes in Psychiatry*. Boca Raton, FL: CRC Press, p. 642.

Question 76 Answer: d, Mood reactivity
Explanation: Melancholia is also known as endogenous depression. It has the following symptoms: motor retardation or agitation, anorexia and weight loss, diurnal variation, excessive guilt, absence of mood reactivity, anhedonia, depression that is subjectively different from grief or loss and sleep characterized by

terminal insomnia (early morning waking). The causes of melancholic-type major depressive disorder are believed to be mostly due to biological factors. Sometimes life events and stressful situations can trigger episodes of melancholic depression, although these are not a necessary or sufficient cause. It has also been found that melancholic symptoms are common in people who suffer from bipolar I disorder and may often be present in people with bipolar II disorder. Psychotic symptoms are also more common in this disorder. It is more frequent in old age.

Reference: Puri BK, Hall AD, Ho RC (2014). *Revision Notes in Psychiatry*. Boca Raton, FL: CRC Press, p. 380.

Question 77 Answer: a, Supportive reassurance
Explanation: Postnatal blues is a brief psychological disturbance, characterized by tearfulness, emotional lability and confusion in mothers occurring in the first few days after childbirth. It typically occurs in around 50% of women. It is associated with tearfulness, irritability and anxiety. With regard to management, reassurance is recommended. No psychotropic medication is required, and the prognosis is usually quite good.

Reference: Puri BK, Hall AD, Ho RC (2014). *Revision Notes in Psychiatry*. Boca Raton, FL: CRC Press, p. 567.

Question 78 Answer: e, Male gender
Explanation: Tardive dyskinesia is a syndrome of potentially irreversible involuntary hyperkinetic dyskinesias that may occur during long-term treatment with antipsychotic medication. The most important hypotheses concerning the neurochemical pathology of tardive dyskinesia include dopamine hypersensitivity, free-radical-induced neurotoxicity and noradrenergic dysfunction. Risk factors for this include old age, diffuse brain injury, a long duration of antipsychotic treatment and affective psychosis. Tardive dyskinesia is more common in females.

Reference: Puri BK, Hall AD, Ho RC (2014). *Revision Notes in Psychiatry*. Boca Raton, FL: CRC Press, p. 201.

Question 79 Answer: a, Cluster analysis
Explanation: Cluster analysis is a set of methods for constructing sensible and informative classification of an initially unclassified set of data, using the variable values observed in each individual. It involves classifying data into groups (cluster) based on the variable values observed in each individual.

Reference: Everitt BS (2006). *Medical Statistics from A to Z* (2nd edition). Cambridge, UK: Cambridge University Press, p. 48.

Question 80 Answer: b, Berkson's bias
Explanation: Berkson's bias is also known as hospital admission bias. It is the artefactual association between a disease and a risk factor resulting from differential admission rates with respect to the suspected causal factor. Ascertainment bias arises from

a relationship between the exposure to a risk factor and the probability of detecting an event of interest. It occurs particularly in retrospective studies. Recall bias, occurring particularly in retrospective studies, is caused by differential recall amongst cases and controls in general by underreporting of exposure in the control group.

Reference: Everitt BS (2014). *Medical Statistics from A to Z* (2nd edition). Cambridge, UK: Cambridge University Press, pp. 13, 23, 195.

Question 81 Answer: c, Neyman bias
Explanation: Neyman bias occurs when studies based on prevalence produce different results compared with studies based on incidence of disease. In this case, there is a gap between exposure and selection of subjects. By recruiting subjects from the psychosis clinic, he would have missed out on those whose psychosis subsided shortly after taking cannabis, without being referred to the clinic. The gap would reduce the odds ratio of cannabis misuse and psychosis.

Reference: Lewis GH, Sheringham J, Kalim K, Crayford T JB (2008). *Mastering Public Health: A Postgraduate Guide to Examination and Revalidation*. London: Royal Society of Medicine Press, pp. 29–32.

Question 82 Answer: a, Caesarean section
Explanation: Pregnant women with active eating disorders have a greater chance for delivery by caesarean section, and they may develop postpartum depression.

Reference: Franko DL, Blais MA, Becker AE, Delinsky SS, Greenwood DN, Flores AT, Ekeblad ER, Eddy KT, Herzog DB (2001). Pregnancy complications and neonatal outcomes in women with eating disorders. *Am J Psychiatry*, 158: 1461–1466.

Question 83 Answer: e, 6 years old
Explanation: Often, the child has unrealistic persistent worry about possible harm befalling the attachment figures or about the loss of the attachment figures. The child has anticipatory anxiety of separation, such as tantrums, persistent reluctance to leave home, excessive need to talk with parents and desire to return home when going out.

Reference: Puri BK, Hall AD, Ho RC (2014). *Revision Notes in Psychiatry*, Boca Raton, FL: CRC Press, p. 652.

Question 84 Answer: a, Very low birth weight and perinatal insult are risk factors for ADHD
Explanation:
b is incorrect as its half-life is approximately 5 hours.
c is incorrect as atomoxetine is a first-line treatment in patients with ADHD with tics.
d is incorrect as there is no evidence for the use of second-generation antipsychotics to treat hyperactivity, although risperidone may be useful in the treatment of aggression in ADHD in learning disability patients.
e is incorrect. Hyperactivity is often a manifestation of epilepsy.

References: Baker P (2004). *Basic Child Psychiatry* (7th edition). London: Blackwell; Taylor D, Paton C, Kapur S (2009). *The Maudsley Prescribing Guidelines* (10th edition). London: Informa Healthcare.

Question 85 Answer: c, CJD
Explanation: The EEG has been noted to be always abnormal in CJD, showing an increase in slow-wave activity and a reduction in rhythm. With the progression of the disease, there may be bilateral slow spike wave discharges, which may accompany myoclonic jerks.

Reference: Puri BK, Hall AD, Ho RC (2014). *Revision Notes in Psychiatry*. Boca Raton, FL: CRC Press, p. 705.

Question 86 Answer: e, 12 years
Explanation: This is a condition that is genetic in nature and that is characterized by continuous involuntary movements and a slowly progressive dementia. Psychiatric disturbance is variable but common. Initial insight may result in depression. Prodromal personality changes, antisocial behaviour with substance misuse and affective and schizophreniform disorders are sometimes seen. Insight gives way to euphoria with explosive outbursts, irritability and rage. There is slowly progressive intellectual impairment, with some patients profoundly demented in the final stages, whereas others remain reasonably acute. The duration to death has been approximated to be between 12 and 16 years.

Reference: Puri BK, Hall AD, Ho RC (2014). *Revision Notes in Psychiatry*. Boca Raton, FL: CRC Press, p. 707.

Question 87 Answer: e, New variant CJD
Explanation: In this form of the disease, it is characterized by extensive prion plaque formation in the cerebellum. The EEG is always abnormal in CJD, showing an increase in slow-wave activity and a reduction in rhythm. As the disease progresses, bilateral slow spike wave discharges may accompany myoclonic jerks. Gross atrophy is seen in the fronto-temporal regions in Pick disease, but the diagnosis cannot be made on this evidence alone.

Reference: Puri BK, Hall AD, Ho RC (2014). *Revision Notes in Psychiatry*. Boca Raton, FL: CRC Press, p. 701.

Question 88 Answer: c, 5–6 years
Explanation: Boys enter puberty at an average age of 11 years (1–2 years later than girls), but it may occur anytime between 9 and 14 years.

Reference: Puri BK, Treasaden I (eds) (2010). *Psychiatry: An Evidence-Based Text*. London: Hodder Arnold, pp. 120–121.

Question 89 Answer: e, Delusional disorders tend to be worsened in pregnancy
Explanation: Option (e) is incorrect. It is incorrect to say that pregnancy has any effect on chronic delusional states.

Reference: Puri BK, Treasaden I (eds) (2010). *Psychiatry: An Evidence-Based Text*. London: Hodder Arnold, pp. 718–721.

Question 90 Answer: c, Petechial haemorrhages in the periaqueductal grey matter
Explanation: With the above presentation, Wernicke's encephalopathy should be suspected. The important clinical features include ophthalmoplegia, nystagmus, ataxia and clouding of consciousness. The following changes are routinely detected, and they include petechial haemorrhages in the periaqueductal grey matter as well as in the mammillary bodies.

Reference: Puri BK, Hall AD, Ho RC (2014). *Revision Notes in Psychiatry*. Boca Raton, FL: CRC Press, p. 513.

Question 91 Answer: d, Confounder does not lead to false association between exposure and outcome, but bias does
Explanation: Confounder is a variable that is both associated with the exposure and also independently associated with the outcome that will distort observation. Bias is a systematic error in the design or conduct of a study. Confounder is caused by the third factor independently related to the exposure and outcome, while bias is introduced by the researcher. Both bias and confounder can lead to false association between exposure and outcome. They can also be countered at the design stage and adjusted for at the analysis stage.

Reference: Lewis GH, Sheringham J, Kalim K, Crayford T JB (2008). *Mastering Public Health: A Postgraduate Guide to Examination and Revalidation*. London: Royal Society of Medicine Press, pp. 27–34.

Question 92 Answer: b, I
Explanation: Clinical trial is a prospective study involving human subjects designed to determine the effectiveness of a treatment administered to patients with a specific disease. There is a well-established categorization of such studies into phases I–IV. This question describes phase I trial. The main purpose of the phase I trials is to determine several things about a drug candidate, including its toxicity, side effects, interaction with the body and proper dosage levels.

Reference: Everitt BS (2006). *Medical Statistics from A to Z* (2nd edition). Cambridge, UK: Cambridge University Press, p. 46.

Question 93 Answer: d, III
Explanation: Clinical trial is a prospective study involving human subjects designed to determine the effectiveness of a treatment administered to patients with a specific disease. There is a well-established categorization of such studies into phases I–IV. This question describes phase III trial. These trials involve large subject groups and are designed to be the final assessment of a drug's efficacy and side effects.

Reference: Everitt BS (2006). *Medical Statistics from A to Z* (2nd edition). Cambridge, UK: Cambridge University Press, p. 46.

Question 94 Answer: b, Approximately, 50% of males are considered to be homosexuals
Explanation: The condition that this individual is suffering from is known as fetishism. It is the reliance on some non-living object as a stimulus for sexual arousal and gratification. It is often an extension of the human body, such as clothing or footwear. It is often characterized by textures such as plastic, rubber or leather. This condition is more common in men, and 20% of them are considered to be homosexual. The behaviour is caused by classical conditioning. It is associated with temporal lobe dysfunction. It is diagnosed only if the fetish is the most important source of sexual stimulation. Fantasies are common, but do not amount to disorder unless they are so compelling that they interfere with sexual intercourse and lead to distress. Treatment involves behavioural therapy focusing masturbatory reconditioning and response prevention.

Reference: Puri BK, Hall AD, Ho RC (2014). *Revision Notes in Psychiatry*. Boca Raton, FL: CRC Press, p. 600.

Question 95 Answer: c, Solvents
Explanation: Volatile substances are inhaled to experience their psychoactive effects. Chronic usage might lead to the development of Goodpasture's syndrome, hypokalaemia and optic neuropathy. High doses could also cause stupor and death. Aspiration of vomit could also occur at any time.

Reference: Puri BK, Hall AD, Ho RC (2014). *Revision Notes in Psychiatry*. Boca Raton, FL: CRC Press, p. 550.

Question 96 Answer: d, After you write the medical report, she is likely to be unhappy with the fact that you did not support her claim of having nervous shock and will lodge a formal complaint to the chief executive through her lawyer
Explanation: This is a case of compensation neurosis, and her unreasonable request may stop after being informed by her own lawyer that the chance of success is low and that there is a high cost to pay if she pursues the case. Option A is incorrect, as more than 50% of cases are not able to work after settlement. She does not meet the criteria for both nervous shock and post-traumatic stress disorder (PTSD). Nervous shock is a legal concept where the patient must be suffering from a positive psychiatric illness, and there is a clear and reasonable chain of causation between the negligent act and psychiatric illness. In this case, the chain of causation is not clear.

Reference and Further Reading: Gunn J, Taylor PJ (1993). *Forensic Psychiatry. Clinical, Legal and Ethical Issues*. Oxford, UK: Butterworth-Heinemann; *Further Reading*: Puri BK, Treasaden I (eds) (2010). *Psychiatry: An Evidence-Based Text*. London: Hodder Arnold, p. 660.

Question 97 Answer: e, Later age of onset
Explanation: Later age of onset is a poor prognostic factor. Other poor prognostic factors include long duration of illness, severe weight loss, substance misuse and obsessive-compulsive personality.

Reference and Further Reading: Ratnasuriya RH, Eisler I, Szmukler GI, Russell GF (1991). Anorexia nervosa: Outcome and prognostic factors after 20 years. *Br J Psychiatry*, 58: 495–502; Puri BK, Treasaden I (eds) (2010). *Psychiatry: An Evidence-Based Text*. London: Hodder Arnold, pp. 687–703, 1063.

Question 98 Answer: b, 15%
Explanation: Fifteen percent of individuals convicted of child sexual abuse are reconvicted in England and Wales, while up to 35%–45% may reoffend on the basis of self reports. Recidivism is associated with early onset, length of history, variety of sexual offending, offending against both sexes and deviant arousal to paedophile images on penile plethysmography. Untreated, such individuals may abuse large numbers of victims. Even with treatment, recidivism rates are high and do not decrease with time.

Reference: Puri BK, Treasaden I (eds) (2010). *Psychiatry: An Evidence-Based Text*. London: Hodder Arnold, pp. 767–769, 772, 773, 1242.

Question 99 Answer: b, Blinding of intervention group but not the observer who collects the measurements
Explanation: A bias is a systematic error that leads to a difference between the comparison groups with regard to how they are chosen, treated, measured or interpreted. This error leads to an incorrect estimate of the association between the exposure and the risk of disease. Blinding of observers who collect measurements or analyse results is necessary to avoid observer and ascertainment bias.

Reference: Lewis GH, Sheringham J, Kalim K, Crayford T JB (2008). *Mastering Public Health: A Postgraduate Guide to Examination and Revalidation*. London: Royal Society of Medicine Press, pp. 26–31.

Question 100 Answer: e, Psychopathic traits
Explanation: About 25% of people exposed to extreme trauma develop PTSD. Having psychopathic traits is a protective factor against development of PTSD. Viewing the dead body of a relative after a disaster is predictive of lower PTSD. Risk factors include female gender, low IQ, previous history of trauma, severity of trauma, perceived life threat, peri-traumatic dissociation, impaired social support and low socioeconomic status. In terms of the course of PTSD, half of patients still have the condition decades later.

Reference: Puri BK, Hall AD, Ho RC (2014). *Revision Notes in Psychiatry*. Boca Raton, FL: CRC Press, p. 427.

Question 101 Answer: c, Frank hallucinations

Explanation: Ganser syndrome is a rare dissociative disorder described by Ganser in 1898 in three prisoners, which is characterized by approximate or absurd answers (vorbeireden), clouding of consciousness, somatic conversion, pseudohallucinations and subsequent amnesia. A neurological consult may be indicated to rule out any organic cause.

Reference: Puri BK, Hall AD, Ho RC (2014). *Revision Notes in Psychiatry*. Boca Raton, FL: CRC Press, 2014, p. 434.

Question 102 Answer: a, Delirium

Explanation: This patient presents with agitation, aggression, confusion and hallucinations.

Reference: Puri BK, Treasaden I (eds) (2010). *Psychiatry: An Evidence-Based Text*. London: Hodder Arnold, p. 880.

Question 103 Answer: b, Low potassium

Explanation: It should be high potassium. The female-to-male gender ratio is 2:1. The neuropsychiatric symptoms include fatigue, weakness, apathy and memory impairment. Psychosis occurs in 20% of patients.

Reference: Puri BK, Hall AD, Ho RC (2014). *Revision Notes in Psychiatry*. Boca Raton, FL: CRC Press, p. 477.

Question 104 Answer: d, 50%

Explanation: About 50% of restrictive patients with anorexia nervosa may develop bulimia after 5 years. The course and outcome for anorexia nervosa are variable. Some patients recover fully after a single episode. Some exhibit fluctuating patterns of weight gain followed by a relapse. For adolescents with anorexia, around 80% recover in 5 years, and 20% may develop chronic anorexia. For adults in anorexia, 50% recover, 25% have an intermediate outcome and 25% have a poor outcome. Anorexia nervosa is associated with a substantially increased mortality rate (5%–20%). The aggregate mortality rate is 5.6% per decade. This is 12 times the annual death rate due to all causes for females aged 15–24 years.

Reference: Puri BK, Hall AD, Ho RC (2014). *Revision Notes in Psychiatry*. Boca Raton, FL: CRC Press, p. 581.

Question 105 Answer: b, SSRI

Explanation: Previous studies have demonstrated that SSRI can cause pulmonary hypertension (especially after 20 weeks) in the newborn. The newborn might experience withdrawal such as agitation and irritability, especially with medications like paroxetine and venlafaxine.

Reference: Puri BK, Hall AD, Ho RC (2014). *Revision Notes in Psychiatry*. Boca Raton, FL: CRC Press, p. 561.

Question 106 Answer: b, Old age at onset of illness
Explanation: Young age at onset of illness is a risk factor for suicide in multiple sclerosis. Other risk factors for suicide include male gender, current or previous history of depression, social isolation and substance abuse. Suicidal ideation is very common in multiple sclerosis. Suicide in this group of patients is 7.5 times higher than in the general population: 15% of mortality of this illness is related to suicide. Depression is seen in about 14%–27% of patients, and this is often associated with interferon treatment. Individuals with advanced multiple sclerosis are much more likely to experience clinically significant depressive symptoms than those with minimal disease. Shorter duration of multiple sclerosis is also associated with a greater likelihood of significant depressive symptoms, but the pattern of illness progression is not. Psychological and social factors are also known to play a role in depression.

Reference: Jefferies K (2006). The neuropsychiatry of multiple sclerosis. *Adv Psychiat Treatment*, 12: 214–220.

Question 107 Answer: c, 20%
Explanation: Twenty percent of patients with ischemic heart disease (IHD) have comorbid depression. Major depression is an independent risk factor for IHD. After an acute myocardial infarction, major depression predicts mortality in the first 6 months. The impact of a depressive disorder is equivalent to the impact of a previous infarct.

Reference: Puri BK, Hall AD, Ho RC (2014). *Revision Notes in Psychiatry*. Boca Raton, FL: CRC Press, p. 468.

Question 108 Answer: b, National Adult Reading Test (NART)
Explanation: The NART is a reading test consisting of phonetically irregular words that have to be read aloud by the subject. If a patient suffers deterioration in intellectual abilities, their premorbid vocabulary may remain less affected (or unaffected). The NART can therefore be used to assess for premorbid IQ.

Reference: Puri BK, Hall AD, Ho RC (2014). *Revision Notes in Psychiatry*. Boca Raton, FL: CRC Press, p. 96.

Question 109 Answer: b, 10 times
Explanation: A previous study studied the proportion of deaths attributed to suicide. Compared with the general population, the odds of a death due to suicide have been estimated to be around 8.2 times that of the general population in the United States.

Reference: Schoenfeld M (1984). Increased rate of suicide amongst patients with Huntington's disease. *J Neurol Neurosurg Psychiatry*, 47(12): 1283–1287.

Extended match items

Theme: Learning Disability

Question 110 Answer: f, 40
Explanation: Turner syndrome occurs secondary to non-disjunction of paternal XY chromosomes resulting in sex chromosomal monosomy (XO, phenotypically female). Fifty percent have karyotype consisting of 45X or 46XX mosaicism, and 50% have 46 chromosomes with one normal X and other X being abnormal in the form of a ring, a long arm isochromosome or a partially deleted X chromosome. Patients with this syndrome have an increased incidence of internal anomalies, especially renal malformations in 40% and coarctation of the aorta in 15%. Learning disability is rare.

Question 111 Answer: d, 20
Explanation: In adults with Turner syndrome, the incidence of hypothyroidism is about 20%.

Question 112 Answer: c, 15
Explanation: In Turner syndrome, coarctation of the aorta occurs in 15%.

Question 113 Answer: i, 80
Explanation: Approximately 50% of women with Turner syndrome have a 45X karyotype, and in 80% of these, the meiotic error would have occurred in a paternal meiotic division. Most of the remaining 50% have a karyotype consisting of either 45X/46XX mosaicism or 46 chromosomes with one normal X and the other X being abnormal in the form of a ring or long-arm isochromosome or a partially deleted X chromosome.

Reference: Young ID (2010). *Medical Genetics*. Oxford, UK: Oxford University Press, p. 60.

Theme: Research Methodology

Question 114 Answer: a, Cox regression
Explanation: This form of multivariate regression is based on proportional hazards assumptions (i.e. that the ratio of hazards in both groups remains the same). It is used to produce the hazard ratio. It is the multivariate extension of the log-rank test. It is used to assess the impact of treatment on survival or other time-related events and adjusts for the effects of other variables.

Question 115 Answer: b, Linear regression
Explanation: It is estimated using the statistical technique of fitting a straight line (line of best fit) to a scatter plot of variables using the method of least squares. For simple linear regression, it is concerned with describing the linear relationship between a dependent (outcome) variable, Y, and single explanatory (independent or predictor) variable, X. Standard errors can be estimated, and CIs can be determined.

Question 116 Answer: d, Multiple linear regression
Explanation: For multiple linear regression (multivariate regression), there is a regression model in which the dependent outcome variable is predicted from two or more independent variables. The independent variables can be continuous or categorical. The objective of this regression is to adjust for confounding and understand which variables are associated with an outcome.

References: Lewis GH, Sheringham J, Kalim K, Crayford TJ (2008). *Mastering Public Health*. London: Royal Society of Medicine Press, p. 100; Gosall N, Gosall G (2012). *The Doctor's Guide to Critical Appraisal*. Cheshire, UK: PasTest, pp. 142–143.

Theme: Research Methodology

Question 117 Answer: d, Matched random sampling
Explanation: In matched random sampling, individuals or groups are first matched according to baseline data – matching them on as many variables as possible. The intervention is then randomly allocated to one member of the pair, with the other member of the pair receiving the control.

Question 118 Answer: i, Systematic sampling
Explanation: A sampling frame is required for all studies that aim to make an inference about the population (i.e. a complete list of the population from which the sample is to be drawn). In systematic sampling, start with the sampling frame and then calculate the sampling interval: number in population/number in sample. Then, draw every *n*th person from the sampling frame. It is more convenient than random sampling and allows calculation of sampling error. However, there is potential for bias if there are underlying patterns to the sampling frame.

Question 119 Answer: c, Event sampling
Explanation: Event sampling is a form of sampling method that allows the study of ongoing experiences and events by taking assessments one or more times per day in the naturally occurring environment. Because of the frequent sampling of events inherent in event sampling, it enables researchers to measure the typology of activity and detect the temporal and dynamic fluctuations of work experiences. The strengths of this form of sampling include the following: (1) It highlights the possible situations and roles that behaviour may be contingent upon. Thus, it serves as a demonstration of the interaction between the person and the context and provides insight to the contingencies of behaviour. (2) It provides ecological validity due to the fact that the data are collected in the participant's natural environment, and this allows greater generalisability of the resulting data.

Question 120 Answer: e, Panel sampling
Explanation: Panel sampling is the method of first selecting a group of participants through a random sampling method and then asking that group for the same information again several times over a period. This longitudinal sampling method allows estimates of changes in the population.

Question 121 Answer: b, Convenience sampling
Explanation: Convenience sampling is a non-probability sampling (whereby the sampling frame is not known) where subjects are chosen on basis of being readily available. It is useful for preliminary research as it is extremely efficient. However, the sampling error cannot be calculated, and there may be volunteer bias.

Question 122 Answer: h, Snowball sampling
Explanation: Snowball sampling is a non-probability sampling (whereby the sampling frame is not known) where subjects are asked to recommend acquaintances who meet the sample criteria. It is very cost effective and useful where no sample frame exists. It also enables the researcher to reach to groups that are otherwise hard to reach. However, sampling error cannot be calculated, and there may be volunteer bias.

Question 123 Answer: a, Cluster sampling
Explanation: Cluster sampling is used when there are 'natural' clusters in the population. A random sampling technique is used to choose which clusters to include in the study. In single-stage cluster sampling, all the elements from each of the selected clusters are used. In two-stage cluster sampling, elements from each of the selected clusters are selected at random. This method is convenient for fieldwork, cost-efficient and allows calculation of sampling error. However, it may lead to increased sampling error.

Reference: Lewis GH, J Sheringham, K Kalim, TJB Crayford (2008). *Mastering Public Health: A Postgraduate Guide to Examination and Revalidation*. London: Royal Society of Medicine Press, pp. 45, 46.

Theme: Neuroimaging in the Elderly

Question 124 Answer: a, Alzheimer's dementia, b, Frontal lobe dementia, f, CJD
Explanation: It has been known that cortical dementia arises from the cerebral cortex, which plays a key role in memory and language. The examples of cortical dementia include Alzheimer dementia, frontal lobe dementia and CJD.

Question 125 Answer: c, HIV-related dementia, d, Huntington chorea, e, Parkinson disease dementia
Explanation: Subcortical dementia results from dysfunction in neuroanatomical structures that are beneath the cortex. Memory impairments and language difficulties are not the early signs of subcortical dementias. Examples include all the above.

Question 126 Answer: g, Vascular dementia, and h, LBD
Explanation: The examples of mixed cortical and subcortical dementia include vascular dementia, LBD and neuropsychiatric sequelae after carbon monoxide poisoning.

Reference: Puri BK, Hall AD, Ho RC (2014). *Revision Notes in Psychiatry*. Boca Raton, FL: CRC Press, p. 693.

Theme: Forensic Psychiatry

Question 127 Answer: a, 1

Explanation: The prevalence of prisoners with chronic epilepsy has been found in a meta-analysis (Fazel et al. 2002) to be about 1%. The prevalence rate in the general populations is also approximately 1% for men aged 25–35 years, according to community-based surveys.

Question 128 Answer: k, 80

Explanation: The peak age for arson is 17 years for men and 45 years for women. There is an increased incidence amongst people with learning disabilities and those with alcohol-dependence syndrome.

Question 129 Answer: h, 50

Explanation: The percentage of psychiatric patients released from medium secure units who re-offend is approximately 50%. Offence predictors include male gender, younger age, early-onset offending, previous convictions and a comorbid or primary diagnosis of personality disorder. Longer in-patient stay and being subject to a restriction order on discharge are protective.

Question 130 Answer: g, 45

Explanation: The heritability of antisocial behaviour in prisoners has been estimated to be about 45%. The heritable form of criminality is, however, associated with petty recidivism and property offences rather than violent crime.

Question 131 Answer: f, 35

Explanation: Thirty-five percent of prisoners screened positive for adult ADHD, with 17% of the sample meeting criteria for a full diagnosis (Moore et al., 2013). Having such a diagnosis is associated with substance abuse disorders and other psychiatric comorbidities.

Question 132 Answer: d, 20

Explanation: About 50% of all male prisoners and 20% of female prisoners have antisocial personality disorder. Antisocial personality disorder is the most prevalent personality disorder diagnosis in prisoners.

References: Fazel S, Vassos E, Danesh J (2002 Jun). Prevalence of epilepsy in prisoners: Systematic review. *BMJ*, 324(7352): 1495; Puri BK, Treasaden I (eds) (2010). *Psychiatry: An Evidence-Based Text*. London: Hodder Arnold, p. 1183; Coid J, Hickey N, Kahtan N, Zhang T, Yang M (2007). Patients discharged from medium secure forensic psychiatry services: Reconvictions and risk factors. *Br J Psychiatry*, 190: 223–229.

Theme: Dementia

Question 133 Answer: e, Mini Mental State Examination (MMSE)

Explanation: The Mini Mental State Examination (MMSE) is used as a screening test for dementia and can be helpful in the diagnosis and monitoring of the course of the disease. The test takes about 10 minutes but will detect subtle memory difficulties, especially in well-educated people. The MMSE provides measures of orientation, registration (immediate memory), short-term memory (but not long-term memory) and language functioning. A score of 26 or less may indicate significant cognitive impairment.

Question 134 Answer: c, Cambridge Neuropsychological Test Automated Battery (CANTAB)

Explanation: The Cambridge Neuropsychological Test Automated Battery (CANTAB) offers a sensitive and specific cognitive assessment for dementia. The standard CANTAB consists of 13 computerized tasks: motor screening, big/little circle, delayed matching to sample, intra-dimensional (ID)/extra-dimensional (ED) shift, matching to sample visual search, paired associates learning, pattern recognition information processing, reaction time, spatial recognition memory, spatial span, spatial working memory and stockings of Cambridge.

Question 135 Answer: b, Cambridge Examination for Mental Disorders of the Elderly (CAMDEX)

Explanation: The Cambridge Examination for Mental Disorders of the Elderly (CAMDEX) is an interview schedule that consists of a structured clinical interview with the person to obtain systematic information about the present state, history and family history; a range of objective cognitive tests, including a mini-neuropsychological battery, known as the Cambridge Cognitive Examination (CAMCOG); and a structured interview with a relative to obtain independent information about the subject's present state, history and family history. The assessment also includes a brief physical and neurological examination.

References: Puri BK, Hall AD, Ho RC (2014). *Revision Notes in Psychiatry*. Boca Raton, FL: CRC Press, pp. 98–100; Puri BK, Treasaden I (eds) (2010). *Psychiatry: An Evidence-Based Text*. London: Hodder Arnold, pp. 1101–1102.

Theme: Management of PTSD

Question 136 Answer: a, CBT

Question 137 Answer: a, CBT, b,eye movement desensitization reprocessing

Question 138 Answer: e, Fluoxetine, f, paroxetine, g, sertraline, h, venlafaxine

Question 139 Answer: i, Carbamazepine, j, Clonidine

Question 140 Answer: k, Buspirone

Explanation: National Institute for Health and Care Excellence (NICE) guidelines recommend that trauma-focused CBT should be offered to people with severe PTSD within 3 months of the trauma, with fewer sessions in the first month after the trauma. The duration of trauma-focused CBT is between 8 and 12 sessions, with approximately one session per week. In terms of medications, fluoxetine, paroxetine, sertraline and venlafaxine are beneficial in PTSD. It should be noted that the drugs require at least 8 weeks of duration before the effects are evident. Carbamazepine and clonidine reduce both hyper-arousal and intrusive symptoms. In addition, fluoxetine and lithium help to reduce explosiveness and to improve mood. Buspirone may help to reduce the fear-induced startle response. It has been also noted that involuntary multi-saccadic eye movements occur during the disturbing thoughts. It is claimed that inducing these eye movements while experiencing intrusive thoughts helps to stop the symptoms of PTSD.

Reference: Puri BK, Hall AD, Ho RC (2014). *Revision Notes in Psychiatry*. Boca Raton, FL: CRC Press, p. 426.

Theme: Learning Disability

Question 141 Answer: d, 10
Explanation: Down syndrome is the most common genetic cause of mental retardation with a reported prevalence of epilepsy of 1%–13%. Infantile spasms or West syndrome is the most frequent epilepsy syndrome in children with Down syndrome. Infantile spasms occur in 0.6%–13% of children with Down syndrome, representing 4.5%–47% of seizures in these children.

Question 142 Answer: f, 40
Explanation: People with Down syndrome are at higher risk of developing Alzheimer disease. The risk for 50- to 59-year-olds is 36%–40% and for 60- to 69-year-olds is 55%. For those over the age of 40 years, there is a higher incidence of neurofibrillary tangles and plaques with an increase in P300 latency.

Question 143 Answer: h, 55
Explanation: People with Down syndrome are at higher risk of developing Alzheimer disease. The risk for 60- to 69-year-olds is 55.

Question 144 Answer: c, 5
Explanation: Ninety-four percent of Down syndrome cases are caused by meiotic nondisjunction or trisomy 21 (47 chromosomes). Five percent of cases are caused by Robertson translocation, that is, a fusion between chromosomes 21 and 14 (46 chromosomes), although fusions between 21 and 13 or 15 or 22 are described. One percent of cases are caused by mosaicism, which is nondisjunction occurring after fertilisation in any cell division.

Question 145 Answer: i, 66
Explanation: The average life expectancy of people with Down syndrome is between 58 and 66 years. The most common cause of death is chest infection.

Question 146 Answer: d, 10
Explanation: Ten percent of people with Down syndrome have leukaemia.

Question 147 Answer: g, 50
Explanation: Hearing loss occurs in 50% of people with Down syndrome.

Question 148 Answer: b, 2
Explanation: Two percent of people with Down syndrome have obsessive-compulsive disorder, presenting especially with a need for excessive order or tidiness. Other psychiatric comorbidities include depression, autism, bipolar disorder and psychosis.

References: Arya R, Kabra M, Gulati S (2011). Epilepsy in children with Down syndrome. *Epileptic Disord*, 13(1): 1–7; Puri BK, Hall AD, Ho RC (2014). *Revision Notes in Psychiatry*. Boca Raton, FL: CRC Press, pp. 664–665.

Theme: Research Methods and Statistics

Question 149 Answer: c, Error variance
Explanation: Error variance is the variance that is unrelated to the exogenous (observed) variable.

Question 150 Answer: d, Exogenous (observed) variable
Explanation: The variables, such as 'being online immediately after waking up' or 'feel energized online', are exogenous or observed variables in Internet addiction questionnaires. The variables measure observed behaviours of the participants.

Question 151 Answer: a, Correlation coefficient estimated by confirmatory factor analysis
Explanation: III refers to the correlation coefficient estimated by confirmatory factor analysis between the exogenous (observed) variable and the endogenous (latent) variable. The correlation coefficient needs to be larger than 0.30. In Figure 5.4, all endogenous (observed) variables demonstrate satisfactory correlation with endogenous (latent) variable ($p > 0.30$).

Question 152 Answer: b, Correlation coefficient estimated by confirmatory factor analysis
Explanation: This variable is identified by confirmatory factor analysis and groups, common exogenous (observed) variables, which share similar characteristics.

Theme: Psychiatry and Endocrine Disorders

Question 153 Answer: b, Hypothyroidism
Explanation: Hypothyroidism is the one of the most common endocrine disorders in the United Kingdom. Twenty percent of patients have psychiatric disorders. Fatigue is usually accompanied by mental and physical slowness. Depression and anxiety are commonly associated.

Question 154 Answer: a, Hyperthyroidism
Explanation: Hyperthyroidism affects 2%–5% of all women mostly between the ages of 20 and 45 years, with a female-to-male ratio of 5:1. Fifty percent of individuals have associated psychiatric disorders. Anxiety and depression are common. Depressive symptoms are not linearly correlated with the levels of the thyroid hormones.

Question 155 Answer: c, Cushing syndrome

Explanation: Cushing syndrome is most commonly caused by exogenous administration of corticosteroids. Fifty to eighty percent of individuals suffer from depression with moderate-to-severe symptoms. Suicide has been reported in 3%–10% of patients. Cognitive impairment such as amnesia and attention deficits is common.

Question 156 Answer: d, Addison disease

Explanation: This is a condition that is more common in females than in males. Fatigue, weakness and apathy are common in the early stage. Ninety percent of patients have psychiatric disorders. Memory impairment is the most common. Depression, anxiety and paranoia tend to have a fluctuating course with symptom-free intervals. Psychosis can occur in 20% of patients.

Question 157 Answer: g, Diabetes insipidus

Explanation: Central causes include those caused by post-head injury, cranial surgery, radiotherapy and CNS infection. Nephrogenic is usually caused by renal disorder.

Reference: Puri BK, Hall AD, Ho RC (2014). *Revision Notes in Psychiatry*. Boca Raton, FL: CRC Press, pp. 476–478.

Theme: Learning Disability

Question 158 Answer: d, 35

Explanation: The prevalence rate of a diagnosable psychiatric disorder is 36% in children and adolescents with learning disabilities, compared with 8% of those who do not have a learning disability. These young people were also 33 times more likely to be on the autistic spectrum and were much more likely to have emotional and conduct disorders.

Question 159 Answer: c, 20

Explanation: The prevalence of dementia is much higher amongst older adults with learning disabilities compared with the general population (21.6% vs 5.7% aged 65). People with Down syndrome are at particularly high risk of developing dementia, with an age of onset 30–40 years younger than in the general population.

Question 160 Answer: a, 7

Explanation: Around 15%–25% of people with learning disability have a history of seizures, compared with 5% in the general population, of whom 0.5%–1% suffer from epilepsy, that is, recurrent seizures. The prevalence increases with the severity of learning disability, with a lifetime history of epilepsy estimated to be 7%–15% in mild-to-moderate learning disability, 45%–67% in severe learning disability and up to 80% in profound learning disability.

Question 161 Answer: f, 70

Explanation: About 70% of children with autism have mental retardation, with 30% having mild-to-moderate and 50% severe-to-profound mental retardation.

References: Cowen P, Harrison P, Burns T (2012). *Shorter Oxford Textbook of Psychiatry* (6th edition). Oxford, UK: Oxford University Press, p. 686; Puri BK, Hall AD, Ho RC (2014). *Revision Notes in Psychiatry*. Boca Raton, FL: CRC Press, p. 627; Cooper, SA (1997). High prevalence of dementia amongst people with learning disabilities not attributable to Down's syndrome. *Psychological Medicine*, 27: 609–616; Mental Health Nursing of Adults with Learning Disabilities. Royal College of Nursing. http://www.rcn.org.uk/__data/assets/pdf_file/0006/78765/003184.pdf

Theme: Side Effects of Anti-Dementia Medications

Question 162 Answer: a, Donepezil
Explanation: Donepezil is the medication that is contraindicated in individuals diagnosed with asthma.

Question 163 Answer: a, Donepezil, b, Rivastigmine, c, Galantamine
Explanation: These above medications tend to lead to excessive cholingeric effects such as nausea, diarrhoea, dizziness, urinary incontinence and insomnia.

Reference: Puri BK, Hall AD, Ho RC (2014). *Revision Notes in Psychiatry*. Boca Raton, FL: CRC Press, p. 697.

Theme: Sleep Disorders

Question 164 Answer: b, Narcolepsy
Explanation: Narcolepsy usually due to the loss of hypo-cretin in the hypothalamus. The first symptom is almost always daytime sleepiness and occurs during adolescence. Based on the *Diagnostic and Statistical Manual of Mental Disorders, Fifth Edition* (*DSM-5*), there must be the presence of hypersomnia and recurrent sleep attacks that have been occurring at least three times per week over the last 3 months.

Question 165 Answer: c, Obstructive sleep apnoea (OSA)
Explanation: The prevalence has been estimated to be between 1% and 10% of the adult population. There is a higher prevalence of OSA in older people.

Question 166 Answer: e, Restless leg syndrome
Explanation: The prevalence of restless leg syndrome is between 2% and 10% of the general population and up to 30% in people with chronic medical illnesses. The prevalence increases with age. It is a condition that is associated with the following medical conditions: Autoimmune thyroid disorders, iron deficiency and diabetes mellitus. The DSM-5 specifies the following: there must be an urge to move the legs as a result of unpleasant sensation, worsening of symptoms during periods of rest and at night and no relief of symptoms by movement. The minimum duration of restless leg syndrome is 3 months.

Question 167 Answer: g, Sleep terrors
Explanation: Sleep terrors tend to occur more commonly in males than in females. The aetiological factors responsible include stress, previous loss of sleep, familial

(10-fold increase in the prevalence in first-degree relatives) and induction by benzo-diazepine antagonist. It can also be caused by upper airway obstruction in children.

Reference: Puri BK, Hall AD, Ho RC (2014). *Revision Notes in Psychiatry*. Boca Raton, FL: CRC Press, p. 620.

Theme: Genetic Risk of Schizophrenia
Question 168 Answer: h, 35%–50%

Question 169 Answer: c, 10%–14%

Question 170 Answer: e, 20%–24%

Question 171 Answer: a, 0%–4%

Question 172 Answer: a, 0%–4%

Question 173 Answer: a, 0%–4%

Question 174 Answer: a, 0%–4%

Question 175 Answer: j, 70%–75%

Question 176 Answer: k, 80%–85%
Explanation: The prevalence of schizophrenia amongst relatives of patients with schizophrenia is as follows:

- MZ twin: 46%

- DS twin: 16%

- Children: 13%

- Siblings: 9%

- Parents: 45.6%

- Grandchildren: 3.7%

The heritability of schizophrenia has been estimated to be between 83% and 85%. An estimated 40%–60% of patients with schizophrenia have been known to be non-concordant with their medications

Reference: Puri BK, Hall AD, Ho RC (2014). *Revision Notes in Psychiatry*. Boca Raton, FL: CRC Press, p. 365.

Theme: Statistical Tests
Question 177 Answer: g, Paired *t*-test
Explanation: This test is used to determine the equality of the means of one group before and after intervention or two groups using matched samples. It assumes the

differences between the pairs are normally distributed. The null hypothesis is that there is no difference between paired observations.

Question 178 Answer: h, Wilcoxon's rank sum test
Explanation: This test is used to test the differences of the pair of observations in the two samples. This is ranked according to size of differences between observations. It is a distribution-free method with non-normal distribution. The null hypothesis is that there is no median difference between pairs of observation.

Question 179 Answer: c, Chi-square, test and e, Mann–Whitney *U* test
Explanation: Option (e) is appropriate given that we are testing the ranked homocystine levels between two independent patients: with and without dementia.

The chi-square test is a good test to test for the equality of proportion of two groups. The Mann–Whitney *U* test helps to test the equality of the location of two groups with ranking of observations in each group. It is a distribution-free method, and normal distribution is not assumed.

Question 180 Answer: a, One-way analysis of variance (ANOVA)
Explanation: To test the equality of the means of ≥ 2 independent groups by comparing the differences in means between the several groups and differences between subjects in each group. The equality of means is assessed by F-test. The method behind ANOVA is the same as the method used in multiple linear regression.

Question 181 Answer: d, Kruskal–Wallis
Explanation: To test the equality of the median in more than two independent groups, it is a distribution-free method, and measurement variable does not meet the normality assumption of ANOVA. It uses H statistics.

Question 182 Answer: h, Wilcoxon rank sum test, and i, median and range
Explanation: To test the differences of the pair of observations in the two samples. This is ranked according to size of differences between observations (the smallest difference getting a rank of 1, the next larger difference getting a rank of 2, etc.). It is a distribution-free method with non-normal distribution. The null hypothesis is that there is no median difference between pairs of observation.

Median = values that divides the data into two parts of equal size.

Reference: Puri BK, Hall AD, Ho RC (2014). *Revision Notes in Psychiatry*. Boca Raton, FL: CRC Press, pp. 307–314.

Theme: Substance Misuse in Forensics
Question 183 Answer: e, 50%

Question 184 Answer: f, 60%

Question 185 Answer: f, 60%

Question 186 Answer: a, 10%

Question 187 Answer: d, 40%

Question 188 Answer: f, 60%
Explanation: Anxiety disorder, based on previous research, has been associated with major depressive as well as addictive disorders. This is especially so for social and simple phobia.

References: Crawford V (2005). Addiction psychiatry: Dual diagnoses. MRCPsych Part II. Guildford MRCPsych Course; Regier DA, Rae DS, Narrow WE et al. (1998). Prevalence of anxiety disorders and their comorbidity with mood and addictive disorders *Brit J Psychiatry*, 173, 24–28.

MRCPYSCH PAPER B MOCK EXAMINATION 4: QUESTIONS

GET THROUGH MRCPSYCH PAPER B MOCK EXAMINATION

Total number of questions: 192 (111 MCQs, 81 EMIs)
Total time provided: 180 minutes

Question 1
Referring to Table 7.1, which of the following moderators explains heterogeneity?
  a. Current smokers among patients with COPD.
  b. Gender distribution of patients with COPD, female.
  c. FEV_1 status of patients with COPD.
  d. Mean age of patients with COPD.
  e. No moderator could explain heterogeneity.

Question 2
Interpret the results in Table 7.2, and choose the correct statement.
  a. Patients with COPD rated by clinicians demonstrated significantly higher prevalence of depression compared with self-rating by them.
  b. Patients with COPD reported significantly higher prevalence of depression compared with assessment by clinicians.
  c. Patients with COPD residing in non-Western countries demonstrated significantly higher prevalence of depression compared with Western countries.
  d. Patients with COPD residing in Western countries demonstrated significantly higher prevalence of depression compared with non-Western countries.
  e. The prevalence of depression rated by clinicians and patients with COPD demonstrates no significant difference.

Question 3
Referring to the 95% CI of clinician rating of depression in Table H, which of the following statements about 95% CIs is most accurate?
  a. There is a probability of 5% or less of happening by chance if the true prevalence of depression in patients with COPD lies outside the interval (21.2%–35.2%).
  b. There is a 95% probability that the pooled prevalence of depression (27.6%) lies within the interval of 21.2%–35.2%.

Table 7.1 Results for random-effects meta-regression of demographic and clinical moderators for patients with chronic obstructive pulmonary disease (COPD)

Moderators	No. of studies used	Univariate coefficient	z value	p value	Estimated tau²	R²
Mean age of patients with COPD (years)	7	0.044	2.027	0.086	0.076	0
FEV₁ status of patients with COPD (%)	6	0.571	0.366	0.715	0.108	0
Current smokers among patients with COPD (%)	4	−0.581	−0.493	0.622	0.036	0
Gender distribution of patients with COPD, female (%)	7	0.832	0.709	0.478	0.145	0

Source: Zhang MW, Ho RC, Cheung MW, Fu E, Mak A (2011). Prevalence of depressive symptoms in patients with chronic obstructive pulmonary disease: A systematic review, meta-analysis and meta-regression. *Gen Hosp Psychiatry*, 33(3) : 217–223.

Table 7.2 Subgroup effect size analysis of pooled prevalence of depression in patients with COPD

Subgroups		No. of studies	Pooled prevalence (%)	95% confidence interval (CI)	p-value between group comparison
Clinician rated assessment of depression		4	27.6	21.2–35.2	0.163
Self-rated assessment of depression		4	21.0	15.6–27.7	
	Overall	8	24.6	21.0–28.6	
Country sampled: Western		6	25.3	21.2–29.9	0.435
Country sampled: non-Western		2	21.3	13.9–31.1	
	Overall	8	24.6	21.0–28.6	

c. There is a 95% probability that the true prevalence of depression in patients with COPD lies within the interval of 21.2%–35.2%.

d. There is a 95% probability that the interval (21.2%–35.2%) covers the true prevalence of depression in COPD.

e. There is a 95% probability that the prevalence of depression from further studies involving patients with COPD will fall within the interval (21.2%–35.2%).

Question 4

Publication biases exist in meta-analytical study A, B, C, D and E. Classic fail-safe test was performed, and the results are summarized in Table 7.3.

Which of the studies has the most convincing results?

a. Study A

b. Study B

c. Study C

d. Study D

e. Study E

Table 7.3 Summary of classic fail-safe test results

Meta-analytical study	Classic fail-safe test results
A	484 missing studies
B	976 missing studies
C	32 missing studies
D	47 missing studies
E	709 missing studies

Question 5

Violence in patients with schizophrenia is uncommon, but they do have a higher risk compared with the general population. Which of the following is the most common form of violence demonstrated by these individuals?
a. Verbal aggression
b. Physical violence towards objects
c. Violence towards others
d. Violence towards self
e. Violence towards self and others

Question 6

Post-schizophrenia depression refers to a depressive episode that arises after a schizophrenic illness. Schizophrenic illness should have occurred within the past 12 months, with some symptoms still being present. Very often, it is tough to differentiate post-schizophrenia depression with that of schizophrenia with prominent negative symptoms. Which of the following is a characteristic feature of post-schizophrenia depression?
a. Presence of low mood for a total duration of 2 weeks
b. Marked reduction in interest
c. Sleep difficulties with significant early morning awakening
d. Presence of thoughts of worthlessness
e. Marked reduction in energy

Question 7

With regard to the prognosis for mood disorder, which of the following is not a factor that predicts a prolonged time to recovery?
a. Long duration of the initial index episode
b. Severe initial episode
c. Having a prior history of affective disorder
d. Low family income
e. Being married during the index episode

Question 8

A 5-year-old girl presents with compulsive acts, without any prior or concomitant obsessions. Which of the following conditions is most likely?
a. Learning disability
b. Basal ganglia lesion

c. Autism
d. Attention-deficit hyperactivity disorder (ADHD)
e. Rett syndrome

Question 9
What is the estimated prevalence of dementia among individuals with human immunodeficiency virus (HIV)?
a. 5%
b. 10%
c. 20%
d. 30%
e. 50%

Question 10
Which of the following clinical features is most dominant during the early stages of onset of general paralysis of the insane?
a. Cognitive impairment
b. Cognitive dulling
c. Depression
d. Hypomanic features
e. Hallucinations

Question 11
Which of the following is a contraindication for psychodynamic psychotherapy?
a. Addiction
b. Adequate ego strength
c. Anxiety disorders
d. Childhood abuse and trauma
e. Relationship and personality problems

Question 12
A 45-year-old man was scolded by his boss at work in the morning. In the evening, when he returns home, he shouts at his wife for misplacing his toothbrush. Which of the following defence mechanisms is this man exhibiting?
a. Acting out
b. Displacement
c. Reaction formation
d. Undoing
e. Sublimation

Question 13
A 15-year-old boy presents with an annular rash (ring-shaped lesion) on the palm, and he also presents with low mood. Which of the following is the most likely diagnosis?
a. Atopic dermatitis
b. Contact dermatitis

c. Infectious mononucleosis
d. Erythema migrans
e. Secondary syphilis

Question 14

A woman with chronic active addiction problems gives birth to a baby boy. At birth, he is found to be irritable and restless. He is small for his age and has growth retardation and also has a small head with small eye openings. Which one of the following substances is implicated?
 a. Alcohol
 b. Benzodiazepine
 c. Cocaine
 d. Opiate
 e. Tobacco

Question 15

A 50-year-old man with alcohol dependency presents to the emergency department with lethargy, giddiness, tremors and anxiety. He admits to drinking large amounts of alcohol just 1 day ago. Which one of the following is the most likely metabolic abnormality?
 a. Hypoglycaemia
 b. Hyponatraemia
 c. Hypokalaemia
 d. Hypocalcaemia
 e. Hyperkalaemia

Question 16

A 6-year-old boy is referred to the Child and Adolescent Mental Health Services for slow learning. He is pleasant and cooperative. On physical examination, he has a small mouth, small teeth and a high-arched palate and has low-set ears with hearing difficulty. He also has oblique palpebral fissures with epicanthic folds. Which of the following disorders is he most likely to have?
 a. Down syndrome
 b. Fragile X syndrome
 c. Hurler syndrome
 d. Phenylketonuria
 e. XYY syndrome

Question 17

Which of the following statements is incorrect about people with XYY syndrome?
 a. It affects approximately 1 in 1,000 males.
 b. They may have mild learning disability and delayed verbal skills.
 c. They have delayed sexual development and infertility.
 d. They have increased susceptibility to develop acne.
 e. They show a three fold increased rate of petty crime compared with the general population.

Question 18
An 18-year-old boy is seen in the clinic for severe self-hurting, including biting of the lips and fingers. He is aggressive and throws tantrums easily. There are delayed secondary sexual developments. His maternal uncle and grandfather also suffered from this disorder. Which one of the following disorders would most likely be present?
a. Fragile X syndrome
b. Hunter syndrome
c. Hurler syndrome
d. Lesch–Nyhan syndrome
e. XXY syndrome

Question 19
An 8-year-old boy has been recently been diagnosed with ADHD. He was initially started on a stimulant, but it was terminated, as he was unable to tolerate the medications. All the following non-stimulants and alternative medications are appropriate for treatment of his underlying condition, as recommended by National Institute for Health and Care Excellence (NICE), with the exception of
a. Atomoxetine
b. Imipramine
c. Bupropion
d. Clonidine
e. Omega-3 fatty acids

Question 20
A 15-year-old boy is referred for assessment of Gilles de la Tourette's syndrome. The following are all common symptoms of Tourette's syndrome, except for
a. Tremor
b. Echolalia
c. Echopraxia
d. Coprolalia
e. Coprophagia

Question 21
A 13-year-old boy presents with bilateral involuntary movements after pharyngeal infection 2 weeks ago. His emotion is labile. What is the most likely diagnosis?
a. Meningitis
b. Huntington's chorea
c. Sydenham's chorea
d. Myoclonic epilepsy
e. Tourette's syndrome

Question 22
With regard to the treatment of childhood-onset depressive disorder, which of the following is incorrect?

a. Psychotherapy is usually the recommended first-line treatment.
b. Fluoxetine could be considered if psychotherapy has not worked out after 3 months.
c. Antidepressants do increase the risk of suicide behaviours in children.
d. Tricyclic antidepressants are usually not used for the treatment of depressive disorder.
e. Very early-onset depressive disorder is associated with good prognosis, as treatment could help recovery.

Question 23

Which one of the following is not a feature of Consolidated Standards of Reporting Trials (CONSORT) guidelines?
a. Inclusion and exclusion criteria are clearly specified.
b. Method of blinding is clearly specified.
c. Pre-study power calculations are provided.
d. There is per-protocol analysis.
e. The randomization procedure is clearly specified.

Question 24

Which of the following is not a proper randomization method used in randomized controlled trials (RCTs)?
a. Centralized randomization
b. Minimization
c. Quasi-randomization
d. Stratified randomization
e. Stepped wedge randomization

Question 25

Children who have Pediatric autoimmune neuropsychiatric disorders associated with streptococcal infections (PANDAS) are likely to have all the following conditions with the exception of which one?
a. Obsessive-compulsive disorder
b. Tourette syndrome
c. ADHD
d. Anxiety
e. Psychosis

Question 26

Which of the following psychiatric conditions is elective mutism associated with?
a. Autistic disorder
b. Childhood disintegrative disorder
c. Hyperkinetic disorder
d. Generalized anxiety disorder
e. Social phobia

Question 27

Approximately what percentage of adult bipolar patients experience their first episode of mania prior to the age of 20 years?

a. 5%
b. 10%
c. 20%
d. 30%
e. 50%

Question 28

Which of the following statements about narcolepsy is false?

a. Automatic behaviour is not common.
b. Peak incidence is around 14 years old.
c. There is excessive sleepiness, but the person wakes up refreshed.
d. The duration of cataplexy is usually short.
e. Selective serotonin re-uptake inhibitor (SSRI) antidepressant is helpful with cataplexy.

Question 29

A 40-year-old man who was previously morbidly obese underwent a successful surgical resection of the stomach 6 months ago. He lost a total of 15 kg over this period. He now presents with symptoms of depression and neuropathy. Which of the following conditions is most likely to be responsible?

a. Bipolar disorder – depressed state
b. Body image disorder
c. Hyperthyroidism
d. Thiamine deficiency
e. Toxic neuropathy

Question 30

A 50-year-old man with rapidly progressive Guillain–Barré syndrome was admitted to the hospital following shortness of breath and difficulty breathing. He does not have any psychiatric history. On the second day in the ward, he develops sudden severe anxiety, confusion and agitation and is referred to you by the ward team for assessment. Which one of the following statements is false regarding his condition?

a. Antipsychotics should be given cautiously and judiciously to reduce respiratory depression.
b. Electrolyte disturbances, in particular hyponatraemia, can cause these symptoms.
c. He can be given doses of benzodiazepine to alleviate his anxiety and uptitrate in response to his anxiety symptoms.
d. Hypoxia and hypercapnia may be the cause of his symptoms as a result of chest and diaphragm wall paresis.
e. Symptoms are not caused by central nervous system dysfunction resulting directly from Guillain–Barré syndrome.

Question 31
Which of the following statements regarding acute intermittent porphyria is false?
a. It is an autosomal dominant disorder of porphyrin metabolism.
b. Phenytoin may exacerbate an attack.
c. Psychiatric symptoms are seen in about 10% of attacks.
d. Urine is red during an attack.
e. There is increased urinary porphobilinogen and 5-aminolevulinic acid in urine.

Question 32
You see a 14-year-old boy with Tourette's syndrome, who also has hyperkinetic disorder. The most effective treatment for this boy would be
a. Tricyclic antidepressant medication
b. Risperidone
c. Pemoline
d. Methylphenidate
e. Atomoxetine

Question 33
Which of the following statements about HIV-related dementia is false?
a. Brain scans usually show cerebral atrophy and white-matter abnormalities.
b. It occurs early in the course when there is minimal immunosuppression.
c. Prevalence of dementia is 30% among HIV-infected patients.
d. Neuropathies are seen in these patients.
e. There is mild protein elevation in cerebrospinal fluid.

Question 34
With regard to ADHD, which of the following percentages is incorrect?
a. The heritability is 90%.
b. 80% concordance rate for monozygotic twins.
c. 40% concordance rate for dizygotic twins.
d. 30% show residual symptoms in adulthood.
e. If a parent has ADHD, there is 50% chance that the child will develop ADHD.

Question 35
Which of the following randomization methods is the least likely to produce bias in a randomized control trial (RCT)?
a. Allocation of patients by their month of birth
b. Allocation of patients by hospitalization status (inpatient versus outpatient)
c. Allocation of patients by gender (subdivided into strata and individuals within each striatum undergo further randomization)
d. Allocation of patients by laboratory results (e.g. blood cholesterol status)
e. Allocation of patients by order of arrival time in clinic

Question 36
Which of the following does not increase the power of a randomized controlled trial?
a. Comparison of active treatment with placebo
b. High compliance rate with treatment

c. High potency of an antidepressant

d. An increase in the number of collaborating centres instead of the number of subjects

e. Using observer rated questionnaires instead of self-reported questionnaires

Question 37

Based on your understanding of the clinical antipsychotic trials of intervention effectiveness (CATIE) trial, which of the following antipsychotics has been shown to be associated with the lowest rate of discontinuation?

a. Olanzapine

b. Quetiapine

c. Risperidone

d. Ziprasidone

e. Perphenazine

Question 38

Which of the following is not a feature associated with Parkinson disease?

a. Characterized pathologically by Lewy bodies

b. Depression has a unimodal age of onset

c. Prevalence increases with age

d. Postural instability

e. Resting and pill-rolling tremor of 4–6 Hz

Question 39

Which of the following is not a feature of Steele–Richardson–Olszewski syndrome?

a. Early postural instability

b. Good eye contact

c. Midline more than appendicular rigidity

d. Monotonous speech

e. Poor response to levodopa

Question 40

Which of the following statements regarding Huntington disease is false?

a. Electroencephalogram (EEG) shows absence of rhythmic background activity along with low-voltage intermittent random activities.

b. Genetic counselling for family members should be offered.

c. It is not commonly associated with psychiatric comorbidity.

d. Tetrabenazine helps to reduce the movement disorder.

e. There is marked atrophy of head of caudate nucleus and putamen.

Question 41

A 31-year-old woman is charged in court for homicide. She pleads that, at the time of the offence, she had epilepsy. Which of the following statements about this phenomenon is false?

a. Her behaviour was involuntary.

b. Her plea is known as sane automatism.

c. The automatism plea is generally restricted to homicide cases.

d. The mind was not conscious of what the body is doing.
e. There are two types of automatism pleas.

Question 42
What is the increase in likelihood of a male with learning disability committing an offence compared with a male with no disorder?
a. Two times more likely
b. Three times more likely
c. Four times more likely
d. Five times more likely
e. Six times more likely

Question 43
Which of the following can be used to assess psychopathy in a non-forensic population?
a. Historical Clinical Risk 20 (HCR-20)
b. Psychopathy Checklist – Revised (PCL-R)
c. Psychopathy Checklist – Screening Version (PCL-SV)
d. Static-99
e. Violence Risk Appraisal Guide (VRAG)

Question 44
An infarct in which of the following regions of the brain is most likely to result in depression?
a. Occipital lobe
b. Basal ganglia
c. Medulla
d. Cerebellum
e. Parietal lobe

Question 45
Which of the following statements is false regarding the relationship between psychiatric disorders and criminal behaviour?
a. Antisocial behaviour may appear before any sign of psychiatric or neurological disturbance in Huntington disease.
b. Offending is more likely in mild and moderate learning disability than in severe learning disability.
c. Prisoners with epilepsy have committed more violent crimes than those without epilepsy.
d. Patients with schizophrenia have similar rates of offending to the general population.
e. Patients with schizophrenia are six times more likely to be charged for violence.

Question 46
Which of the following statements is false regarding the conduction of an RCT?
a. A multi-centred trial is preferred to assess effects of trial drug in different ethnic groups because of variation in pharmacokinetics.
b. A patient can withdraw from the RCT at any time, and a valid reason is required.

c. Placebo treatment is not recommended in chronic and severe illnesses.
d. The RCT needs to obtain ethic committee approval beforehand.
e. The RCT should be guided by the uncertainty principle, and both investigators and subjects should not know the efficacy of trial drug and gold-standard treatment.

Question 47

For depression, relapse refers to the return of depressive symptoms. The risk has been estimated to be particularly high within how many months following the initial withdrawal of antidepressants?
a. 1 month
b. 2 months
c. 3 months
d. 4 months
e. 6 months

Question 48

A 30-year-old woman has been diagnosed with depression, and she has been researching more about depression online. She finds out about a previous trial, called STAR*D, which was conducted. She wants to know more about the trial. Which of the following statements about the trial is incorrect?
a. A third of the patients managed to reach a remission or virtual absence of the symptoms during the initial phase of the study.
b. The remission rate was 10%.
c. One in three depressed patients who previously did not achieve remission using an antidepressant became symptom free with the help of augmenting with another antidepressant.
d. One in four depressed patients became symptom free after 9 weeks.
e. The level 4 findings suggested that either venlafaxine or mirtazapine treatment may be a better choice than a monoamine oxidase inhibitor (MAOI).

Question 49

Which of the following statements about the pharmacological treatment of delirium is incorrect?
a. Benzodiazepines should be avoided because they can exacerbate delirium.
b. Behaviour, not amenable to other interventions such as gentle reassurance, may respond to treatment like antipsychotics.
c. Haloperidol is the most frequently used in this situation, as it is generally effective and safe.
d. Second-generation antipsychotics are indicated for patients who are prone to extrapyramidal side effects.
e. Psychotropic medications should be commenced for the treatment of hypoactive delirium.

Question 50

Approximately what percentage of elderly patients suffer from somatization disorders?

a. 1%
b. 2%
c. 3%
d. 4%
e. 5%

Question 51
Which of the following statements regarding the work of Hayflick is true?
a. Cells double at a rate that is inversely proportional to age.
b. Cells double at a rate that is proportional to age.
c. Cells triple at a rate that is proportional to age.
d. Death of a cell line is not usually caused by faulty laboratory techniques.
e. No human cell may be immortal.

Question 52
A 40-year-old woman was scolded by her boss for being slow and for making mistakes at work. Her boss threatens to dismiss her. At home that night, she tells her husband all the details involving her boss scolding her and her thinking about what she could have done. Which of the following defence mechanisms is this?
a. Displacement
b. Intellectualization
c. Rationalization
d. Regression
e. Undoing

Question 53
Which of the following is not a characteristic of Milieu Group Therapy?
a. Communalism
b. Democratization
c. Permissiveness
d. Psychodrama
e. Reality confrontation

Question 54
Which of the following is the most important factor for effective psychotherapy?
a. Age of patient
b. Empathy of therapist
c. Frequency of sessions
d. Psychological mindedness
e. Therapeutic alliance

Question 55
Childhood-onset bipolar disorder has been known to be rare. Which of the following psychiatric comorbidities is it commonly associated with?
a. ADHD
b. Autistic spectrum disorder

c. Separation anxiety disorder

d. Enuresis

e. Selective mutism

Question 56

A 50-year-old woman has strong family history of depression, and she is being prescribed with venlafaxine 225 mg ON and mirtazapine 45 mg ON for 6 months. She is admitted for severe depressive episode, but she refuses electroconvulsive therapy (ECT) and psychotherapy. She does not have any other medical illnesses. Which of the following treatment strategies is recommended?

a. Augment with mianserin, continue with venlafaxine and mirtazapine

b. Augment with mianserin, continue with venlafaxine but stop mirtazapine

c. Augment with lithium, continue with venlafaxine and mirtazapine

d. Augment with lithium, continue with venlafaxine but stop mirtazapine

e. Augment with lamotrigine, continue with venlafaxine and mirtazapine

Question 57

A 20-year-old woman suffers from anorexia nervosa, and she is 30 weeks' pregnant. The neonatologist consults you on the potential complications for her foetus. Which of the following is not known to be found in foetuses born by mothers suffering from anorexia nervosa?

a. Appearance, Pulse, Grimace, Activity, Respiration (APGAR) score of 2 at 1 minute and 3 at 5 minutes

b. Small head circumference

c. Low birth weight

d. Small for gestational age

e. Microcephaly at 3 years old

Question 58

A core trainee has informed you that a patient taking quetiapine has developed amenorrhoea with raised prolactin. Which one of the following actions is correct?

a. Reassure the patient that it is due to quetiapine

b. No further intervention and check the prolactin level in 3 months

c. Order a computed tomography (CT) brain scan

d. Order a magnetic resonance imaging (MRI) brain scan

e. Prescribe bromocriptine

Question 59

A 55-year-old woman was admitted to the psychiatric ward after the accidental death of her son, which occurred 3 months ago. She complains of low mood, poor sleep, poor appetite and hearing her son's voice. What is the diagnosis?

a. Bereavement – phase I: shock and protest

b. Bereavement – phase II: preoccupation

c. Bereavement – phase III: disorganization
d. Major depressive disorder
e. Pathological grief

Question 60

A 20-year-old university student attested to the consumption of cannabis out of curiosity. He has just consumed it around 4 hours again. Which of the following is not one of the symptoms he would experience?
a. Decreased appetite
b. Conjunctival injection
c. Impaired reaction time
d. Impaired judgement and attention
e. Paranoid ideations

Question 61

Interpersonal psychotherapy (IPT) is a form of talking therapy for treating depression. Which of the following is not a component of this therapy?
a. Grief
b. Interpersonal disputes
c. Interpersonal deficits
d. Psychodynamic conflicts
e. Role transitions

Question 62

Behaviour activation in psychotherapy includes which of the following?
a. Identifying maladaptive core belief
b. Formulate alternative positive belief
c. Graded assignment on exposure
d. Pleasure and mastery
e. Activity scheduling

Question 63

A 67-year-old man with terminal lung cancer consciously puts his illness 'out of his mind' and tries to enjoy life to the maximum by doing voluntary work. Which of the following defence mechanisms is he using?
a. Displacement
b. Reaction formation
c. Repression
d. Sublimation
e. Suppression

Question 64

Approximately what percentage of adolescent males will kill themselves within 5 years after their first episode of suicide attempt?
a. 1%
b. 5%

c. 7%
d. 9%
e. 11%

Question 65

Which of the following is not one of the biological factors commonly associated with children who are diagnosed with conduct disorder?
a. Low plasma serotonin level
b. High plasma dopamine level
c. Excess testosterone excess
d. Low cholesterol
e. Low skin tolerance

Question 66

Which of the following EEG findings is most typical of patients with delirium?
a. Delta bursts
b. Diffuse slowing
c. Frontocentral spikes
d. High-voltage fast activity
e. Intermittent high and low voltage activities

Question 67

Which of the following helps to differentiate hyperactive from hypoactive delirium?
a. EEG shows diffuse increased activity for hyperactive delirium and diffuse slowing for hypoactive delirium.
b. Patients with hyperactive delirium are more responsive to neuroleptics than those with hypoactive delirium.
c. Patients with hyperactive delirium have higher mortality rates than those with hypoactive delirium.
d. Patients with hyperactive delirium have global cognitive deficits, while those with hypoactive delirium have selected cognitive deficits.
e. Patients with hyperactive delirium demonstrate features of restlessness, agitation and hyper vigilance, while patients with hypoactive delirium present with lethargy, sedation and respond slowly to questioning.

Question 68

Which of the following cancers is not generally associated with a significantly higher risk of depression?
a. Brain cancer
b. Lung cancer
c. Oropharyngeal cancer
d. Pancreatic cancer
e. Skin cancer

Question 69

Which of the following antidepressants would you prescribe for a medically ill patient who is depressed and suffers from insomnia and poor appetite?

a. Bupropion
b. Methylphenidate
c. Moclobemide
d. Mirtazepine
e. Venlafaxine

Question 70

Which of the following statements about epileptic psychosis is false?
a. Chronic interictal psychosis is more common than postictal psychosis.
b. Mesial temporal focus is a risk factor for interictal psychosis.
c. Postictal psychosis follows an increase in seizure frequency.
d. Psychotic symptoms are more common with left-sided seizure foci or temporal lobe lesions.
e. Postictal psychotic symptoms occur immediately following a seizure.

Question 71

A woman was arrested after killing her 10-month-old daughter. The infant is described to be very noisy and cried excessively. Which of the following conditions is the most common predisposing factor?
a. Battering father
b. Battering mother
c. Elder brother with conduct disorder
d. Mother suffering from depression
e. Father suffering from depression

Question 72

A 25-year-old married woman with a history of anorexia nervosa of 8 years of duration presents to an obstetrician asking for help with infertility. She wants medication to induce ovulation as she does not have menses. She keeps her body mass index (BMI) strictly at 12, eats mainly vegetables and jogs 2 km every day. She is determined that she will not gain weight. The obstetrician is worried by her request. He seeks a consultation from you. Which of the following recommendations is inappropriate?
a. To highlight to the obstetrician the ambivalence inherent in her request.
b. To explore the symbolic significance of bypassing the normal conception to achieve motherhood.
c. To take a full developmental history, paying particular attention to her psychosexual development and conflicts with her own parents.
d. To explore the psychodynamic issues relating to the patient and her partner.
e. To respect her request to become pregnant and offer the best intervention to induce ovulation.

Question 73

A 20-year-old university student presents for a consultation. She is very concerned that she might acquire schizophrenia, as her distant relative has been recently

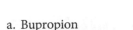

diagnosed with the condition. She is keen to know the average age of onset of schizophrenia. Which of the following is true?
a. 15–20 years
b. 21–30 years
c. 31–40 years
d. 40–50 years
e. 50–60 years

Question 74

A patient on follow-up with the cardiologist for heart problems complains of low mood and seeing yellow rings around objects in his visual field. Which of the following medications could possibly be responsible for his symptoms?
a. Alpha-blocker
b. Beta-blocker
c. Clonidine
d. Digoxin
e. Reserpine

Question 75

For which of the following conditions would speech therapy be useful for symptomatic relief?
a. Cyclic vomiting
b. Functional abdominal pain
c. Gastroesophageal reflux
d. Globus
e. Inflammatory bowel syndrome

Question 76

Which of the following antidepressants has been shown to be of most benefit in irritable bowel syndrome (IBS)?
a. Dopaminergic antidepressant
b. Monoamine oxidase inhibitors
c. Selective serotonin reuptake inhibitors
d. Selective noradrenaline reuptake inhibitors
e. Tricyclic antidepressants

Question 77

A 35-year-old woman is 12 weeks pregnant. She is having a relapse of her depression. Which of the following antidepressants is contraindicated for her?
a. Citalopram
b. Fluoxetine
c. Fluvoxamine
d. Duloxetine
e. Paroxetine

Question 78

Melancholic depression has been considered to be of biological origin. All the following are characteristic symptoms of this condition, with the exception of

a. Motor agitation
b. Excessive guilt
c. Loss of interest
d. Excessive guilt
e. Initial insomnia

Question 79
Which of the following options describes the most frequently reported psychiatric symptoms reported by the elderly?
a. Anxiety and depression
b. Anxiety and insomnia
c. Depression and fatigue
d. Depression and insomnia
e. Insomnia and fatigue

Question 80
Which of the following statements regarding suicide in the elderly is true?
a. The highest rate is in black men above the age of 70 years.
b. The highest rate is in white men above the age of 70 years.
c. It is inversely correlated with age.
d. It is associated with cognitive impairment in the elderly.
e. It is not preventable.

Question 81
With regard to the cognition changes involved in ageing, which of the following statements is not true?
a. Intelligence peaks at the age of 25 years and levels off until the age of 60–70 years before declining further.
b. Memory tests, such as the Wechsler Adult Intelligence Scale (WAIS) Revised inventory, show a classical pattern of intellectual decline, with verbal intelligence quotient (IQ) declining more than performance IQ.
c. Tasks that have been learnt over a lifetime, relying on over-learned abilities, are more resistant to age-related changes.
d. The ability to abstract a concept and apply it to a new situation declines with age, most prominently after the age of 70 years.
e. Reaction time is noted to increase with ageing.

Question 82
All the following are characteristic diagnostic features for patients with fronto-temporal lobe dementia, with the exception of
a. Severe apathy
b. Disinhibition
c. Presence of primitive reflexes
d. Relatively mild impairment in construction
e. Hyper-sexuality

Question 83

All the following statements about the psychopathology of old-age psychotic disorder are true, with the exception of which one?

a. Almost all have at least one type of delusional belief.
b. Approximately 45% of them have first-rank symptoms.
c. The most common type of hallucination in the elderly is visual hallucinations.
d. Thought disorder and catatonic symptoms rarely develop.
e. Negative symptoms might be seen but tend to be very mild.

Question 84

Which of the following statements regarding Graves disease and psychiatric symptoms is false?

a. Anti-thyroid therapy is associated with improvement in depressive symptoms.
b. Common symptoms reported by patients with Graves disease include tremors, irritability and anxiety.
c. Graves disease is associated with hypomania.
d. Hyperthyroidism with anxious dysphoria is more common in older patients.
e. The severity of psychiatric symptoms correlates poorly with thyroid hormone levels in patients with Graves disease.

Question 85

Which of the following symptoms is not typical of a patient presenting with depression associated with Cushing syndrome?

a. Hypersomnia
b. Insomnia
c. Irritability
d. Poor concentration
e. Poor energy

Question 86

Which of the following types of cancer is least associated with depression?

a. Breast cancer
b. Lung cancer
c. Lymphoma
d. Oropharyngeal cancer
e. Pancreatic cancer

Question 87

A 25-year-old woman has been diagnosed with depression and has been started on an older generation of medication known as an MAOI. She is aware that there are certain foods she needs to avoid. She was taken ill recently and consulted a physician at the emergency services. In view of her persistent abdominal pain, she was administered a dose of opioid analgesic. This increases the incidence of her having which of the following conditions?

a. Serotonin syndrome
b. Neuroleptic malignant syndrome
c. Opioid toxicity
d. Acute liver impairment
e. Cardiac arrhythmia

Question 88
All the following antidepressants are safe for use in mothers who are breastfeeding with the exception of?
a. Fluoxetine
b. Paroxetine
c. Sertraline
d. Imipramine
e. Nortriptyline

Question 89
Based on current research, a maintenance strategy using lithium carbonate mono-therapy in bipolar disorder is likely to result in remission in approximately what percentage of individuals?
a. 5%
b. 10%
c. 20%
d. 30%
e. 50%

Question 90
Which of the following symptoms of obsessive-compulsive disorder is most resistant to treatment?
a. Checking
b. Counting
c. Washing
d. Doubting
e. Hoarding

Question 91
Clomipramine and SSRIs antidepressants are commonly being used to treat obsessive-compulsive disorder. What is the approximate response rate?
a. 10%
b. 20%
c. 30%
d. 50%
e. 90%

Question 92
With regard to the pharmacological management of post-traumatic stress disorder (PTSD), which of the following medications would be helpful in reducing the amount of fear-induced startle?
a. Buspirone
b. Carbamazepine
c. Fluoxetine
d. Paroxetine
e. Sertraline

Question 93

Which of the following defence mechanisms has the highest degree of adaptivity?
a. Delusional projection
b. Humour
c. Idealization
d. Psychotic denial
e. Reaction formation

Question 94

Which of the following is uncommonly associated with pica?
a. Learning disability
b. Psychosis
c. Eating non-nutritive substances
d. Iron deficiency anaemia
e. Lead poisoning

Question 95

A 20-year-old man admits to the occasional use of 'coke'. His last use was just yesterday. How long would 'coke' remain in the urine sample, for the sample to be test positive?
a. 6–8 hours
b. 24 hours
c. 72 hours
d. 8 days
e. 1 week

Question 96

With regard to the genetic disorder known commonly as Digeorge syndrome, which of the following psychiatric disorders is a common comorbidity?
a. Obsessive-compulsive disorder
b. Generalized anxiety disorder
c. Depressive disorder
d. Schizophrenia
e. Attention deficit hyperactivity disorder

Question 97

Fragile X syndrome is known to be the most common inherited cause of learning disability. It accounts for around 10%–12% of mental retardation in men. Which of the following statements about the condition is incorrect?
a. It is an X-linked dominant genetic disorder with low penetrance.
b. The disorder is due to the presence of more than 200 tri-nucleotide CGG repeats.
c. The presence of tri-nucleotide repeats would lead to hyper-methylation at the fragile X mental retardation gene.
d. Only males are affected by this disorder.
e. The length of the repeats is inversely related to the intelligence quotient.

Question 98

What is the incidence of epilepsy in Rett syndrome?

a. 10%
b. 20%
c. 40%
d. 50%
e. 60% and higher

Question 99
Which of the following statements is false regarding Lesch–Nyhan disease?
a. Hyperuricaemia is a rare feature in the variant form.
b. Hypoxanthine–guanine phosphoribosyl transferase activity is grossly reduced or absent.
c. It is associated with movement disorder.
d. It is an X-linked recessive disorder.
e. The variant form presents later and is less severe and without any self-mutilation.

Question 100
Which of the following is the most frequent cutaneous manifestation of tuberous sclerosis?
a. Adenoma sebaceum
b. Axillary freckles
c. Butterfly rash
d. Café au lait spots
e. Hypomelanotic macules

Question 101
A 10-year-old girl is noted to be always happy and smiling. She has jerking movement and ataxic gait. She has a history of epilepsy, and she studies in a special school. Which chromosome would be affected in her presentation?
a. Chromosome 5
b. Chromosome 9
c. Chromosome 10
d. Chromosome 15
e. Chromosome 22

Question 102
Children who are depressed tend to present more with which of the following symptoms, compared with adults?
a. Low depressed mood
b. Marked loss of interest
c. Poor appetite
d. Mood congruent psychotic symptoms
e. Somatic complaints

Question 103
Which of the following statements is false about the findings from multimodal treatment study (MTA) on ADHD?
a. There is a small but detectible reduction in overall growth in height for children who remain on stimulants.
b. Loss of growth is maximal in the first year of treatment.

c. 35% showed a moderate and gradual improvement, and 50% showed significant improvement over the 3-year study period.
d. 15% initially responded well but deteriorated over 3 years.
e. Drug treatment reduces the rate of delinquency and substance abuse in children with ADHD to the rate found in normal controls.

Question 104
For adolescent-onset bipolar disorder, what percentage of adolescents has first-rank symptoms?
a. 2%
b. 5%
c. 10%
d. 15%
e. 20%

Question 105
What is the approximate heritability of autism?
a. 10%
b. 50%
c. 70%
d. 80%
e. 90%

Question 106
A medical student is currently on attachment to the Child and Adolescent Mental Health Services (CAMHS) unit. Of note, he has seen two children been diagnosed with chronic motor and vocal tics. With regard to the prognosis of the condition, you will advise the medical student that the disorder usually lasts for approximately how long before eventually stopping?
a. 6 months
b. 8 months
c. 1 year
d. 2 years
e. 4 years

Question 107
Which one of the following statements regarding conduct disorder is false?
a. It begins in early childhood.
b. It is associated with a low plasma 5-hydroxytryptamine (5-HT) level.
c. It is associated with reading difficulty.
d. It is associated with overcrowding (>four children) environment.
e. Male-to-female ratio is 3:1.

Question 108
With regard to the pharmacological treatment of PTSD, which of the following medications would be helpful in reducing the hyper-arousal and intrusive symptoms?

a. Buspirone
b. Carbamazepine
c. Fluoxetine
d. Lithium
e. Propranolol

Question 109

Which of the following statements about the aetiological factors pertaining to PTSD is false?
a. The exaggerated physiological responses are mediated by both the noradrenergic and dopaminergic neurotransmitter systems.
b. There is an increase in the glucocorticoid receptors in the hippocampus.
c. There is a corresponding reduction in the peripheral cortisol.
d. There is a possible catecholaminergic mediation of PTSD symptoms.
e. Opioid functions have been proposed to be disturbed in PTSD.

Question 110

An 8-year-old boy has frequent loss of temper, arguments with parents and feels irritable at home but not at school. These symptoms have persisted for 8 months. Which of the following treatments would you recommend?
a. Cognitive behavioural therapy (CBT)
b. Fluoxetine
c. Multisystemic therapy
d. Parent management training
e. Risperidone

Question 111

Which of the following is a 3-year-old child able to do if he or she has normal motor developmental milestones?
a. Build a tower of 10 cubes
b. Copy a square
c. Stand on one foot
d. Build a tower of 10 cubes and copy a square
e. Build a tower of 10 cubes and stand on one foot

Extended Match Items

Theme: Research Methodology

Options:
a. Level 1A
b. Level 1B
c. Level 1C
d. Level 2A
e. Level 2B
f. Level 2C
g. Level 3A

h. Level 3B
i. Level 4
j. Level 5

Lead in: Match one correct hierarchy of research evidence with each of the following study types. Each option may be used once, more than once or not at all.

Question 112
Individual cohort study. (Choose one option.)

Question 113
Individual randomized controlled trials. (Choose one option.)

Question 114
Individual case–control studies. (Choose one option.)

Theme: Research Methodology

Options:
   a. Case–control study
   b. Cohort study
   c. Cross-sectional study
   d. Ecological study
   e. RCT

Lead in: Select one appropriate study design to match each scenario below. Each option may be used once, more than once or not at all.

Question 115
A study aims to determine the effects of cannabis misuse on the incidence of schizophrenia in a community. (Choose one option.)

Question 116
A study aims to find out if alcohol dependence is a risk factor for morbid jealousy in a community. (Choose one option.)

Question 117
A study examines the data from 23 member states of the European Union and investigates whether television exposure is related to fear of terrorism. This study is controlled for population size, education level, age distribution and income. (Choose one option.)

Question 118
A study aims to find out if long-term aspirin use in patients with ischaemic heart disease protects against dementia. (Choose one option.)

Question 119
A study aims to find out the prevalence of schizophrenia in San Francisco. (Choose one option.)

Theme: Dementia

Options:
a. Alzheimer's disease
b. Binswanger disease
c. Cerebral autosomal dominant arteriopathy with subcortical infarcts and leukoencephalopathy (CADASIL)
d. Fronto-temporal lobe dementia (Pick disease)
e. Korsakoff psychosis
f. Lewy body dementia
g. Normal pressure hydrocephalus
h. Psychogenic fugue
i. Pseudodementia
j. Vascular dementia
k. Wernicke encephalopathy

Lead in: Match one appropriate diagnosis to each clinical scenario. Each option may be used once, more than once or not at all.

Question 120
A 35-year-old woman presents with irritability and increasing inability to concentrate. She is also getting more forgetful, and she finds herself having difficulty walking. She has had two seizures over the last 3 months. On further enquiry, her aunt also has similar problems. (Choose one option.)

Question 121
A 54-year-old man presents with a gradual change in behaviour over the past 2 years. He was previously soft-spoken and reserved but is now very vocal and argumentative. He insists on driving despite having previously knocked into curbs because of poor judgement. He does not consider himself to be forgetful. (Choose one option.)

Question 122
A 45-year-old woman lost her husband in a fire 2 months ago. Since then, she has been complaining of persistent memory loss and forgetfulness. She is also lethargic, has no appetite and is not sleeping well. When she is asked to perform the Mini Mental State Examination, most of her answers are 'I don't know'. (Choose one option.)

Question 123
A 55-year-old man fell off a ladder and knocked his head against a wall about 2 weeks ago. Since then, he has been having memory problems, difficulty walking and difficulty passing urine. (Choose one option.)

Theme: Dementia

Options:
a. Alzheimer's disease
b. Binswanger disease

c. CADASIL
d. Fronto-temporal lobe dementia (Pick disease)
e. Korsakoff psychosis
f. Lewy body dementia
g. Normal pressure hydrocephalus
h. Psychogenic fugue
i. Pseudodementia
j. Vascular dementia
k. Wernicke encephalopathy

Lead in: Match one appropriate diagnosis to each clinical scenario. Each option may be used once, more than once or not at all.

Question 124

A 60-year-old woman is brought in by the police for psychiatric assessment, as she was found wandering around the streets. She is unable to provide any personal details about herself and appears to be in a daze. Her son, with whom she is very close, died in a road traffic accident a few days ago. All physical investigations are normal. (Choose one option.)

Question 125

A 65-year-old man presents with fluctuating memory loss with mood swings. He has slurred speech and left-sided muscle weakness. He has multiple medical comorbidities, including poorly controlled hypertension and diabetes. (Choose one option.)

Question 126

A 75-year-old woman presents with memory loss, fluctuating consciousness and poor gait. She has very few facial expressions and appears to be stiff on walking. She has had several falls over the course of 6 months. She also mentions that she sees little children running across the ward in the middle of the night. (Choose one option.)

Question 127

A 60-year-old man is brought in by the police to the hospital for assessment, as he was found wandering the streets. When the doctor speaks to him, he says that he is here to meet a friend who was hospitalized and that he has seen the doctor before. Medical records show that he has been a chronic heavy alcohol drinker. (Choose one option.)

Question 128

A 25-year-old woman with a diagnosis of anorexia nervosa is brought in to the hospital after she fainted while running on the treadmill for 2 hours. Her BMI is 15. According to her family, she has been refusing food and taking medication to induce vomiting. She is given intravenous dextrose solution for fluid replacement in the emergency department. She subsequently becomes confused, and neurological examination reveals horizontal diplopia and ataxia. Her family says that she does habitually drink alcohol. (Choose one option.)

Theme: Gender Ratios

Options:
  a. 1:1
  b. 1:2
  c. 2:1
  d. 3:1
  e. 1:3
  f. 1:10
  g. 10:1

Lead in: Match one male-to-female ratio to each of the following questions. Each option may be used once, more than once or not at all.

Question 129
Anorexia nervosa. (Choose one option.)

Question 130
Bulimia nervosa. (Choose one option.)

Question 131
Post-traumatic stress disorder. (Choose one option.)

Question 132
Social phobia. (Choose one option.)

Question 133
Suicide. (Choose one option.)

Question 134
Depressive disorder. (Choose one option.)

Question 135
Schizophrenia. (Choose one option.)

Theme: Learning Disability

Options:
  a. Cri du chat syndrome
  b. Homocystinuria
  c. Phenylketonuria
  d. Prader–Willi syndrome
  e. Neurofibromatosis

Lead in: Match one correct syndrome to each of the following clinical phenotypes. Each option may be used once, more than once or not at all.

Question 136
Short stature. (Choose one option.)

Question 137
Tall stature. (Choose one option.)

Question 138
Microcephaly. (Choose one option.)

Question 139
Macrocephaly. (Choose one option.)

Question 140
Hyperactivity and aggression. (Choose one option.)

Theme: Liver Impairment and Medications
Options:
a. Haloperidol
b. Chlorpromazine
c. Paroxetine
d. Citalopram
e. Tricyclic antidepressant
f. Fluoxetine
g. Lithium
h. Carbamazepine
i. Valproate

Lead in: For patients with liver impairment, match the correct drugs to the following statements. Each option may be used once, more than once or not at all.

Question 141
Which antipsychotic is not recommended for patients with liver impairment? (Choose one option.)

Question 142
Which antidepressants could be used for patients with liver impairment? (Choose two options.)

Question 143
Which mood stabilizers are indicated for patients with liver impairment? (Choose one option.)

Question 144
Which mood stabilizers are not indicated for patients with liver impairment? (Choose two options.)

Theme: Infectious Disease and Psychiatry
Options:
a. Acute stress reaction
b. Adjustment disorder

c. Depressive disorder
d. Mania
e. Cognitive impairment
f. Dementia

Lead in: Match one diagnosis to each of the following statements. Each option may be used once, more than once or not at all.

Question 145
The prevalence of this psychiatric condition in patients with HIV is around 1.5%. If it presents early in the course of the infection, it is usually associated with social problems. If it presents late in the course of the HIV infection, it is usually associated with HIV dementia. Which psychiatric condition is this? (Choose one option.)

Question 146
This is a common psychiatric condition that usually occurs immediately after the diagnosis of HIV infection. The patient may present in a state of shock, with depersonalization and de-realization. (Choose one option.)

Question 147
The prevalence of this psychiatric condition in people with HIV is around 30%. It is more frequent in the period following the identification of the seropositive HIV infection or even in the initial stages of HIV dementia. (Choose one option.)

Question 148
This usually occurs late into the course of the illness, especially when there is significant immunosuppression. (Choose one option.)

Theme: Prevalence of Mental Retardation
Options:
   a. 1%
   b. 2%
   c. 3%
   d. 5%
   e. 10%
   f. 20%
   g. 50%
   h. 80%
   i. 90%

Lead in: Match one number to each of the following statements. Each option may be used once, more than once or not at all.

Question 149
Mild mental retardation accounts for approximately what percentage of all learning disabilities? (Choose one option.)

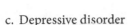

Question 150

Moderate mental retardation accounts for approximately what percentage of all learning disabilities? (Choose one option.)

Question 151

Severe mental retardation accounts for approximately what percentage of all learning disabilities? (Choose one option.)

Question 152

Profound mental retardation accounts for approximately what percentage of all learning disabilities? (Choose one option.)

Theme: Features of Learning Disabilities

Options:
   a. Conductive deafness
   b. Almond-shaped eyes slanting laterally upwards
   c. Prominent epicanthic folds
   d. Macrocephaly
   e. Gaze aversion
   f. High-arched palate
   g. Wide sandal gap between first and second toes
   h. Shield-shaped thorax
   i. Widely spaced nipples
   j. Rudimentary ovaries
   k. Testicular atrophy and infertility

Lead in: Match the correct features to each of the following statements. Each option may be used once, more than once or not at all.

Question 153

Which is a characteristic feature of Klinefelter syndrome? (Choose one option.)

Question 154

Which are characteristic features of fragile X syndrome? (Choose three options.)

Question 155

Which are characteristic features of Down syndrome? (Choose four options.)

Question 156

Which are characteristic features of Turner syndrome? (Choose four options.)

Theme: Research Methodologies and Statistics

Options:
   a. Fixed-effect meta-regression
   b. Mixed-effects meta-regression
   c. Multivariate meta-regression
   d. Simple meta-regression
   e. Univariate meta-regression

Lead in: Match one regression model with each of the following descriptions. Each option may be used once, more than once or not at all.

Question 157
This model allows for within-study variability only. (Choose one option.)

Question 158
This model allows for within- and between-study variation and adds in the effects of moderators. (Choose one option.)

Question 159
This model does not allow specification of within-study variation. (Choose one option.)

Theme: Immune-Related Disorders

Options:
a. Encephalopathy
b. Limbic encephalitis
c. Multiple sclerosis
d. Systemic lupus erythematosus
e. Sclerosis
f. Rheumatoid arthritis
g. Sarcoidosis

Lead in: Which of the above-mentioned immune-mediated disorders is most likely to be the cause for each of the following?

Question 160
A 35-year-old man has a long-standing history of chronic cough as well as associated dyspnoea. He has not been a smoker all his life and has not been exposed to passive smoking. Recently, he decided to seek a consult, as he finds that he has been having difficulties with his memories. In addition, he has been having some fixed and unshakable beliefs.

Question 161
A 25-year-old university student is here for a consultation with the General Psychiatry service. She reports feeling increasingly low in her mood with associated symptoms of marked lethargy. She shared that a few months ago, her friends and family commented that she has had a malar rash on her face.

Question 162
A 25-year-old woman has been having symptoms of hypersomnolence despite having a good night's rest. Her general practitioner (GP) has ran some routine labs, and it was noted that she has elevated calcium levels.

Theme: Consultation Liaison Psychiatry

Options:
  a. Huntington's disease
  b. Multiple sclerosis
  c. Amyotrophic lateral sclerosis (ALS)
  d. Parkinson disease
  e. Progressive supranuclear palsy (PSP)
  f. Spinocerebellar ataxia

Lead in: Which of the above-mentioned immune-mediated disorders is most likely to be the cause for each of the following?

Question 163
A 65-year-old man has been referred to the psycho-geriatrics service for worsening visual hallucinations. On clinical examination, the core trainee noted that the patient has rather severe tremors, which are predominantly on the right side. In addition, reduced arm swing and a typical gait (small steps and shuffling gait) were noted.

Question 164
A 38-year-old man has been referred to the psychiatrist for an evaluation by his neurologist. Of note, his family has noted that he would cry uncontrollably at times without any reasons. Of late, he has been requiring more assistance in his activities of daily living from his family members.

Question 165
A 60-year-old woman has been referred as she has been having much memory impairment of late. In addition, she has been having frequent falls as well.

Question 166
A 26-year-old man has been referred to the psychiatrist for an assessment. Of late, his wife has noted that he has a marked change in terms of his personality. At times, he has been noted to be irritable and impulsive. In addition, he has been noted to be increasingly clumsy.

Theme: Schizophrenia and Psychosis

Options:
  a. No increase in risk
  b. Two fold increment
  c. Four fold increment
  d. Six fold increment
  e. Ten fold increment

Lead in: Please select the correct option for each of the following:

Question 167
What is the increase in risk of acquiring schizophrenia if a person is of the male gender?

Question 168
What is the increase in risk of acquiring schizophrenia if an individual is of Afro-Caribbean ethnicity in the United Kingdom?

Question 169
What is the increase in risk of an individual acquiring schizophrenia if he has been using cannabis on a long-term basis?

Question 170
What is the increase in risk of an individual acquiring psychosis if he has been using cannabis on a long-term basis?

Theme: Mood and Affective Disorders

Options:
a. Step 1
b. Step 2
c. Step 3
d. Step 4
e. Step 5

Lead in: Based on your understanding of the NICE stepped care model for depressive disorder, please select from the above-mentioned options for each of the following questions.

Question 171
In this particular step, only assessment is involved.

Question 172
In this particular step, ECT is indicated.

Question 173
In this particular step, complex psychological interventions are recommended.

Question 174
In this particular step, watching waiting is recommended

Question 175
In this particular step, computerized CBT is an indication.

Theme: General Adult Psychiatry – Treatment

Options:
a. Listen to loud stimulating music to drown out the auditory hallucinations not responding to antipsychotic treatment
b. Maintenance in antipsychotic treatment
c. Psychoeducation about schizophrenia
d. Reduction in perinatal trauma
e. Reduction in stress associated with migration

f. Successful treatment of middle-ear disease in childhood
g. Teaching problem-solving skills

Lead in: The Department of Health has devised various strategies to prevent schizophrenia in the United Kingdom. Classify the above-mentioned prevention strategies into the following type of prevention. Each option may be used once, more than once or not at all.

Question 176
Primary prevention. (Choose three options.)

Question 177
Secondary prevention. (Choose two options.)

Question 178
Tertiary prevention. (Choose one option.)

Theme: Psychotherapy
Options:
 a. Aversive conditioning
 b. Chaining
 c. Flooding
 d. Habituation
 e. Insight learning
 f. Latent learning
 g. Penalty
 h. Premack's principle
 i. Reciprocal inhibition
 j. Shaping
 k. Systematic desensitization
 l. Token economy

Lead in: From the above-mentioned list of behavioural techniques, select the option that best matches each of the following examples. Each option might be used once, more than once or not at all.

Question 179
The staff of a hostel for learning disability patients want to train their clients to clean up the tables after meals. They develop a successive reinforcing schedule to reward their clients. The clients will be rewarded successively over time for removing their utensils from the dining table into the kitchen. Then they need to wash and dry the utensils and put them back into the right drawers. (Choose one option.)

Question 180
A 2-year-old son of a woman is scared of dogs. His mother tries to reduce his fear by bringing him to see the dogs in the park. The fear-provoking situation is coupled and opposed by putting him on her lap and allowing him to drink his favourite juice. (Choose one option.)

Question 181
A 40-year-old woman staying in London develops fear of the tube (underground metro), and she sees a psychologist for psychotherapy. The psychologist has drafted a behavioural programme in which the patient is advised to start with travelling between two tube stations with her husband and gradually increase this to more stations without her husband. At the end of the hierarchy, she will travel alone on the long journey from a Heathrow terminal station to Cockfosters station along almost the entire length of the Piccadilly line. (Choose one option.)

Theme: Effect on the Newborn Due to Substance Abuse
Options:
  a. Alcohol
  b. Benzodiazepine
  c. Opiate
  d. Tobacco

Lead in: Match the above-mentioned substance misuse to the following situations where the mothers took the substance throughout the pregnancy. Each option might be used more than once.

Question 182
The neonate developed floppy baby syndrome after he was born. On physical examination, it was noted to have cleft palate.

Question 183
The 4-year-old child developed attention deficit and hyperactivity.

Question 184
The infant was noted to be irritable. On physical examination, he has a small head with short eye openings. The cardiovascular examination reveals a heart murmur. The health visitor measures his length regularly, and it is obvious that the infant has growth retardation.

Question 185
The infant develops fever, inability to sleep, and poor feeding 3 days after birth. Due to repeating vomiting and diarrhoea, he appears to be dehydrated with poor weight gain since birth. On physical examination, he appears to be irritable and exhibits yawning and sneezing. The tone in upper limbs and lower limbs is increased.

Theme: Eating Disorders
Options:
  a. Anorexia nervosa
  b. Coeliac disease
  c. Crohn's disease
  d. Hyperthyroidism
  e. Iatrogenic cause
  f. Whipple's disease

Lead in: Match the above-mentioned causes of weight loss to the following situations. Each option might be used more than once.

Question 186

A 68-year-old woman with history of diabetes was referred by the geriatrician for assessment for depression. She complains of low mood and weight loss. Physical examination reveals oedema in her lower limbs. Echocardiogram shows congestive heart failure. Her medications include fluoxetine, metformin and furosemide.

Question 187

A 40-year-old Irish woman was referred by her GP for assessment of depression. She complains of having lethargy, frequent diarrhoea with offensive stool and weight loss. She appears to be pale, and physical examination shows clubbing, abdominal distension and oral ulceration. Barium follow-through is abnormal. Her medications include iron and vitamin D supplements.

Question 189

A 16-year-old girl was referred by the paediatrician for assessment of depression. She was admitted due to fever, weight loss, diarrhoea and abdominal pain. She appears to be thin and pale. Physical examination shows clubbing, aphthous ulceration, abdominal tenderness and perianal skin tags. She is a smoker. Her medication includes paracetamol, and she is currently nil by mouth.

Question 190

A 40-year-old man was referred by the rheumatologist for assessment of depression. He complains of weight loss and migratory polyarthritis and appears to be pale. Physical examination reveals clubbing and pigmentation. His medications include sulphamethoxazole and trimethoprin.

Question 191

A 30-year-old woman was referred by her GP for the management of depression and anxiety. She complains of loose stool, palpitations and tremor. Her hair appears to be very wet, as if she has just washed her hair without drying. Her medication includes alprazolam 0.25 mg thrice a day (TDS).

Question 192

A 16-year-old male adolescent was referred to you by the paediatrician after a suicide attempt. He had recently broken up with his girlfriend. He was criticized of being too fat. He has rapid weight loss, and he is still very dissatisfied with his body shape. He is very preoccupied with the amount of calories consumed and tries to avoid all carbohydrate- or lipid-rich foods.

MRCPYSCH PAPER B MOCK EXAMINATION 4: ANSWERS

GET THROUGH MRCPSYCH PAPER B MOCK EXAMINATION

Question 1 Answer: e, No moderator could explain heterogeneity
Explanation: The authors performed meta-regression and found that mean age ($p = 0.086$), mean forced expiratory volume in 1 second (FEV$_1$)($p = 0.715$), proportion of gender ($p = 0.478$) and proportion of current smokers ($p = 0.622$) among patients with chronic obstructive pulmonary disease (COPD) were not significant moderators and did not explain the heterogeneity in prevalence of depressive symptoms among patients with COPD, because the p values are larger than 0.05. As a result, none of the moderators explain heterogeneity.

Reference: Zhang MW, Ho RC, Cheung MW, Fu E, Mak A (2011). Prevalence of depressive symptoms in patients with chronic obstructive pulmonary disease: A systematic review, meta-analysis and meta-regression. *Gen Hosp Psychiatry*, 33(3): 217–223.

Question 2 Answer: e, The prevalence of depression rated by clinicians and patients with COPD demonstrates no significant difference
Explanation: In meta-analysis, studies can be further classified, and pooled results are compared based on different subgroups. There is no difference in prevalence of depression between clinician-rating versus self-rating ($p = 0.163$) and Western countries versus non-Western countries ($p = 0.435$). As a result, the prevalence of depression rated by clinicians and patients with COPD demonstrates no significant difference.

Question 3 Answer: a, There is a probability of 5% or less of happening by chance if the true prevalence of depression in patients with COPD lies outside the interval (21.2%–35.2%)
Explanation: MRCPsych candidates and researchers often have misunderstanding of the 95% interval. In fact, the 95% confidence interval reflects a significance level of 0.05. In Table 7.2, there is a probability of 5% or less of happening by chance if the true prevalence of depression in patients with COPD lies outside the interval (21.2%–35.2%). A 95% confidence interval does not mean that there is a 95% probability that the true prevalence of depression in patients with COPD lies within the interval, nor that there is a 95% probability that the interval covers the true prevalence of depression

in patients with COPD. A 95% confidence interval does not mean that there is a 95% chance the pooled prevalence of depression lies within the interval. A 95% confidence interval does not mean that there is a 95% probability that the prevalence of depression has a 95% chance to fall within this interval in future studies.

Question 4 Answer: b, Study B

Explanation: When there is publication bias, researchers will perform classic fail-safe tests to identify the number of missing studies required to nullify the results in a meta-analysis. As a rule of thumb, the larger the number of missing studies required, the stronger the results. Among the five studies, study B requires 976 missing studies to nullify its results, and its results should be most convincing and strongest. It takes a long time and a lot of effort to conduct 976 studies to nullify the result. In contrast, studies C and D have weak results, as they require 32 and 47 missing studies, respectively, to nullify the results.

Question 5 Answer: a, Verbal aggression

Explanation: The prevalence of recent aggressive behaviour among outpatients with schizophrenia is around 5%. The types of violence and aggression are classified as follows: verbal aggression (45%), physical violence towards objects (30%), violence towards others (20%) and self-directed violence (10%). Family members are involved in around 50% of the assaults.

Reference: Puri BK, Hall AD, Ho RC (2014). *Revision Notes in Psychiatry*. Boca Raton, FL: CRC Press, p. 370.

Question 6 Answer: d, Presence of thoughts of worthlessness

Explanation: Option (d), in accordance to the research done by Siris et al. (2000), could help to differentiate between schizophrenia with prominent negative symptoms with post-schizophrenia depression. To diagnose post-schizophrenia depressive, it should be noted that the depressive symptoms need to fulfil at least the criteria for a depressive episode and should be present for a minimum duration of 2 weeks. Due to the presence of thoughts of worthlessness, there is an increased risk of suicide.

References: Puri BK, Hall AD, Ho RC (2014). *Revision Notes in Psychiatry*. Boca Raton, FL: CRC Press, p. 355; Siris SG (2000). Depression in schizophrenia: Perspective in the era of atypical antipsychotic agents. *AM J Psychiatry*, 17: 1379–1389.

Question 7 Answer: c, Having a prior history of affective disorder

Explanation: Depression is a chronic and recurrent condition. It has become increasingly clear that a significant proportion of the patients followed in the long term after suffering from depression remains chronically ill, despite the previously held belief that patients tend to recover fully between depressive episodes. Factors that predict a prolonged time to recovery include longer duration and the increased severity of the index episode, a history of non-affective psychiatric disorder, lower family income and married status during the index episode.

Reference: Puri BK, Hall AD, Ho RC (2014). *Revision Notes in Psychiatry*. Boca Raton, FL: CRC Press, p. 397.

Question 8 Answer: c, Autism
Explanation: This could be the stereotyped behaviour associated with autism.

Reference: Puri BK, Treasaden I (eds) (2010). *Psychiatry: An Evidence-Based Text*. London: Hodder Arnold, pp. 109, 1066–1067, 1088–1090.

Question 9 Answer: d, 30%
Explanation: HIV dementia is one of the most prominent features of human immunodeficiency virus (HIV) encephalopathy. The prevalence has been estimated to be 30% among those with the active infection. Encephalopathy is thought to be directly caused by HIV, which is a neurotropic virus. The onset of HIV is usually gradual and occurs later in the course with significant immunosuppression. There is noted to be initial lethargy, apathy, cognitive disturbance, reduced libido and general withdrawal. As the condition progresses, there will be more clinical signs suggestive of dementia.

Reference: Puri BK, Hall AD, Ho RC (2014). *Revision Notes in Psychiatry*. Boca Raton, FL: CRC Press, p. 705.

Question 10 Answer: c, Depression
Explanation: This is in itself a rare condition and could be missed. The disease is a terminal consequence of syphilis. The condition develops 5–25 years after the primary infection. The onset has been noted to be gradual, predominantly with depression as the first symptom. This is followed by slowly progressive memory and intellectual impairment. Frontal lobes are particularly involved, and this might result in characteristic personality changes – with disinhibition, uncontrolled excitement and over activity.

Reference: Puri BK, Hall AD, Ho RC (2014). *Revision Notes in Psychiatry*. Boca Raton, FL: CRC Press, p. 707.

Question 11 Answer: a, Addiction
Explanation: Contraindications for psychodynamic psychotherapy include schizophrenia, a tendency for serious self-harm, addiction and extremely poor insight. Indications include depressive and anxiety disorders, childhood abuse and trauma, relationship and personality problems and client factors (adequate ego strength, capacity to form and sustain relationships, motivation for change and psychological mindedness).

Reference: Sadock BJ, Sadock VA (2003). *Kaplan and Sadock's Synopsis of Psychiatry* (9th edition). Philadelphia, PA: Lippincott, Williams & Wilkins, p. 926.

Question 12 Answer: b, Displacement
Explanation: Displacement refers to the shifting of an emotion or drive invested in one idea or object (cathexis) to another that resembles the original in some aspect or quality. Displacement permits the symbolic representation of the original idea or object by one that is less highly cathected or evokes less distress. It is a form of

neurotic defence, which is encountered in obsessive-compulsive and hysterical patients as well as adults under stress.

Reference: Sadock BJ, Sadock VA (2003). *Kaplan and Sadock's Synopsis of Psychiatry* (9th edition). Philadelphia, PA: Lippincott, Williams & Wilkins, p. 208.

Question 13 Answer: d, Erythema migrans
Explanation: Erythema migrans is the earliest sign in Lyme disease at the site of the tick bite. It occurs 7–10 days after the bite. It evolves from an erythematous macule initially to form a large, annular lesion if left untreated.

Secondary syphilis is a possible diagnosis but unlikely in a 15-year-old.

The other possibility is erythema marginatum associated with active carditis, dermatophytes and tinea infection.

Reference: Kaufman DM, Milstein MJ (2013). *Kaufman's Clinical Neurology for Psychiatrists* (7th edition). Philadelphia, PA: Saunders, p. 67.

Question 14 Answer: a, Alcohol
Explanation: The baby is suffering from foetal alcohol syndrome. Diagnostic criteria include prenatal and postnatal growth deficiency; central nervous system (CNS) abnormalities, which include neurological deficits and intellectual disability; facial anomalies, which include short palpebral fissures, thin upper lip, flattened mid-face and indistinct philtrum.

Reference: Puri BK, Hall AD, Ho RC (2014). *Revision Notes in Psychiatry*. Boca Raton, FL: CRC Press, pp. 545–546, 679–680.

Question 15 Answer: a, Hypoglycaemia
Explanation: Alcohol-induced hypoglycaemia occurs in people who are dependent on alcohol after drinking large amounts. Ethanol produces hypoglycaemia by inhibiting gluconeogenesis and hepatic glycogen synthesis. When ethanol is metabolized, it causes changes in co-enzyme systems, resulting in a disturbance of enzymatic control of carbohydrate metabolism. This disturbance causes further glycogen depletion, which in turn increases the vulnerability of the liver to the effects of ethanol. This cycle persists until it is broken by the administration of carbohydrate.

Reference: Truman JC, Picchi J (1965). Ethanol-induced hypoglycemia. *Calif Med*. 103(3): 204–206.

Question 16 Answer: a, Down syndrome
Explanation: This boy has clinical features of Down syndrome. People with Down syndrome have significant learning disability, with intelligence quotient (IQ) between 40 and 45. IQ less than 50 is found in approximately 85% of cases. It is the most common cytogenic cause of learning disability. It accounts for 30% of all children with mental retardation.

Reference: Puri BK, Hall AD, Ho RC (2014). *Revision Notes in Psychiatry*. Boca Raton, FL: CRC Press, pp. 664–665.

Question 17 Answer: c, They have delayed sexual development and infertility
Explanation: People with XYY syndrome have normal sexual development and fertility. They are taller than the average person and have very mild physical abnormalities. Some individuals show muscle weakness with poor coordination.

Reference: Puri BK, Hall AD, Ho RC (2014). *Revision Notes in Psychiatry*. Boca Raton, FL: CRC Press, p. 668.

Question 18 Answer: d, Lesch–Nyhan syndrome
Explanation: Compulsive and severe self-mutilation tends to occur before the age of 3 years. Lips and fingers are often bitten. People with this syndrome also have generalized aggression with tantrums directed towards people and objects. Well-planned behavioural interventions may be helpful in reducing these behaviours.

Reference: Puri BK, Hall AD, Ho RC (2014). *Revision Notes in Psychiatry*. Boca Raton, FL: CRC Press, pp. 668–669.

Question 19 Answer: e, Omega-3 fatty acids
Explanation: The National Institute for Health and Care Excellence (NICE) guidelines do not recommend any particular dietary supplements (such as omega-3 fatty acids) in the treatment of attention-deficit hyperactivity disorder (ADHD). NICE guidelines also do not recommend elimination of artificial colouring and additives from the diet but do advise parents to keep a diary if there are foods or drinks that appear to affect behaviour.

Reference: Puri BK, Hall AD, Ho RC (2014). *Revision Notes in Psychiatry*. Boca Raton, FL: CRC Press, p. 633.

Question 20 Answer: e, Coprophagia
Explanation: Coprophagia refers to eating faeces. Coprolalia refers to the complex vocal tics involving inappropriate social vocalizations. Less than one-third of cases display tremor, echolalia and echopraxia. Mental coprolalia is more common than overt coprolalia.

Reference: Puri BK, Treasaden I (eds) (2010). *Psychiatry: An Evidence-Based Text*. London: Hodder Arnold. pp. 523, 550–551, 1068.

Question 21 Answer: c, Sydenham's chorea
Explanation: Sydenham's chorea occurs in 10% of rheumatic fever triggered by β-haemolytic streptococci.

Reference: Puri BK, Treasaden I (eds) (2010). *Psychiatry: An Evidence-Based Text*. London: Hodder Arnold. pp. 523, 581.

Question 22 Answer: e, Very-early onset depressive disorder is associated with good prognosis as treatment could help recovery
Explanation: Most children do have good prognosis with the exception of very early-onset depression, which is associated with poor prognosis.

Reference: Puri BK, Hall AD, Ho RC (2014). *Revision Notes in Psychiatry*. Boca Raton, FL: CRC Press, p. 649.

Question 23 Answer: d, There is per-protocol analysis
Explanation: The Consolidated Standards of Reporting Trials (CONSORT) statement, most recently updated in March 2010, is an evidence-based minimum set of recommendations, including a checklist and flow diagram for reporting randomized controlled trials (RCTs), and is intended to facilitate the complete and transparent reporting of trials and aid their critical appraisal and interpretation. In CONSORT guidelines, there is intention-to-treat analysis instead of per-protocol analysis. Another feature is that all patients assessed for the trial are accounted for, and the report is accompanied by a diagram that summarizes the outcomes of all patients involved in the trial.

Reference: Turner L, Shamseer L, Altman DG, Weeks L et al. (2012). Consolidated standards of reporting trials (CONSORT) and the completeness of reporting of randomized controlled trials (RCTs) published in medical journals. *Cochrane Database Syst Rev*, 14;11:MR000030.

Question 24 Answer: c, Quasi-randomization
Explanation: Quasi-randomization is not a proper randomization method, as it is based on subjects' characteristics, such as date of birth, and confounders can exert effects. Centralization randomization is done by a remote computer and third party to avoid selection bias. In minimization, to ensure the balance of factors between groups, the next allocation depends on the characteristics of subjects already being allocated. For stratified randomization, subjects are subdivided into strata and individuals within each striatum are then randomized. In stepped wedge randomization, the population is divided into groups, and then the intervention is progressively introduced, in random order, across the groups until every group is receiving it. This is used when other allocation methods would be unfeasible because of widespread belief that the intervention is beneficial.

Reference: Lewis GH, Sheringham J, Kalim K, Crayford TJB (2008). *Mastering Public Health: A Postgraduate Guide to Examination and Revalidation*. London: Royal Society of Medicine Press, pp. 48–49.

Question 25 Answer: e, Psychosis
Explanation: Pediatric autoimmune neuropsychiatric disorders associated with streptococcal infections (PANDAS) is caused by haemolytic streptococcal infection and is associated with obsessive-compulsive disorder (OCD). The association between OCD and tics also suggests the role of basal ganglia lesions. The common

disorders include Tourette syndrome, ADHD, anxiety disorder, depression, bed-wetting, sleep disturbance, psychomotor changes and joint pain.

Reference: Puri BK, Hall AD, Ho RC (2014). *Revision Notes in Psychiatry*. Boca Raton, FL: CRC Press, p. 654.

Question 26 Answer: e, Social phobia

Explanation: Based on *International Classification of Diseases* (ICD)-10 diagnostic criteria, elective mutism is characterized by a marked, emotionally determined selectivity in speaking, such that the child demonstrates language competency in some situations but fails to speak in other situations. The condition must last for a minimum duration of 4 weeks. This condition tends to be associated with social anxiety, withdrawal, sensitivity and resistance.

Reference: Puri BK, Hall AD, Ho RC (2014). *Revision Notes in Psychiatry*. Boca Raton, FL: CRC Press, p. 639.

Question 27 Answer: c, 20%

Explanation: Approximately 20% of adult bipolar patients experience their first episode of mania before the age of 20 years. The prevalence of bipolar disorder in adolescents is 0.5%–1.0%. The clinical features are similar to those of adults. First-rank symptoms are present in 20% of cases. First-line treatment is olanzapine, although valproate and lithium have been shown to be effective in treatment. Family therapy could be helpful in terms of stabilization of symptoms.

Reference: Puri BK, Hall AD, Ho RC (2014). *Revision Notes in Psychiatry*. Boca Raton, FL: CRC Press, p. 651.

Question 28 Answer: a, Automatic behaviour is not common

Explanation: Sleep paralysis, hypnagogic hallucinations, automatic behaviour and nocturnal sleep disruption commonly occur in patients with narcolepsy. The prevalence of this disorder is 3–6 per 100,000, with equal gender ratio. It is due to the loss of hypocretin cells in the hypothalamus, leading to lack of hypocretin (neurotransmitter regulating arousal and wakefulness). Management includes (1) non-pharmacological – lifestyle adjustment and scheduled napping and (2) pharmacological – stimulants such as methylphenidate and modafinil that can reduce daytime sleepiness and (3) rapid eye movement (REM) suppressants such as selective serotonin receptor inhibitors that can treat hypnagogic hallucinations, cataplexy and sleep paralysis.

References: Kaufman DM, Milstein MJ (2013). *Kaufman's Clinical Neurology for Psychiatrists* (7th edition). Philadelphia, PA: Saunders. pp. 370–372; Puri BK, Hall AD, Ho RC (2014). *Revision Notes in Psychiatry*. Boca Raton, FL: CRC Press, p. 616.

Question 29 Answer: d, Thiamine deficiency

Explanation: Post-bariatric surgery as well as various vitamin and electrolyte deficiencies (thiamine, vitamin B12, vitamin E and copper) frequently cause neuropathy and occasionally encephalopathy or myelopathy. This may be accompanied by depression, dementia or other mental state abnormality. Thus, routine postoperative administration of these nutrients is necessary. Thiamine deficiency generally leads to absent deep tendon reflexes and loss of position sensation. In fact, until patients walk in the dark, when they must rely on position sense generated in the legs and feet, their deficits may remain asymptomatic.

Reference: Kaufman DM, Milstein MJ (2013). *Kaufman's Clinical Neurology for Psychiatrists* (7th edition). Philadelphia, PA: Saunders, pp. 65–66.

Question 30 Answer: c, He can be given doses of benzodiazepine to alleviate his anxiety and uptitrate in response to his anxiety symptoms

Explanation: Patients with uncomplicated Guillain–Barré syndrome should not have altered mental status, as it is a peripheral nervous system disorder. Thus, when these patients present with behavioural and mood problems, it is important to look for complications that involve the CNS, such as hypoxia from respiratory depression or electrolyte abnormalities. Furthermore, unless patients are already on respirator, benzodiazepines should be avoided, as they depress respiration.

Reference: Kaufman DM, Milstein MJ (2013). *Kaufman's Clinical Neurology for Psychiatrists* (7th edition). Philadelphia, PA: Saunders, pp. 62–64.

Question 31 Answer: c, Psychiatric symptoms are seen in about 10% of attacks

Explanation: Acute intermittent porphyria is an autosomal dominant genetic disorder of porphyrin metabolism. It causes dramatic attacks of quadriparesis and colicky, often severe, abdominal pain. In about 25%–50% of attacks, patients with acute intermittent porphyria develop a variety of psychiatric symptoms, which include agitation, delirium, depression and psychosis. During attacks, excess porphyrins colour the urine red. Quantitative tests that replace the classic Watson–Schwartz test readily detect urine porphobilinogen and 5-aminolevulinic acid in urine and serum.

Reference: Gonzalez-Arriaza HL, Bostwick JM (2003). Acute porphyrias. *Am J Psychiatry*, 160: 923–926.

Question 32 Answer: e, Atomoxetine

Explanation: Atomoxetine is indicated in the patients with hyperkinetic disorder and Tourette syndrome.

Reference: Puri BK, Treasaden I (eds) (2010). *Psychiatry: An Evidence-Based Text*. London: Hodder Arnold. pp. 523, 550–551, 1068.

Question 33 Answer: b, It occurs early in the course when there is minimal immunosuppression

Explanation: The onset of HIV dementia is usually insidious and occurs later in the course with significant immunosuppression. There is initial lethargy, apathy, cognitive disturbance and general withdrawal. As the condition progresses, evidence of dementia becomes apparent with cognitive impairment, incontinence, ataxia, hyper-reflexia and increased muscle tone.

Reference: Puri BK, Hall AD, Ho RC (2014). *Revision Notes in Psychiatry*. Boca Raton, FL: CRC Press, pp. 705–706.

Question 34 Answer: a, The heritability is 90%
Explanation: The heritability is 75%.

Reference: Puri BK, Treasaden I (eds) (2010). *Psychiatry: An Evidence-Based Text*. London: Hodder Arnold. pp. 1059–1060.

Question 35 Answer: c, Allocation of patients by gender (subdivided into strata and individuals within each striatum undergo further randomization)
Explanation: Option C is stratified randomization, while the other options are quasi-randomization. For stratified randomization, subjects are subdivided into strata, and individuals within each striatum are then randomized. This is less likely to produce bias in RCT compared with quasi-randomization, which is not a proper randomization method as it is based on subjects' characteristics, such as month of birth, hospitalization status and laboratory results.

Reference: Lewis GH, Sheringham J, Kalim K, Crayford T JB (2008). *Mastering Public Health: A Postgraduate Guide to Examination and Revalidation*. London: Royal Society of Medicine Press, pp. 48–49.

Question 36 Answer: d, An increase in the number of collaborating centres instead of the number of subjects
Explanation: The power of an RCT depends on sample size, total number of endpoints, difference in compliance between two groups, increased number of endpoints by selecting a high-risk population or increased duration of follow-up. Having more collaborating centres does not necessarily mean more subjects, which is important in increasing the power of a RCT.

Reference: Lewis GH, Sheringham J, Kalim K, Crayford T JB (2008). *Mastering Public Health: A Postgraduate Guide to Examination and Revalidation*. London: Royal Society of Medicine Press, p. 39.

Question 37 Answer: a, Olanzapine
Explanation: Based on the findings of the trial, which compared second-generation antipsychotics with first-generation antipsychotics, olanzapine has been shown to be the most effective in terms of the rate of discontinuation.

Reference: Puri BK, Hall AD, Ho RC (2014). *Revision Notes in Psychiatry*. Boca Raton, FL: CRC Press, p. 251.

Question 38 Answer: b, Depression has a unimodal age of onset
Explanation: Depression in Parkinson disease has bimodal onset. Patients may become depressed at the time of diagnosis, although it may occur late in the course and be associated with severe bradykinesia and gait disturbances. Depressive

symptoms precede motor symptoms in 30% of cases. The prevalence of major depressive disorder in Parkinson disease is 20%, with prevalence increased to 40% if dysthymia and minor depression are included. Comorbidity with anxiety occurs in two-thirds of cases. Selective serotonin reuptake inhibitors are the first-line treatment for depression in this group of patients. Tricyclic antidepressants should be avoided as they may cause confusion and cognitive impairment.

Reference: Puri BK, Hall AD, Ho RC (2014). *Revision Notes in Psychiatry*. Boca Raton, FL: CRC Press, p. 489.

Question 39 Answer: b, Good eye contact

Explanation: Steele–Richardson–Olszewski syndrome is also known as progressive supranuclear palsy (PSP). It is associated with parkinsonism without prominent tremor, vertical gaze palsy, midline more than appendicular rigidity, early postural instability, frequent falls, poor eye contact and monotonous speech. Unlike in Parkinson disease, there is little or no response to levodopa.

Reference: Blazer DG, Steffens DC (2009). *The American Psychiatric Publishing Textbook of Geriatric Psychiatry* (4th edition). Arlington, VA: American Psychiatric Publishing Inc., pp. 234–235.

Question 40 Answer: c, It is not commonly associated with psychiatric comorbidity

Explanation: Psychiatric disturbance is variable but common. Initial insight may result in depression. There may also be prodromal personality changes, antisocial behaviour with substance misuse and affective and schizoaffective disorders. Mild euphoria with explosive outbursts, irritability and rage may also be noted. In addition, there is a slowly progressive intellectual impairment.

Reference: Puri BK, Hall AD, Ho RC (2014). *Revision Notes in Psychiatry*. Boca Raton, FL: CRC Press, pp. 706–707.

Question 41 Answer: b, Her plea is known as sane automatism

Explanation: Automatism is a plea generally restricted to cases of homicide. The defendant pleads that, at the time of the offence, their behaviour was automatic. The law uses this term to mean a state almost near-unconsciousness. It refers to unconscious, involuntary, non-purposeful acts where the mind is not conscious of what the body is doing. The case law now differentiates sane automatism caused by external factors (extrinsic factors), such as hypoglycaemia owing to insulin use, from insane automatism caused by disease of the mind resulting from illness or brain disease (intrinsic factors), such as diabetes mellitus, epilepsy and even hysterical dissociative fugue states. This case is an example of insane automatism plea.

Reference: Puri BK, Treasaden I (eds) (2010). *Psychiatry: An Evidence-Based Text*. London: Hodder Arnold, pp. 1165–1166.

Question 42 Answer: b, Three times more likely
Explanation: Men with learning disabilities are three times more likely to offend than men with no disorder or handicap and five times more likely to commit a violent offense. Women with learning disabilities are almost four times more likely to offend than women with no disorder or handicap and 25 times more likely to commit a violent offense. As they lack an understanding of the nature of their behaviour and its legal consequences, they are more suggestible and are easier to catch. Learning disabilities may also lead to violence and even homicide. In addition, in panic and frustration, such people may commit arson or sexual offences that relate to their difficulty initiating and sustaining interpersonal and sexual relationships.

References: Hodgins S (1992). Mental disorder, intellectual deficiency, and crime. Evidence from a birth cohort. *Arch Gen Psychiatry*, 49: 476–83; Puri BK, Treasaden I (eds) (2010). *Psychiatry: An Evidence-Based Text*. London: Hodder Arnold, pp. 1092–1094, 1161.

Question 43 Answer: c, Psychopathy Checklist – Screening Version (PCL-SV)
Explanation: The Psychopathy Checklist – Revised (PCL-R) was devised by Hare and is used to measure the presence and level of psychopathy in forensic populations. It has been proven to be a good predictor of risk. A short version, the PCL-SV, can be used in non-forensic populations. The PCL-R has two factors: personality traits (superficial, grandiose, manipulative, lacks remorse, lacks empathy, does not accept responsibility) and deviancy of social behaviour (impulsive, poor behavioural control, lacks goals, irresponsible, adolescent antisocial behaviour, adult antisocial behaviour). The Historical Clinical Risk 20 (HCR-20) and Violence Risk Appraisal Guide (VRAG) measure violence risk, whereas the STATIC-99 is used to assess sexual recidivism among male adult sex offenders.

Reference: Puri BK, Treasaden I (eds) (2010). *Psychiatry: An Evidence-Based Text*. London: Hodder Arnold, pp. 707, 1196, 1241.

Question 44 Answer: b, Basal ganglia
Explanation: Patients with depression have been reported as having a higher number and larger volume of infarcts affecting the prefrontosubcortical circuits, particularly the caudate and pallidum in basal ganglia and genu of internal capsule, with left-sided predominance.

Reference: Vataja R, Pohjasvaara T, Leppävuori A, Mäntylä R, Aronen HJ, Salonen O, Kaste M, Erkinjuntti T (2001). Magnetic resonance imaging correlates of depression after ischemic stroke. *Archives of General Psychiatry*, 58: 925–931.

Question 45 Answer: c, Prisoners with epilepsy have committed more violent crimes than those without epilepsy
Explanation: There is no excess of violent crimes in prisoners with epilepsy. The increase in prevalence of epilepsy in prisoners (two times that of general population) is due to common social and biological adversity, leading to both epilepsy and crime.

Reference: Whitman S, Coleman TE, Patmon C et al. (1984). Epilepsy in prisons: Elevated prevalence and no relationship to violence. *Neurology*, 34: 775–782.

Question 46 Answer: b, A patient can withdraw from the RCT at any time, and a valid reason is required

Explanation: This option is contrary to the Declaration of Helsinki, which states that research subjects can withdraw from study without giving any reason. Steps involved in the conduction of RCT include identify and engage investigational sites, develop trial governance procedures, develop trial procedures according to good clinical practice, apply and obtain funding, develop recruitment strategies and methods to identify and overcome recruitment problems, develop data capture methods, engage in oversight of trial progress, develop procedures for adverse event reporting and complete trial termination procedures.

References: Lewis GH, Sheringham J, Kalim K, Crayford T JB (2008). *Mastering Public Health: A Postgraduate Guide to Examination and Revalidation*. London: Royal Society of Medicine Press, pp. 48–49; Smith A, Palmer S, Johnson DW, Navaneethan S et al. (2010). How to conduct a randomized trial. *Nephrology (Carlton)*, 15(8): 740–746.

Question 47 Answer: d, 4 months

Explanation: Risk of relapse is particularly high, with rates between 40% and 60% following the withdrawal of antidepressants within the first 4 months of achieving an initial response. The risk is much reduced if antidepressant therapy is continued, to around 10%–30%.

Reference: Puri BK, Hall AD, Ho RC (2014). *Revision Notes in Psychiatry*. Boca Raton, FL: CRC Press, p. 390.

Question 48 Answer: b, The remission rate was 10%

Explanation: A third of the participants reached a remission or virtual absence of their symptoms during the initial phase of the study, with an additional 10%–15% experiencing some improvement. The remission rate was noted to be 30% higher than expected, and this might be due to the systematic and comprehensive approach to care.

Reference: Puri BK, Hall AD, Ho RC (2014). *Revision Notes in Psychiatry*. Boca Raton, FL: CRC Press, p. 392.

Question 49 Answer: e, Psychotropic medications should be commenced for the treatment of hypoactive delirium

Explanation: Hypoactive delirium is characterized by apathy, confusion and lethargy. Hypoactive delirium is often mistaken for depression. Treatment of hypoactive delirium with psychotropic medications is not recommended. In addition, general principles of prescription in delirium include mono-therapy, prescription with lowest dose and tapering off the medications when delirium resolves.

Reference: Puri BK, Hall AD, Ho RC (2014). *Revision Notes in Psychiatry*. Boca Raton, FL: CRC Press, p. 709.

Question 50 Answer: e, 5%
Explanation: The most common somatic complaints in the elderly include pain, constipation, fatigue, headache, impaired balance, dry mouth, nausea, fatigue, headache, impaired balance, dry mouth, change in appetite and difficulty in urinating. Somatic complaints may be a presentation of underlying depressive (masked depression) and anxiety disorders.

Reference: Puri BK, Hall AD, Ho RC (2014). *Revision Notes in Psychiatry*. Boca Raton, FL: CRC Press, p. 715.

Question 51 Answer: a, Cells double at a rate that is inversely proportional to age
Explanation: Several studies have replicated Hayflick's work, which showed that the number of population doublings of cultured human cells is inversely proportional to the person's age. The death of a cell line is usually caused by faulty laboratory techniques. The only human cells that may be immortal are the transformed or abnormal mixoploid cells, such as the HeLa cells. This cell line was derived from cervical cancer cells taken in 1951 from Henrietta Lacks, a patient who eventually died of her cancer.

Reference: Blazer DG, Steffens DC, Busse EW (2004). *The American Psychiatric Publishing Textbook of Geriatric Psychiatry* (3rd edition). Arlington, VA: American Psychiatric Publishing, p. 4.

Question 52 Answer: b, Intellectualization
Explanation: Intellectualization is a defence mechanism whereby a person deals with and avoids emotional difficulties using excessive abstract thinking. The person excessively uses intellectual processes to avoid affective expression or experience. Undue emphasis is focused on the inanimate to avoid intimacy with people, attention is paid to external reality to avoid the expression of inner feelings and stress is excessively placed on irrelevant details to avoid perceiving the whole.

Reference: Sadock BJ, Sadock VA (2003). *Kaplan and Sadock's Synopsis of Psychiatry* (9th edition). Philadelphia, PA: Lippincott, Williams & Wilkins, p. 208.

Question 53 Answer: d, Psychodrama
Explanation: Rapaport described the four characteristics in Milieu Group Therapy: democratization (equal sharing of power); permissiveness (tolerance of others' behaviour); reality confrontation (confronting the views of others); and communalism (sharing of amenities). Most milieu therapy programmes, such as therapeutic communities, emphasize group and social interaction; rules and expectations are mediated by peer pressure for normalization of adaption. When patients are viewed as responsible human beings, adoption of the passive patient role becomes reduced.

Reference: Sadock BJ, Sadock VA (2003). *Kaplan and Sadock's Synopsis of Psychiatry* (9th edition). Philadelphia, PA: Lippincott, Williams & Wilkins, p. 966.

Question 54 Answer: e, Therapeutic alliance

Explanation: Therapeutic alliance is the single best predictor of benefit for psychotherapy. It is key for the therapist to develop trust and respect between the therapist and the client. It is also essential for the therapist to demonstrate empathy.

References: Department of Health (2001). *Treatment Choice in Psychological Therapies and Counselling: Evidence-Based Clinical Practice Guideline*. London: Crown Copyright, 2001; Puri BK, Hall AD, Ho RC (2014). *Revision Notes in Psychiatry*. Boca Raton, FL: CRC Press, p. 332.

Question 55 Answer: a, ADHD

Explanation: Previous research has found an association with that of ADHD. The core clinical features include reduction of sleep. The first-line of treatment is that of olanzapine. In particular, childhood bipolar disorder has been ranked as having the second worst prognosis among all the psychiatric disorders in childhood.

Reference: Puri BK, Hall AD, Ho RC (2014). *Revision Notes in Psychiatry*. Boca Raton, FL: CRC Press, p. 651.

Question 56 Answer: c, Augment with lithium and continue with venlafaxine and mirtazapine

Explanation: Based on NICE guidelines, a trial of lithium augmentation should be considered for patients whose depression has failed to respond to several antidepressants such as venlafaxine and mirtazapine. Augmentation with lithium has better evidence than augmentation with mianserin. Removing the current antidepressants might worsen the patient's existing mood state.

Reference: NICE Guidelines on depression. https://www.nice.org.uk/guidance/cg90

Question 57 Answer: a, Appearance, Pulse, Grimace, Activity, Respiration (APGAR) score of 2 at 1 minute and 3 at 5 minutes

Explanation: The other features are found in foetuses born by mothers with past or active eating disorders. The majority of the women with eating disorders have normal length of pregnancy (mean length = 39 weeks). Their babies usually have normal Apgar score (at 1 and 5 minutes after birth, the scores are 8 and 9 points, respectively).

Reference: Koubaa S, Hallstrom T, Lindholm C, Hirschberg AL (2005). Pregnancy and neonatal outcome in women with eating disorders. *Obstet Gynecol*, 105(2): 255–260.

Question 58 Answer: d, Order a magnetic resonance imaging (MRI) brain scan
Explanation: Quetiapine has a high affinity for muscarinic receptors. It carries the lowest risk for Extra Pyramidal Side Effect (EPSE). It carries the lowest risk of sexual dysfunction. It carries low risk for hyperprolactinaemia.

Reference: Puri BK, Hall AD, Ho RC (2014). *Revision Notes in Psychiatry*. Boca Raton, FL: CRC Press, p. 365.

Question 59 Answer: d, Major depressive disorder
Explanation: It is important to understand and comprehend the differences between depression and bereavement. The following features are more common in depression but not in bereavement, and they include active suicidal ideations, depressive symptoms that are out of proportion with loss, feelings of guilt not related to the deceased, marked functional impairment for longer than 2 months, marked psychomotor changes lasting more than a few days and preoccupation with worthlessness.

Reference: Puri BK, Hall AD, Ho RC (2014). *Revision Notes in Psychiatry*. Boca Raton, FL: CRC Press, p. 380.

Question 60 Answer: a, Decreased appetite
Explanation: In the acute intoxication of cannabis, the clinical signs usually include conjunctival injection, dry mouth, tachycardia as well as increased appetite. Other associated behavioural changes include anxiety or agitation, auditory, visual or tactile illusions, depersonalization, euphoria and dis-inhibition and hallucinations with persevered orientation. There will be impaired judgement, attention or reaction time. There will also be suspiciousness or paranoid ideations. There is also temporal slowing, or a sense that time is passing very slowly, or rapid flow of ideas.

Reference: Puri BK, Hall AD, Ho RC (2014). *Revision Notes in Psychiatry*. Boca Raton, FL: CRC Press, p. 535.

Question 61 Answer: d, Psychodynamic conflicts
Explanation: The components of interpersonal psychotherapy (IPT) include grief, interpersonal disputes, role transitions and interpersonal deficits. This treatment is indicated for depressive disorders, eating disorder and dysthymia.

Reference: Puri BK, Hall A, Ho RC (2014). *Revision Notes in Psychiatry* (3rd edition). Boca Raton, FL: CRC Press, pp. 340–341.

Question 62 Answer: e, Activity scheduling
Explanation: Activity scheduling helps to increase contact with positive activities and decrease avoidance and withdrawal. Other behavioural techniques include rehearsal, assignment, training to be self-reliant, pleasure and mastery and diversion or distraction techniques.

Reference: Puri BK, Hall AD, Ho RC (2014). *Revision Notes in Psychiatry*. Boca Raton, FL: CRC Press, p. 335.

Question 63 Answer: e, Suppression
Explanation: The man is using suppression, a mature defence, by consciously putting the illness out of his mind. This may be contrasted with repression, a neurotic defence, whereby the person involuntarily forgets a painful experience.

Reference: Levenson JL (2004). *The American Psychiatric Publishing Textbook of Psychosomatic Medicine*. Arlington, VA: American Psychiatric Publishing, p. 79.

Question 64 Answer: e, 11%
Explanation: With regard to the prognosis, around 10% of adolescents self-harm in 1 year. Higher risks of repetition are present in those who are older, with a history of suicide attempt, in those with psychotic symptoms, substance misuse and those who used methods other than overdose or self-cutting. With regard to suicide, approximately 4% of females and 11% of boys kill themselves within 5 years after their first episode of suicide attempt.

Reference: Puri BK, Hall AD, Ho RC (2014). *Revision Notes in Psychiatry*. Boca Raton, FL: CRC Press, p. 651.

Question 65 Answer: b, High plasma dopamine level
Explanation: Conduct disorder is associated with the inheritance of antisocial trait from parents who demonstrate criminal behaviours. In terms of biological factors, it is associated with low plasma serotonin level, low plasma dopamine level, low cholesterol, excess testosterone excess, greater right frontal EEG activity and abnormal prefrontal cortex. There might be neurological impairment as well as maternal alcohol and smoking during pregnancy.

Reference: Puri BK, Hall AD, Ho RC (2014). *Revision Notes in Psychiatry*. Boca Raton, FL: CRC Press, p. 635.

Question 66 Answer: b, Diffuse slowing
Explanation: Of those with delirium, 90% have abnormal tracing. Diffuse slowing is the most typical electroencephalogram (EEG) pattern seen in delirium. Delta activity, asymmetry in delta waves and localized spike and sharp wave complexes occur more in those with intracranial pathology. Alpha activity correlates with cognitive functioning, and delta activity correlates with length of illness.

Reference: Puri BK, Hall AD, Ho RC (2014). *Revision Notes in Psychiatry*. Boca Raton, FL: CRC Press, pp. 690–691.

Question 67 Answer: e, Patients with hyperactive delirium demonstrate features of restlessness, agitation and hyper vigilance, while patients with hypoactive delirium present with lethargy, sedation and respond slowly to questioning
Explanation: An electroencephalogram shows diffuse slowing for both types of delirium. Both types of delirium are equally responsive to neuroleptics, and diffuse cognitive deficits are seen in both. Patients with hypoactive delirium

have higher mortality rates than those with hyperactive delirium. Delirium from drug-related causes is most commonly hyperactive, while delirium from metabolic causes is more frequently hypoactive. Clinical features sometimes can help to differentiate between hyper- and hypoactive delirium. For hyperactive delirium, there may be restlessness, agitation, hyper vigilance and often hallucinations and delusions, while for hypoactive delirium, there may be lethargy, sedation and little spontaneous movement.

References: Levenson JL (2004). *The American Psychiatric Publishing Textbook of Psychosomatic Medicine*. Arlington, VA: American Psychiatric Publishing Inc., p. 106; Puri BK, Hall AD, Ho RC (2014). *Revision Notes in Psychiatry*. Boca Raton, FL: CRC Press, p. 709.

Question 68 Answer: e, Skin cancer
Explanation: The prevalence of depression in patients with cancer is 10%–30%. Drastic changes in lifestyle and the fear and anxiety that accompany the chronic and sometimes fatal disease can impact the emotional well-being of patients. Higher rates of depression are associated with certain types of cancer such as brain, lung, oropharyngeal and pancreas tumours. Skin cancer is not generally associated with a significant risk of depression. Studies have shown that patients who exhibited increasing depressive symptoms had a greater probability of receiving chemo/medication therapy than any other treatment.

References: Levenson JL (2004). *The American Psychiatric Publishing Textbook of Psychosomatic Medicine*. Arlington, VA: American Psychiatric Publishing Inc., p. 201; Burton CL, Galatzer-Lew IR, Bonanno GA (2014). Treatment type and demographic characteristics as predictors for cancer adjustment: Prospective trajectories of depressive symptoms in a population sample. *Health Psychol*, 34(6):602–9.

Question 69 Answer: d, Mirtazepine
Explanation: Mirtazepine is the best choice as it is most likely to not only improve mood but also improve sleep and appetite in medically ill patients. This is because its main side effects are sedation and weight gain. It increases norepinephrine and serotonin concentrations through blockage of inhibitory receptors but does not appear to cause the nausea, insomnia, anxiety or sexual dysfunction associated with selective serotonin reuptake inhibitors. As a result of its serotonin3 receptor-blocking antiemetic effects, mirtazapine may be useful in treating medically ill patients who are experiencing nausea. Furthermore, it has minimal drug interactions.

Reference: Levenson JL (2004). *The American Psychiatric Publishing Textbook of Psychosomatic Medicine*. Arlington, VA: American Psychiatric Publishing Inc., p. 206.

Question 70 Answer: e, Postictal psychotic symptoms occur immediately following a seizure
Explanation: Postictal psychosis occurs usually with a non-psychotic period of 1–7 days between the last seizure and the psychosis. It may occur in the background of clouded consciousness. In EEG of postictal psychosis, slow-wave changes that

may last up to a few hours may be seen. Patients may present with fugues (prolonged episode of wandering, altered behaviour, amnesia and impaired consciousness that may last for hours or days) or twilight states (abnormal subjective experiences – perceptual and affective and are associated with cognitive impairment and perseveration).

Interictal psychosis occurs in temporal lobe epilepsy. Risk factors of interictal psychosis include hamartomas, an aura of fear, left-handedness, mesial temporal focus and onset of epilepsy in adolescence. Patients classically present with chronic paranoid hallucinatory psychosis with the presence of first-rank symptoms, with onset 10–15 years after the first episode of epilepsy.

Reference: Puri BK, Hall AD, Ho RC (2014). *Revision Notes in Psychiatry*. Boca Raton, FL: CRC Press, p. 497.

Question 71 Answer: b, Battering mother

Explanation: The battering mother lost her temper and killed the infant in response to her behaviours. In the United Kingdom, the rate of infanticide has remained relatively constant, with about 20 convictions per year. In contrast, if the scenario changes and states that the infant is calm and stable, the common predisposing factor will become severe postpartum mental illness.

Reference: Puri B, Treasaden I (eds) (2010). *Psychiatry: An Evidence-Based Text*. London: Hodder Arnold. pp. 719, 726, 1165.

Question 72 Answer: e, To respect her request to become pregnant and offer the best intervention to induce ovulation

Explanation: The psychiatrist should not accept the problem as presented by the patient but help the obstetrician to explore her denial of chronic illness. The patient may be looking for an untenable solution to a problem that she does not fully understand. Her condition is not optimal to get pregnant at this moment. The complications of an eating disorder on the reproductive system are that it can lead to reduced growth, delayed puberty and amenorrhea. It can also lead to small ovaries and uterus and can cause infertility and breast atrophy.

Reference: Puri BK, Hall AD, Ho RC (2014). *Revision Notes in Psychiatry*. Boca Raton, FL: CRC Press, p. 574.

Question 73 Answer: b, 21–30 years

Explanation: The incidence of schizophrenia is between 15 and 30 new cases per 100,000 of the population per year. The lifetime risk is that of 1%. The age of onset is usually between 15 and 45 years, earlier in men than in women.

Reference: Puri BK, Hall AD, Ho RC (2014). *Revision Notes in Psychiatry*. Boca Raton, FL: CRC Press, p. 356.

Question 74 Answer: d, Digoxin

Explanation: Common neuropsychiatric side effects of digoxin include visual hallucinations (typically yellow rings around objects), delirium, depression, agitation or combativeness, anxiety and sleep disturbances. These side effects may be observed even at therapeutic levels in the elderly. This might be due to digoxin's protein-binding capacity, which for malnourished older people with low albumin, could result in an actual higher plasma level than that measured by serum blood levels. Furthermore, psychotropic side effects of digoxin may be the first and only manifestation of digoxin toxicity, which, if uncorrected, can be fatal.

References: Levenson JL (2004). *The American Psychiatric Publishing Textbook of Psychosomatic Medicine*. Arlington, VA: American Psychiatric Publishing, p. 426; Eisendrath SJ, Sweeney MA (1987). Toxic neuropsychiatric effects of digoxin at therapeutic serum concentrations. *Am J Psychiatry*, 144(4): 506–507.

Question 75 Answer: d, Globus

Explanation: The other conditions are not indicated for speech therapy. Globus is a persistent or intermittent non-painful sensation of a lump or foreign body in the throat. It is commonly encountered, usually long-lasting, difficult to treat and has a tendency to recur. As a first step of managing globus, careful history taking and nasolaryngoscopy are essential. Speech and language therapy, antidepressants and cognitive behavioural therapy can be helpful in patients whose symptoms persist despite negative investigations.

References: Levenson JL (2004). *The American Psychiatric Publishing Textbook of Psychosomatic Medicine*. Arlington, VA: American Psychiatric Publishing p. 472; Lee BE, Kim GH (2012). Globus pharyngeus: A review of its etiology, diagnosis and treatment. *World J Gastroenterol*, 18(20): 2462–2471.

Question 76 Answer: e, Tricyclic antidepressants

Explanation: Irritable bowel syndrome (IBS) is a symptom-based diagnosis characterized by chronic abdominal pain, discomfort, bloating and alteration of bowel habits. As a functional gastrointestinal disorder (FGID), IBS has no known organic cause. It remains a therapeutic challenge in part because of limited understanding of the pathophysiology. A meta-analysis concluded that the tricyclic antidepressants were superior to placebo in IBS, although the individual trial results were variable. Tricyclic antidepressants have been found to be effective in the treatment of IBS at low doses with rapid onset. Selective serotonin reuptake inhibitors are of uncertain benefit to treatment of IBS. Selective serotonin reuptake inhibitor antidepressants seem to promote global well-being in some patients with IBS and, possibly, some improvement in abdominal pain and bowel symptoms, but this effect appears to be independent of improved depression.

References: Levenson JL (2004). *The American Psychiatric Publishing Textbook of Psychosomatic Medicine*. Arlington, VA: American Psychiatric Publishing, p. 475; Talley NJ (2003). Evaluation of drug treatment in irritable bowel syndrome. *Br J Clin Pharmacol*, 56(4): 362–369; Creed F (2006). How do SSRIs help patients with irritable bowel syndrome? *Gut*, 55(8): 1065–1067.

Question 77 Answer: e, Paroxetine
Explanation: In 2007, two studies determined that antidepressants such as paroxetine, if used during the course of a pregnancy, were associated with an increased risk of cardiac defect. It should also be noted that the potential risk associated with antidepressants taken in pregnancy is not just limited to the teratogenicity and issues of neonatal withdrawal and of longer-term effects on cognitive development or behaviour. Previous studies have found an association between exposure to selective serotonin re-uptake inhibitor (SSRI) and a heightened risk of autism.

Reference: Ian Jones and Liz McDonald (2014). Living with uncertainty: Antidepressants and pregnancy. *BJP*, 205: 103–104.

Question 78 Answer: e, Initial insomnia
Explanation: The endogenous form of depression has been thought to be of biological origin. The characteristic symptoms include motor retardation/agitation, anorexia and weight loss, diurnal variation, excessive guilt, lack of reactivity of mood, lost of interest, distinct quality of mood and terminal insomnia.

Reference: Puri BK, Hall AD, Ho RC (2014). *Revision Notes in Psychiatry*. Boca Raton, FL: CRC Press, p. 380.

Question 79 Answer: b, Anxiety and insomnia
Explanation: The most frequently reported psychiatric symptoms are anxiety and problems with sleep.

Reference: Blazer DG, Steffens DC, Busse EW (2004). *The American Psychiatric Publishing Textbook of Geriatric Psychiatry* (3rd edition). Arlington, VA: American Psychiatric Publishing, p. 21.

Question 80 Answer: b, The highest rate is in white men above the age of 70 years
Explanation: The rates are positively correlated with age.

Reference: Blazer DG, Steffens DC, Busse EW (2004). *The American Psychiatric Publishing Textbook of Geriatric Psychiatry* (3rd edition). Arlington, VA: American Psychiatric Publishing, p. 27.

Question 81 Answer: b, Memory tests, such as the Wechsler Adult Intelligence Scale inventory, show a classical pattern of intellectual decline, with verbal IQ declining more than performance IQ
Explanation: It is true that intelligence levels off until the age of 60–70 years and decline thereafter. Many studies have demonstrated an accelerated decline in cognitive functioning in those who are closest to their death, and this has been commonly referred to as terminal drop; poor health may be one of the causes. Using inventories such as the WAIS-R, there is a classical pattern of intellectual decline, with performance IQ noted to be declining more than verbal IQ. Factors that have

been proposed to contribute to this include increased speed of processing and also the concept of familiarity and novelty.

Reference: Puri BK, Hall AD, Ho RC (2014). *Revision Notes in Psychiatry*. Boca Raton, FL: CRC Press, p. 683.

Question 82 Answer: d, Relatively mild impairments in construction
Explanation: Patients with fronto-temporal dementia (FTD) tend to have younger age of onset, with more severe apathy, disinhibition, reduction in speech output, loss of insight and coarsening of social behaviour but less spatial dis orientation compared with that of Alzhemier's dementia (AD). Primitive reflexes may be present. Patients who suffer from AD have more impairment in calculation and constructions, lower MMSE scores and higher prevalence of depression (20%) compared with patients with FTD. Both AD and FTD have insidious onset.

Reference: Puri BK, Hall AD, Ho RC (2014). *Revision Notes in Psychiatry*. Boca Raton, FL: CRC Press, p. 701.

Question 83 Answer: c, The most common hallucination in the elderly is that of visual hallucinations
Explanation: Characteristically, all would have at least one type of delusional belief. Approximately 46% of individuals have one first-rank symptom. Eighty-three percent of individuals experience hallucinations, with the most common hallucinations being auditory. At times, there might be visual, somatic and olfactory hallucinations as well. Thought disorder and catatonic symptoms are rarely seen. Negative symptoms are seen frequently but are usually mild.

Reference: Puri BK, Hall AD, Ho RC (2014). *Revision Notes in Psychiatry*. Boca Raton, FL: CRC Press, p. 713.

Question 84 Answer: d, Hyperthyroidism with anxious dysphoria is more common in older patients
Explanation: Hyperthyroidism affects 2%–5% of all women mostly between the age of 20 and 45 years, with a female:male ratio of 5:1. Common causes include Graves disease, toxic multinodular goitre, solitary adenoma, thyrotoxicosis factitia and drugs such as amiodarone and exogenous iodine. Fifty percent of patients will present with psychiatric symptoms, of which anxiety and depression are more common. Other neuropsychiatric symptoms include hypomania and cognitive deficits that may improve with anti-thyroid therapy. Hyperthyroidism with anxious dysphoria is more common in younger patients. Depressive symptoms are not linearly related to thyroxine levels. Psychosis is rare in hyperthyroidism. If there is no improvement in the neuropsychiatric symptoms by 1 month after treatment with anti-thyroid hormone, psychotropic medication such as antidepressant is required.

References: Levenson JL (2004). *The American Psychiatric Publishing Textbook of Psychosomatic Medicine*. Arlington, VA: American Psychiatric Publishing, pp. 500–501; Puri BK, Hall A, Ho RC (2014). *Revision Notes in Psychiatry* (3rd edition). Boca-Raton, FL: CRC Press, p. 476.

Question 85 Answer: a, Hypersomnia

Explanation: Cushing syndrome is most commonly caused by exogenous administration of corticosteroids. Other causes include adrenocorticotropic hormone (ACTH)–dependent causes (e.g. Cushing disease, ectopic ACTH-producing tumours and ACTH administration), non-ACTH dependent causes (e.g. adrenal adenomas or carcinomas) and alcohol-dependent pseudo-Cushing syndrome. Depression is the most common psychiatric disorder found in patients with Cushing syndrome, with 50%–80% of patients suffering from depression with moderate-to-severe symptoms. It is usually associated with insomnia rather than hypersomnia, irritability, poor energy and concentration, poor memory and suicidal ideation. Suicide has been reported in between 3% and 10% of patients.

References: Levenson JL (2004). *The American Psychiatric Publishing Textbook of Psychosomatic Medicine*. Arlington, VA: American Psychiatric Publishing, p. 503; Puri BK, Hall A, Ho RC (2014). *Revision Notes in Psychiatry* (3rd edition). Boca-Raton, FL: CRC Press, p. 476.

Question 86 Answer: c, Lymphoma

Explanation: Depression is challenging to study because depressive symptoms occur on a spectrum that ranges from sadness to major affective disorder, and mood change may be difficult to evaluate when a patient is confronted by a major threat to life. The prevalence of depression in patients with cancer is similar to that in comparably ill patients with other medical diagnoses. This suggests that it is the degree of illness, irrespective of its underlying cause, that is the primary determinant of depression. When severe depression is present in patients with cancer, it should be treated as aggressively as it is in other medically ill patients. The types of cancer that have been found to be highly associated with depression include breast, pancreatic, lung and oropharyngeal. The prevalence of depression is reported to be lower in patients with other cancers such as colon cancer, lymphoma and gynaecological cancer.

References: Massie MJ (2004). Prevalence of depression in patients with cancer. *J Natl Cancer Inst Monogr*, 32: 57–71; Massie MJ, Gagnon P, Holland JC (1994). Depression and suicide in patients with cancer. *J Pain Symptom Manage*, 9(5): 325–340.

Question 87 Answer: a, Serotonin syndrome

Explanation: Patients who are taking monoamine oxidase inhibitors (MAOIs) should inform their doctor that they are on the medication. Ingestion of food high in dietary tyramine could lead to a hypertensive crisis due to the inhibition of peripheral pressor amines. In addition, some of the commonly used opioid analgesics also serve as weak serotonin re-uptake inhibitors. Hence, they could potentially precipitate serotonin toxicity when administered together with MAOIs.

Reference: Gilman PK et al. (2005). Monoamine oxidase inhibitors, opioid analgesics and serotonin toxicity. *Br J Anaesth*, 95(4): 434–441.

Question 88 Answer: a, Fluoxetine
Explanation: Citalopram and fluoxetine are present in breast milk at relatively high levels and hence contraindicated.

Reference: Puri BK, Hall AD, Ho RC (2014). *Revision Notes in Psychiatry*. Boca Raton, FL: CRC Press, p. 570.

Question 89 Answer: e, 50%
Explanation: Lithium carbonate is commonly used in the prophylaxis of bipolar disorder. It could also be used in the treatment of acute mania. Using it as a mono-therapy in bipolar disorder is likely to result in sustained remission in approximately 50% of individuals. NICE guidelines recommend pharmacological treatment for at least 2 years after an episode of bipolar disorder.

Reference: Puri BK, Hall AD, Ho RC (2014). *Revision Notes in Psychiatry*. Boca Raton, FL: CRC Press, p. 396.

Question 90 Answer: e, Hoarding
Explanation: Hoarding is most commonly found in people with OCD. Around 10%–15% of people with OCD have compulsive hoarding as their most prominent symptom.

Reference: Puri BK, Hall AD, Ho RC (2014). *Revision Notes in Psychiatry*. Boca Raton, FL: CRC Press, p. 425.

Question 91 Answer: d, 50%
Explanation: Clomipramine and SSRI antidepressants are commonly being used to treat OCD. They have demonstrated greater efficacy than antidepressants with no selective serotonergic properties. Concomitant depression is not necessary for serotonergic antidepressants to improve symptoms. The success rates have been estimated to be approximately 50%–79%. If the patient does not continue on the medications, relapse often occurs.

Reference: Puri BK, Hall AD, Ho RC (2014). *Revision Notes in Psychiatry*. Boca Raton, FL: CRC Press, p. 418.

Question 92 Answer: a, Buspirone
Explanation: With regard to the pharmacological treatment for post-traumatic stress disorder (PTSD), medications such as fluoxetine, paroxetine, sertraline, venlafaxine and escitalopram have been considered to be beneficial. To lessen fear-induced startle, medications such as buspirone can be used.

Reference: Puri BK, Hall AD, Ho RC (2014). *Revision Notes in Psychiatry*. Boca Raton, FL: CRC Press, p. 428.

Question 93 Answer: b, Humour
Explanation: In 1993, Vaillant proposed a hierarchy of defence mechanisms that is ranked according to the degree of adaptivity. In this hierarchy, mature defence

mechanisms (such as humour) have the highest degree of adaptivity, followed by neurotic defence mechanisms (such as reaction formation), immature defence mechanisms (such as idealization) and then psychotic defence mechanisms (such as delusional projection and psychotic denial).

Reference: Vaillant GE (1993). *The Wisdom of the Ego*. Cambridge, MA: Harvard University Press.

Question 94 Answer: e, Lead poisoning
Explanation: Pica may lead to lead poisoning but is not common. It may persist into adulthood as geophagy (i.e. eating clay and dirt).

Further Reading: Puri BK, Treasaden I (eds) (2010). *Psychiatry: An Evidence-Based Text*. London: Hodder Arnold. p. 716.

Question 95 Answer: c, 72 hours
Explanation: 'Coke' is the colloquial name for cocaine. The other names include that of snow, girl and lady. It could be detected in the urine between 6 and 8 hours, and its metabolites would last for 2–4 days.

Reference: Puri BK, Hall AD, Ho RC (2014). *Revision Notes in Psychiatry*. Boca Raton, FL: CRC Press, p. 529.

Question 96 Answer: d, Schizophrenia
Explanation: This is a condition that has an incidence of 1 in 4000 live births. More than 50% of patients have mild-to-moderate learning disability. The commonest associated psychiatric feature is that of schizophrenia.

Reference: Puri BK, Hall AD, Ho RC (2014). *Revision Notes in Psychiatry*. Boca Raton, FL: CRC Press, p. 673.

Question 97 Answer: d, Only males are affected by this disorder
Explanation: Fragile X syndrome affects 1 in 4000 men and 1 in 8000 women. 1 in 700 women is a carrier for fragile X syndrome. The prevalence is less common in men because only one in five men affected by the mutations at the fragile site is phenotypically and intellectually unaffected.

Reference: Puri BK, Hall AD, Ho RC (2014). *Revision Notes in Psychiatry*. Boca Raton, FL: CRC Press, p. 661.

Question 98 Answer: e, 60% and higher
Explanation: Rett syndrome is attributable to mutation of the methyl CpG binding protein 2 (MECP2) gene on the X chromosome. The prevalence rate is between 1 in 15,000 and 1 in 22,000 females. The incidence of seizures is 60%–90%. Other features include plateau in social skill development by 6 months, severe impairment in expressive and receptive language and trunk ataxia and apraxia.

Reference: Puri BK, Hall AD, Ho RC (2014). *Revision Notes in Psychiatry*. Boca Raton, FL: CRC Press, pp. 629–630.

Question 99 Answer: a, Hyperuricaemia is a rare feature in the variant form
Explanation: Hyperuricaemia is a constant feature of this disease in both classic and variant forms. Tophaceous gout and gouty nephropathy may appear in adolescence. It is caused by defect in hypoxanthine guanine phosphoribosyl-transferase resulting in accumulation of uric acid. Allopurinol reduces uric acid levels but offers no therapeutic benefits in behavioural symptoms.

Reference: Moore DP, Puri BK (2012). *Textbook of Clinical Neuropsychiatry and Behavioral Neuroscience* (3rd edition). London: Hodder Arnold, p. 463.

Question 100 Answer: e, Hypomelanotic macules
Explanation: Skin findings are very common in tuberous sclerosis. In most cases, the presence of hypomelanotic macules is the first sign of tuberous sclerosis, which is present in 90% or more of the affected infant. These hypopigmented lesions are described as ash-leaf spots and are best observed using a Wood's lamp.

Reference: Moore DP, Puri BK (2012). *Textbook of Clinical Neuropsychiatry and Behavioral Neuroscience* (3rd edition). London: Hodder Arnold, p. 456.

Question 101 Answer: d, Chromosome 15
Explanation: The girl has Angelman syndrome, which is deletion of maternal chromosome 15. It is an autosomal dominant disorder with prevalence of 1/20,000–1/30,000. Clinical features include paroxysms of laughter, cheerful disposition, ataxia, axial hypotonia, jerky movements, epilepsy, gastrointerstinal problems and severe or profound learning disability.

Reference: Puri BK, Treasaden I (eds) (2010). *Psychiatry: An Evidence-Based Text*. London: Hodder Arnold, p. 471.

Question 102 Answer: e, Somatic complaints
Explanation: Childhood depression is less common compared with that of childhood dysthymia. The clinical features tend to include that of growth impairment, boredom, low motivation to play, poor academic performance, poor feeding and somatic complaints. Mood symptoms are similar to adults, and severe cases may present with mood congruent psychotic features. There tends to be more anxiety and anger but fewer vegetative symptoms compared with adults.

Reference: Puri BK, Hall AD, Ho RC (2014). *Revision Notes in Psychiatry*. Boca Raton, FL: CRC Press, p. 648.

Question 103 Answer: e, Drug treatment reduces the rate of delinquency and substance abuse in children with ADHD to the rate found in normal controls
Explanation: The MTA study shows that children with ADHD continue to show higher than normal rates of delinquency (four times) and substance use (two times). In the MTA study, 485 children took part in the 3-year follow-up study. Their mean age was 12 years. The primary outcome measures were ADHD and oppositional defiant disorder symptoms, reading scores, social skills, level of

impairment and diagnosis. At the end of the first year, the research protocol was dropped, which allowed for more naturalistic and personalized treatment.

Reference: Bates G (2009). Drug treatments for attention-deficit hyperactivity disorder in young people. *Adv Psychiatr Treat*, 15: 162–171.

Question 104 Answer: e, 20%
Explanation: The prevalence of bipolar disorder in adolescents is 0.5%–1.0%. There may be either a genetic predisposition or a drug-induced cause. The clinical features are similar to those of adults. First-rank symptoms are present in around 20% of patients. The first-line treatment is still olanzapine, although valproate and lithium are effective. Family therapy may be indicated and helpful for stabilization of symptoms.

Reference: Puri BK, Hall AD, Ho RC (2014). *Revision Notes in Psychiatry*. Boca Raton, FL: CRC Press, p. 651.

Question 105 Answer: e, 90%
Explanation: The heritability for autism is around 90%, with concordance rates around 60% in identical twins and 0%–10% in fraternal twins. The recurrence rate in siblings is roughly 3% for narrowly defined autism but is about 10%–20% for milder variants. The loci may involve chromosomes 2q and 7q.

Reference: Puri BK, Hall AD, Ho RC (2014). *Revision Notes in Psychiatry*. Boca Raton, FL: CRC Press, p. 623.

Question 106 Answer: e, 4 years
Explanation: Chronic motor or vocal tic disorder usually lasts for 4–6 years and stops in early adolescence.

Reference: Puri BK, Hall AD, Ho RC (2014). *Revision Notes in Psychiatry*. Boca Raton, FL: CRC Press, p. 642.

Question 107 Answer: a, It begins in early childhood
Explanation: Conduct disorder begins in middle childhood. In terms of biological factors, low plasma 5-hydroxytryptamine (5-HT) level, excess testosterone, low cholesterol and low skin tolerance are all associated risks. In terms of social factors, uncaring school, parental psychiatric disorder, parental criminality, hostility towards the child, single parent and overcrowded (>four children) environment are all associated risks.

References: Golubchik P, Mozes T, Vered Y, Weizman A (2009). Platelet poor plasma serotonin level in delinquent adolescents diagnosed with conduct disorder. *Prog Neuropsychopharmacol Biol Psychiatry*, 33: 1223–1225; Puri BK, Hall AD, Ho RC (2014). Revision Notes in Psychiatry. Boca Raton, FL: CRC Press, pp. 635–639.

Question 108 Answer: b, Carbamazepine
Explanation: One of the core symptoms in PTSD is that of having intrusion symptoms such as recurrent distressing dreams, dissociative reactions and prolonged stress. Medications such as carbamazepine, propranolol and clonidine could help to reduce all these symptoms.

Reference: Puri BK, Hall AD, Ho RC (2014). *Revision Notes in Psychiatry*. Boca Raton, FL: CRC Press, p. 428.

Question 109 Answer: b, There is an increase in the glucocorticoid receptors in the hippocampus
Explanation: Previous research demonstrated an increase in the glucocorticoid receptors in the hypothalamus and a reduction in the peripheral cortisol. The initial mobilization and the subsequent depletion of noradrenaline following shock in animals indicate a possible catecholaminergic mediation of PTSD symptoms. In view of the similarities between PTSD symptoms and opioid withdrawal, there has been much speculation that opioid functioning is disturbed in PTSD. It has been noted that stress-induced analgesia is reversible by naloxone in PTSD veterans exposed to traumatic stimulus.

Reference: Puri BK, Hall AD, Ho RC (2014). *Revision Notes in Psychiatry*. Boca Raton, FL: CRC Press, p. 427.

Question 110 Answer: d, Parent management training
Explanation: The boy has oppositional defiant disorder. Parent management training and family therapy are possible treatments. In parental training, the aim is to eliminate harsh and punitive parenting and to increase positive parent–child interactions. As for behavioural therapy, it aims to discourage oppositional defiant behaviour and to encourage appropriate and adaptive behaviour; parents can coach the children to develop adaptive responses.

Reference: Puri BK, Hall AD, Ho RC (2014). *Revision Notes in Psychiatry*. Boca Raton, FL: CRC Press, p. 639.

Question 111 Answer: e, Build a tower of 10 cubes and stand on one foot
Explanation: By the age of 3 years, a child is able to stand on one foot, dance and jump and build a tower of 10 cubes. At the age of 5 years, the child can copy a square.

Reference: Wiener JM, Dulcan MK (2003). *The American Psychiatric Publishing Textbook of Child and Adolescent Psychiatry* (3rd edition). Arlington, VA: American Psychiatric Press, p. 17.

Extended Match Items

Theme: Research methodology

Question 112 Answer: e, Level 2B

Question 113 Answer: b, Level 1B

Question 114 Answer: h, Level 3B
Explanation: The Centre for Evidence-Based Medicine (CEBM) has ranked the different types of research evidence based on how likely they are to be true. The strongest evidence comes from a systematic review that demonstrates consistent findings from several high-quality RCTs. This is termed as level 1 evidence, and recommendations based on level 1 results are called grade A. Further down the hierarchy comes more heterogeneous findings and evidence from less robust sources.

Reference: Lewis GH, Sheringham J, Kalim K, Crayford TJ (2008). *Mastering Public Health*. London: Royal Society of Medicine Press, p. 62.

Theme: Research Methodology

Question 115 Answer: b, Cohort study
Explanation: In a cohort study, a group of individuals is selected who do not initially have the outcome of interest. A range of exposures is quantified for cohort members, and at the end of the study, those people who have developed the outcome of interest are compared (according to the exposure of interest) with those who have not. The strengths of such a study include able to follow temporal relationships, well suited to rare exposures, multiple effects of a single exposure, minimize selection bias and useful for diseases with long latency periods. The weaknesses of such a study include that it is time consuming, expensive, with a risk of loss of follow-up, is inefficient for rare diseases and records may be inadequate for ascertainment.

Question 116 Answer: a, Case–control study
Explanation: In a case–control study, individuals with the outcome of interest (cases) are matched with individuals who do not have the outcome of interest (controls). The strengths of such a study include that it is rapid and cheap, ideal for rare diseases/outcomes, useful for diseases with long latent periods and can simultaneously examine a large number of potential exposures. The weaknesses of such a study include selection bias (as exposure and disease have already occurred); that temporal relationships may be difficult to establish; that recall bias (of information on exposure and disease) cannot compare incidence rates and there may be misclassification of exposure/disease status.

Question 117 Answer: d, Ecological study
Explanation: Ecological study is characterized by the unit of observation being a group (e.g. a population or community) rather than an individual. It describes disease patterns for an entire population with regard to another parameter. It can be used for international comparisons, study of group-level effects (e.g. legislation) and hypothesis formulation. The strengths of such a study include rapid results and low cost. The weaknesses of the study include inability to control for unknown confounders; that it considers only average exposure, so would not be able to detect a J-shaped curve; there may be spatial autocorrelation (analysis assumes that all

areas are independent but may not be); leakage of exposures through migration; no information on individuals and risk of ecological fallacy. An ecological fallacy is an error of logic that occurs when inferences are made regarding individuals, based on aggregate data from the population to which the individuals belong.

Question 118 Answer: a, Case–control study
Explanation: In a case–control study, individuals with the outcome of interest (cases) are matched with individuals who do not have the outcome of interest (controls). The strengths of such a study include that it is rapid and cheap, ideal for rare diseases/outcomes, useful for diseases with long latent periods and can simultaneously examine a large number of potential exposures. The weaknesses of such a study include selection bias (as exposure and disease have already occurred), that temporal relationships may be difficult to establish, recall bias (of information on exposure and disease), that it cannot compare incidence rates and there may be misclassification of exposure/disease status.

Question 119 Answer: c, Cross-sectional study
Explanation: In a cross-sectional study, all the variables (exposures and outcomes) are measured at the same time. It determines the simultaneous prevalence of exposure and disease. It also measures prevalence of various diseases, characteristics and health-care usage and makes comparisons. The strengths of such a study include that it can examine multiple exposures and outcomes, is rapid and cheap and useful for rare diseases. The weaknesses of such a study include that findings cannot differentiate the determinants of aetiology and survival because it is measuring prevalence, not incidence.

Reference: Lewis GH, Sheringham J, Kalim K, Crayford TJB (2008). *Mastering Public Health: A Postgraduate Guide to Examination and Revalidation*. London: Royal Society of Medicine Press, pp. 34–38.

Theme: Dementia

Question 120 Answer: c, Cerebral autosomal dominant arteriopathy with subcortical infarcts and leukoencephalopathy (CADASIL)
Explanation: This patient suffers from cerebral autosomal dominant arteriopathy with subcortical infarcts and leukoencephalopathy (CADASIL). It may start with attacks of migraine with aura or subcortical transient ischemic attacks or strokes or a mood disorder between 35 and 55 years of age. The disease progresses to subcortical dementia associated with pseudobulbar palsy and urinary incontinence.

Question 121 Answer: d, Fronto-temporal lobe dementia (Pick disease)
Explanation: This patient suffers from fronto-temporal lobe dementia (Pick disease). It has an average onset of 53 years. It is characterized by disinhibition, apathy, loss of empathy, perseverative or compulsive behaviours, hyperorality and impaired executive ability.

Question 122 Answer: i, Pseudodementia

Explanation: This patient suffers from pseudodementia. Depression is most commonly responsible for pseudodementia. Depression does not significantly impair performance on cognitive testing if the assessor provides enough time and encouragement. However, depression in the elderly may well be associated with cognitive deficits, and those with dementia may develop depression.

Question 123 Answer: g, Normal pressure hydrocephalus

Explanation: This patient suffers from normal pressure hydrocephalus. He has the symptoms of dementia, gait apraxia and urinary incontinence. This dementia conforms to the subcortical classification because it entails slowing of thought and gait but spares language skills. Gait apraxia is generally the initial, most consistent and most prominent feature of normal pressure hydrocephalus. Dilation of the cerebral ventricles, especially the third ventricle, and normal cerebrospinal fluid (CSF) pressure on lumber puncture are found. Prompt treatment may result in reversibility.

Reference: Kaufman DM, Milstein MJ (2013). *Clinical Neurology for Psychiatrists*. Philadelphia, PA: Saunders, pp. 122–125, 127–128, 133.

Theme: Dementia

Question 124 Answer: h, Psychogenic fugue

Explanation: This patient suffers from a psychogenic fugue as she exhibits features of dissociative amnesia and an apparently purposeful journey away from home. Self-care and social interaction are maintained during a fugue. It is usually precipitated by severe stress. It lasts for hours to days, but recovery is abrupt and complete.

Question 125 Answer: j, Vascular dementia

Explanation: This patient suffers from vascular dementia. He had multiple risk factors for stroke. Vascular dementia is characterized by a stepwise deteriorating course with a patchy distribution of neurological ad neuropsychological deficits. There is usually evidence of vascular disease on physical examination (hypertension, carotid bruits, enlarged heart, focal neurological deficits suggestive of stroke). Depression and/or episodes of affective lability are common.

Question 126 Answer: f, Lewy body dementia

Explanation: This person suffers from Lewy body dementia. It is characterized by cognitive impairment, fluctuating consciousness, extrapyramidal signs and motor features of parkinsonism, hallucinations, especially recurrent well-formed and detailed visual hallucinations, and neuroleptic sensitivity. It is the third most common cause of late-onset dementia and a less common cause of early-onset dementia.

Question 127 Answer: e, Korsakoff psychosis

Explanation: This person suffers from Korsakoff psychosis. It is characterized by anterograde and retrograde amnesia, sparing of immediate recall, disorientation in time, inability to recall temporal sequence of events and confabulation.

Question 128 Answer: k, Wernicke encephalopathy
Explanation: This person suffers from Wernicke encephalopathy, which is characterized by an acute confusional state, ophthalmaplegia, nystagmus and an ataxic gait. It is associated with peripheral neuropathy. It is caused by severe deficiency of thiamine, which is usually caused by alcohol abuse. Other causes include starvation (in this scenario) lesions in stomach and small intestine disorders causing malabsorption. The administration of sugars before replacing thiamine can precipitate Wernicke encephalopathy, as in this case.

Reference: Puri BK, Hall AD. Ho RC (2014). *Revision Notes in Psychiatry*. Boca Raton, FL: CRC Press, pp. 433, 699, 702–703, 517–518.

Theme: Gender Ratios
Question 129 Answer: f, 1:10

Question 130 Answer: f, 1:10

Question 131 Answer: b, 1:2

Question 132 Answer: a, 1:1

Question 133 Answer: d, 3:1

Question 134 Answer: b, 1:2

Question 135 Answer: a, 1:1
Explanation: For schizophrenia, there is an equal male-to-female ratio. Women tend to show a bimodal peak of incidence in their late 20s and 50s. For depressive disorder, the ratio is 1:2. The peak age of first onset of depression is 30. In the United Kingdom, the male-to-female ratio of self-harm and suicide has been estimated to be 3:1, and the rate for women is raising. For social phobia, there is an equal gender ratio. The first onset is between 11 and 15 years. In PTSD, the male-to-female ratio is 1:2. Men's trauma is mainly due to combat experience, and women's trauma is related to assault or rape. The gender ratio for anorexia nervosa and bulimia nervosa is also 1:10.

Reference: Puri BK, Hall AD, Ho RC (2014). *Revision Notes in Psychiatry*. Boca Raton, FL: CRC Press, p. 295.

Theme: Learning Disability
Question 136 Answer: d, Prader–Willi syndrome
Explanation: Other syndromes than Prader–Willi Syndrome that can cause short stature include Williams syndrome, foetal alcohol syndrome, Cornelia de Lange syndrome, Rubinstein–Taybi syndrome and Sanfillipo syndrome.

Question 137 Answer: b, Homocystinuria
Explanation: Other syndromes than homocystinuria that can cause tall stature include XYY syndrome and Klinefelter syndrome.

Question 138 Answer: a, Cri du chat syndrome
Explanation: Other syndromes than cri du chat that can cause microcephaly include Wolf–Hirschhorn syndrome, Di George syndrome, Rubinstein–Taybi syndrome, Cornelia de Lange syndrome and Angelman syndrome.

Question 139 Answer: e, Neurofibromatosis
Explanation: Features of neurofibromatosis other than macrocephaly include short stature, optic nerve glioma, hypertension, tumours arising from the connective tissue of nerve sheaths, café au lait spots, cutaneous neurofibromas, freckling of groin or armpit, skeletal deformities and lisch nodules.

Question 140 Answer: c, Phenylketonuria
Explanation: Syndromes other than phenylketonuria that are associated with hyperactivity and aggression include Hurler syndrome, Soto syndrome, fragile X syndrome and tuberous sclerosis.

Reference: Puri BK, Hall AD, Ho RC (2014). *Revision Notes in Psychiatry*. Boca Raton, FL: CRC Press, p. 673.

Theme: Liver Impairment and Medications

Question 141 Answer: b, Chlorpromazine
Explanation: Only low doses of haloperidol should be used for patients with liver impairment. It is important to avoid antipsychotic drugs that have extensive hepatic metabolism, such as chlorpromazine, which is also associated with anti-cholinergic side effects.

Question 142 Answer: c, Paroxetine, d, Citalopram
Explanation: Paroxetine and citalopram are indicated for use in patients with liver impairment. It is essential to avoid tricyclic antidepressants and also to avoid fluoxetine due to it having a long half-life and the risk of accumulation of metabolites.

Question 143 Answer: g, Lithium
Explanation: Lithium is the correct answer, as it is mainly metabolized by the renal system.

Question 144 Answer: h, Carbamazepine, i, Valproate
Explanation: It is essential to avoid carbamazepine, as it induces hepatic metabolism. It is also essential to avoid valproate because it is highly protein-bound and metabolized by the liver.

Reference: Puri BK, Hall AD, Ho RC (2014). *Revision Notes in Psychiatry*. Boca Raton, FL: CRC Press, p. 475.

Theme: Infectious Disease and Psychiatry

Question 145 Answer: d, Mania

Explanation: The prevalence increases as the disease progresses. If it presents early in the course of the HIV infection, it is usually associated with social problems. If it presents late in the course of the HIV infection, it is usually associated with HIV dementia. Other causes of mania may be drug induced or due to the direct effect of HIV infection on the CNS. Metabolic disturbances may be another causative factor.

Question 146 Answer: a, Acute stress reaction

Explanation: Acute stress reaction is common immediately after the diagnosis of HIV infection. The patient may present in a state of shock with depersonalization and de-realization. Other psychological reactions include anger, withdrawal, guilt, denial, fear of death and despair.

Question 147 Answer: c, Depressive disorder

Explanation: The prevalence of depression in people living with HIV has been estimated to be round 30%. Depressive disorder is more frequent in the period following the identification of the seropositive HIV infection or in the initial stages of HIV dementia. SSRIs are generally suitable for patients infective with HIV because SSRIs do not affect the CD4 counts.

Question 148 Answer: f, Dementia

Explanation: Early cognitive impairment occurs in 20% of patients infected with HIV. It can be classified into cognitive, behavioural and motor symptoms. The prevalence of dementia in patients suffering from acquired immune deficiency syndrome (AIDS) is around 25%. The onset of AIDS-associated dementia is usually insidious and occurs later in the course of the illness when there is significant immunosuppression.

Reference: Puri BK, Hall AD, Ho RC (2014). *Revision Notes in Psychiatry*. Boca Raton, FL: CRC Press, pp. 485–487.

Theme: Prevalence of Mental Retardation

Question 149 Answer: h, 80%

Explanation: Those with mild mental retardation have an IQ range of 50–69. There has been noted to be delayed understanding and usage of language. There are possible difficulties in gaining independence. Work is possible in practical occupations, and any behavioural, social and emotional difficulties are similar to the normal.

Question 150 Answer: e, 10%

Explanation: Those with moderate mental retardation have an IQ range of 35–49. There are varying profiles of abilities. Language use and development are variable. They often have associated epilepsy and neurological and other disabilities. There are delays in the achievement of self-care. Simple practical work is possible. Independent living is rarely achieved.

Question 151 Answer: c, 3%
Explanation: Those with severe mental retardation have an IQ range of between 20 and 34. There are more marked motor impairments than in those with moderate mental retardation. Achievements tend to be at the lower end of those with moderate mental retardation.

Question 152 Answer: b, 2%
Explanation: Those with profound mental retardation have an IQ that is difficult to measure but is usually less than 20. It accounts for approximately 2% of learning difficulties. There are severe limitations in ability to understand or comply with requests or instructions. There is little or no self-care. Mostly severe mobility restricted. Basic or simple tasks may be acquired.

Reference: Puri BK, Hall AD, Ho RC (2014). *Revision Notes in Psychiatry*. Boca Raton, FL: CRC Press, p. 663.

Theme: Features of Learning Disabilities

Question 153 Answer: k, Testicular atrophy and infertility
Explanation: The clinical features include tall stature (4 cm taller than average), poor beard growth, gynaecomastia, osteoporosis and testicular atrophy and infertility.

Question 154 Answer: d, Macrocephaly, e, Gaze aversion, f, High arched palate
Explanation: The clinical features include macrocephaly, gaze aversion, large floppy ears, mid-face hypoplasia, high arched palate and long thin face with prominent jaw.

Question 155 Answer: a, Conductive deafness, b, Almond-shaped eyes slanting laterally upwards, c, Prominent epicanthic folds, g, Wide sandal gap between first and second toes
Explanation: For individuals with Down syndrome, on examination, there will be more conductive rather than sensori-neural deafness. There is the presence of almond-shaped eyes slanting laterally upwards with Brushfield spots on the iris. There will be prominent epicanthic folds, with low-set simple external ears and hearing impairments. There is the presence of wide sandal gap between the first and second toes with increased congenital heart disease.

Question 156 Answer: h, Shield-shaped thorax, i, Widely spaced nipples, j, Rudimentary ovaries
Explanation: Other features include short stature, low hairline, poor breast development and elbow deformity.

Reference: Puri BK, Hall AD, Ho RC (2014). *Revision Notes in Psychiatry*. Boca Raton, FL: CRC Press, p. 667.

Theme: Research Methodologies and Statistics

Question 157 Answer: a, Fixed-effect meta-regression

Question 158 Answer: b, Mixed-effects meta-regression

Question 159 Answer: d, Simple meta-regression

Explanation: In meta-analysis, meta-regression is mainly used to examine the impact of different variables on study effect size and to identify moderators that explain heterogeneity. There are three models of meta-regression: simple, fixed-effect and mixed-effects. The simple meta-regression model is not commonly used because it does not allow specification of within-study variation. The fixed-effect meta-regression model allows for within-study variability but not between-study variability, because all studies have an identical expected fixed-effect size. The fixed-effect meta-regression model does not allow generalization of results to the population. The mixed-effects meta-regression model allows for within-and between-study variations and adds in the effects for moderators. The mixed-effects meta-regression model is the most appropriate model to apply in most situations.

Reference: Bellavance F, Dionne G, Lebeau M (2009). The value of a statistical life: A meta-analysis with a mixed effects regression model. *Journal of Health Economics*, 28(2): 444–464.

Theme: Immune-Related Disorders

Question 160 Answer: g, Sarcoidosis

Explanation: The typical age of onset is that of 20–30 years old. The age of onset is very often gradual. Most of the cases are detected via chest X-rays. More than 90% of individuals do have chest involvement with symptoms such as cough and difficulties breathing. In addition, there might be a dementia-like clinical picture. At times, there is frontal lobe involvement with resultant frontal lobe syndrome.

Question 161 Answer: d, Systemic lupus erythematosus (SLE)

Explanation: SLE is a condition that affects females predominantly. The age of onset is usually between puberty and 40 years old. SLE is a systemic disease, and it could affect multiple systems. In particular, cerebral lupus could always manifest as depression, mania, psychosis, delirium or even dementia.

Question 162 Answer: g, Sarcoidosis

Explanation: In this condition, hypercalcaemia is a common presentation. There might also be cerebral involvement, which are usually characterized by the presenece of multiple granulomas.

Reference: Puri BK, Treasaden I (eds) (2010). *Psychiatry: An Evidence-Based Text*. London: Hodder Arnold, pp. 586–590.

Theme: Consultation Liaison Psychiatry

Question 163 Answer: d, Parkinson disease
Explanation: The diagnosis is typical of that of Parkinson disease. Their gait is characteristic in that the patients are able to take only small steps.

Question 164 Answer: c, Amyotrophic lateral sclerosis (ALS)
Explanation: The condition that he is having is that of emotional incontinence. Patients tend to present initially with weakness in the upper emtremities, and this would limit their ability to carry out activities of daily living.

Question 165 Answer: e, Progressive supranuclear palsy (PSP)
Explanation: This condition usually presents itself in the sixth decade with frequent unexplained falls, mainly due to marked postural instability. Dementia would occur in approximately one half of all the patients.

Question 166 Answer: a, Huntington's disease
Explanation: This is an example of the above disorder. It is an autosomal-dominant diorder and hence a positive family history is usually found.

Reference: Puri BK, Treasaden I (eds) (2010). *Psychiatry: An Evidence-Based Text*. London: Hodder Arnold, pp. 541–552.

Theme: Schizophrenia and Psychosis

Question 167 Answer: a, No increase in risk
Explanation: Schizophrenia is a disorder that has been known to be equally common among males and females. There is no increment in the risk.

Question 168 Answer: b, Twofold increment
Explanation: Afro-Carribbean immigrants to the United Kingdom tend to have higher risk of acquiring schizophrenia. This phenomenon is seen in the second generation.

Question 169 Answer: b, Twofold increment
Explanation: Cannabis leads to a twofold increment in the risk of schizophrenia. This is also dependent on genetic factors such as the alleles that he possesses.

Question 170 Answer: c, Fourfold increase
Explanation: Cannabis usage leads to a fourfold increase in the risk of psychosis.

Reference: Puri BK, Hall AD, Ho RC (2014). *Revision Notes in Psychiatry*. Boca Raton, FL: CRC Press, p. 359.

Theme: Mood and Affective Disorders

Question 171 Answer: a, Step 1

Question 172 Answer: e, Step 5

Question 173 Answer: d, Step 4

Question 174 Answer: b, Step 2

Question 175 Answer: b, Step 2
Explanation (Questions 171 through 175): In accordance to the NICE guidelines, in Step 1, the doctor needs to assess and provide support and monitor accordingly. In Step 2, when there are persistent subthrehold depressive symptoms or mild-to-moderate depression, low-intensity psychological interventions, psychological interventions and medications are recommended. In Step 3, when there are persistent subthreshold depressive symptoms or mild-to-moderate depression with inadequate response to initial interventions and moderate or severe depression, medication, high-intensity psychological interventions and combined treatments are recommended. In Step 4, the depression is usually deemed to be severe and complex with risk to life and severe self-neglect. Medication, high-intensity psychological interventions, electroconvulsive therapy, crisis service and combined treatments are recommended.

Reference: http://www.nice.org.uk/guidance/cg90/chapter/1-recommendations#stepped-care, last assessed on 22 Aug 2015.

Theme: General Adult Psychiatry—Treatment

Question 176 Answer: d, Reduction in perinatal trauma, e, Reduction in stress associated with migration, Successful treatment of middle-ear disease in childhood
Explanation: Primary prevention targets people before the onset of schizophrenia, and it includes reduction of schizophrenia-like psychosis, prevention of perinatal trauma and targeting adverse social factors (e.g. stress associated with migration). Successful treatment of middle ear disease in childhood may reduce the risk of temporal lobe epilepsy and schizophrenia-like psychosis.

Question 177 Answer: b, Maintenance in antipsychotic treatment, c, Psychoeducation about schizophrenia
Explanation: Secondary prevention targets people who have developed schizophrenia. Secondary prevention strategies include drug treatment and social treatment (e.g. psychoeducation of schizophrenia).

Question 178 Answer: a, Listen to loud stimulating music to drown out the auditory hallucinations not responding to antipsychotic treatment
Explanation: Tertiary prevention is designed to reduce the severity and disability associated with schizophrenia such as auditory hallucination not responding to treatment.

Reference: Paykel ES, Jenkins R (1994). *Prevention in Psychiatry*. London: Gaskell.

Theme: Psychotherapy

Question 179 Answer: j, Shaping
Explanation: This phenomenon is known as shaping.

Reference And Further Reading: Puri BK, Treasaden I (eds) (2010). *Psychiatry: An Evidence-Based Text*. London: Hodder Arnold, p. 204.

Question 180 Answer: i, Reciprocal inhibition
Explanation: Reciprocal inhibition is a concept developed by Joseph Wolpe. Opposing emotions cannot exist simultaneously.

Reference: Puri BK, Treasaden I (eds) (2010). *Psychiatry: An Evidence-Based Text*. London: Hodder Arnold, pp. 655, 990.

Question 181 Answer: k, Systematic desensitization
Explanation: Systemic desensitization was developed by Wolpe.

Reference And Further Reading: Puri BK, Treasaden I (eds) (2010). *Psychiatry: An Evidence-Based Text*. London: Hodder Arnold p. 990.

Theme: Effect on the Newborn Due to Substance Abuse

Question 182 Answer: b, Benzodiazepine
Explanation: Benzodiazepine is contraindicated in the first trimester. It leads to floppy baby syndrome if taken near term.

Question 183 Answer: d, Tobacco
Explanation: Tobacco also causes intra-uterine growth retardation (IUGR), low birth weight and developmental delay.

Question 184 Answer: a, Alcohol
Explanation: The diagnostic criteria of Fetal Alcohol Syndrome (FAS) include (1) pre- or post-natal growth deficiency; (2) CNS abnormalities: neurological abnormality, developmental delay, intellectual impairment and structural abnormalities and (3) facial anomalies: short palpebral fissures, thin upper lip, flattened mid-face and indistinct philtrum.

Question 185 Answer: c, Opiate
Explanation: 90% of infants born to dependent mothers show signs of withdrawal.
   Other drugs such as cocaine cause low birth weight, inverse dose-dependent relationship with brain circumference and brain weight with motor abnormalities.

Reference: Puri BK, Hall AD, Ho RC (2014). *Revision Notes in Psychiatry*. Boca Raton, FL: CRC Press, pp. 561–562.

Theme: Eating Disorders

Question 186 Answer: e, Fluoxetine
Explanation: The three medications mentioned above can cause unintentional weight loss in elderly. Fluoxetine is stronger than other SSRIs in causing anorectic effect.

Reference: Brymer C, Winograd CH (1992). Fluoxetine in elderly patients: Is there cause for concern? *J Am Geriatr Soc*, 40: 902–905.

Question 187 Answer: b, Coeliac disease
Explanation: This patient suffers from coeliac disease. Investigations include full blood count (FBC) ($\downarrow$Hb) and detection of antigliaden antibody. Treatment involves a gluten-free diet, iron supplementation and immunosuppression.

Reference: Firth JD, Collier JD (2001). *Medical Masterclass: Gastroenterology and Hepatology*. London: Royal College of Physicians.

Question 189 Answer: c, Crohn's disease
Explanation: This patient suffers from Crohn's disease. Investigations include FBC ($\downarrow$Hb), $\uparrow$C Reactive protein (CRP), $\uparrow$erythrocyte sedimentation rate (ESR), $\downarrow$B$_{12}$ and folate. Sigmoidoscopy and colonoscopy show patch inflammation, and biopsy may show granuloma. Small bowel follow-through may show fistulae. Corticosteroids and azathioprine are prescribed for short term and long term, respectively.

Reference: Firth JD, Collier JD (2001). *Medical Masterclass: Gastroenterology and Hepatology*. London: Royal College of Physicians.

Question 190 Answer: f, Whipple's disease
Explanation: The patient suffers from Whipple's disease, which is caused by *Tropheryma whippelli*. Jejunal biopsy shows large foamy macrophages in lamina propria, which contain positive periodic acid-Schiff staining material. Treatment is to continue sulphamethoxazole and trimethoprin for 1 year. Other causes of malabsorption include chronic pancreatitis, tropical sprue (rare in the United Kingdom), giardiasis (with travelling history), small bowel syndrome and postgastric surgery.

Reference: Firth JD, Collier JD (2001). *Medical Masterclass: Gastroenterology and Hepatology*. London: Royal College of Physicians.

Question 191 Answer: d, Hyperthyroidism
Explanation: This affects commonly between 2% and 5% of all women mostly between the age of 20 and 45 years with a female-to-male ratio of 5:1. Fifty percent present with psychiatric symptoms. Anxiety and depression are common. Depressive symptoms are not linearly related to thyroxine levels.

Reference: Puri BK, Hall AD, Ho RC (2014). *Revision Notes in Psychiatry*. Boca Raton, FL: CRC Press, p. 476.

Question 192 Answer: a, Anorexia nervosa
Explanation: The ICD-10 diagnostic criteria requires the presence of the following: (a) Body weight that is maintained at 15% below expected, (b) weight loss self-induced by avoidance of fattening food and one or more of the following: self-induced vomiting, self-induced purging, excessive exercise, (c) body image distortion and (d) amenorrhoea.

Reference: Puri BK, Hall AD, Ho RC (2014). *Revision Notes in Psychiatry*. Boca Raton, FL: CRC Press, p. 577.

MRCPYSCH PAPER B MOCK EXAMINATION 5: QUESTIONS

GET THROUGH MRCPSYCH PAPER B MOCK EXAMINATION

Total number of questions: 174 (116 MCQs, 58 EMIs)
Total time provided: 180 minutes

Question 1
Which of the following is not a feature of Consolidated Standards of Reporting Trials (CONSORT) guidelines?
  a. Inclusion and exclusion criteria are clearly specified.
  b. Method of blinding is clearly specified.
  c. Pre-study power calculations are provided.
  d. There is per-protocol analysis.
  e. The randomization procedure is clearly specified.

Question 2
Which of the following is not a proper randomization method used in randomized controlled trials (RCTs)?
  a. Centralized randomization
  b. Minimization
  c. Quasi-randomization
  d. Stratified randomization
  e. Stepped wedge randomization

Question 3
What percentage of patients diagnosed with human immunodeficiency virus (HIV) have HIV-associated neurocognitive impairment?
  a. Less than 5%
  b. Between 5% and 15%
  c. Between 16% and 30%
  d. Between 30% and 50%
  e. More than 50%

Question 4

Which of the following complications best describes a man who recovered from herpes encephalitis and subsequently develops very good appetite, weight gain and high sexual drive?

a. Churg Strauss syndrome
b. Devic syndrome
c. Kluver Bucy syndrome
d. Hallervorden–Spatz disease
e. Tolosa–Hunt syndrome

Question 5

The court decision is that the murder charge is reduced to manslaughter in view of diminished responsibility as a result of the abnormality of the mind. Which of the following terminologies correctly describes the above?

a. Lawful homicide
b. Unlawful homicide
c. Involuntary manslaughter
d. Voluntary manslaughter
e. Gross negligence

Question 6

Which of the following statements regarding various types of offenders is correct?

a. A hepatologist refers a patient with hepatitis B to you. She is a 55-year-old woman with no previous offences and is an active member of her church. She has just been convicted of shoplifting. In this case, the most likely cause is depression.
b. In the United Kingdom, homicide of the father is more common than that of the mother.
c. Castration of violent offenders and reduction of testosterone have shown resultant significant reductions in violent offending.
d. Cautioning is not a common disposal method for female offenders.
e. Research studies have suggested that raised levels of serotonin turnover and alterations in dopamine metabolism occur in violent offenders.

Question 7

Which of the following is a characteristic feature of Lesch–Nyhan syndrome?

a. Café au lait spots
b. Hepato-splenomegaly
c. Macrocephaly
d. Micrognathia
e. Self-injurious behaviours

Question 8

Which of the following would you not expect to observe in the electroencephalogram (EEG) reading of an elderly person with normal ageing?

a. No significant increase in delta activity
b. A significant increase in delta and theta frequency
c. A small decrease in alpha frequency
d. A small increase in theta activity
e. A small increase in beta frequency

Question 9
The presence of eosinophilic inclusion bodies is most likely to be found in which of the following types of dementia?
a. Alzheimer's disease
b. Frontotemporal lobe dementia
c. Lewy body dementia
d. Huntington's disease
e. Vascular dementia

Question 10
Which personality disorder (PD) is associated with suicide in the elderly?
a. Anxious PD
b. Dependent PD
c. Histrionic PD
d. Paranoid PD
e. Schizoid PD

Question 11
What is the percentage of children with autistic disorder also suffering from mental retardation?
a. 10%
b. 20%
c. 35%
d. 50%
e. 70%

Question 12
Which of the following statements regarding personality changes across adulthood is false?
a. Personality retains stable over long periods.
b. Personality changes greatly over long periods.
c. There is an increase in the dimension of agreeableness.
d. There is a decline in the dimensions of extraversion.
e. There is a decline in the dimensions of openness to experience.

Question 13
Which of the following statements regarding coping in the elderly is true?
a. Involvement in religion and having spiritual beliefs do not help.
b. The elderly have less emotional reactivity when encountering stress compared with younger adults.

c. Minority groups use less religious coping when faced with difficulties.
d. The elderly have the same level of internal control as younger adults.
e. Retirement increases the risk of psychiatric disorders and leads to poorer coping in the elderly.

Question 14
A 35-year-old man who has been diagnosed with acquired immune deficiency syndrome (AIDS) is on follow-up with you for depression. He is keen to have psychological treatment in addition to medication. Which of the following therapies would you recommend?
a. Cognitive behavioural stress management
b. Family therapy
c. Psychodynamic psychotherapy
d. Hypnosis
e. Interpersonal psychotherapy

Question 15
Which of the following psychiatric disorders is least commonly seen in patients with chronic fatigue syndrome?
a. Anxiety
b. Cognitive dysfunction
c. Depression
d. Mania
e. Psychosis

Question 16
Which of the following is a defence mechanism associated with obsessions?
a. Denial
b. Projection
c. Reaction formation
d. Reversal into the opposite
e. Splitting

Question 17
Which of the following randomization methods is the least likely to produce bias in a randomized controlled trial?
a. Allocation of patients by their month of birth
b. Allocation of patients by hospitalization status (inpatient versus outpatient)
c. Allocation of patients by gender (subdivided into strata and individuals within each striatum undergo further randomization)
d. Allocation of patients by laboratory results (e.g. blood cholesterol status)
e. Allocation of patients by order of arrival time in clinic

Question 18
Which of the following does not increase the power of a randomized controlled trial?
a. Comparison of active treatment with placebo
b. High compliance rate with treatment

c. High potency of an antidepressant

d. An increase in the number of collaborating centres instead of the number of subjects

e. Using observer-rated questionnaires instead of self-reported questionnaires

Question 19

In the brief intervention for alcohol dependency with the acronym FRAMES, what does the 'E' stand for?

a. Expectation

b. Explanation

c. Evidence

d. Empathetic style

e. Empowerment

Question 20

A 20-year-old man was brought in by his parents, as he insists on waiting for a man to take revenge on him at the bus station. He appears to be odd in his speech and behaviour. Which of the following supports the diagnosis of schizotypal disorder?

a. Abnormal ideas but consistent with cultural norms.

b. Compulsive checking behaviour.

c. First-rank symptoms.

d. Good rapport with the interviewer.

e. The onset of symptoms occurs at the age of 14 years.

Question 21

Which of the following statements regarding vitamin B_{12} deficiency is false?

a. It increases with age.

b. It may present with macrocytic anaemia and neuropathy.

c. Psychosis may occur with the deficiency.

d. Measurement of vitamin B_{12} should be done in an elderly man presenting with cognitive impairment.

e. Serum homocysteine level is not a good indicator of vitamin B_{12} or folate status.

Question 22

A 68-year-old man presents to your clinic with worsening memory impairment and difficulty in finding words. You diagnose him to have Alzheimer's disease. His family has read up on apolipoprotein E (APOE) testing and is keen for him to undergo the test to confirm the diagnosis and guide treatment. Which one of the following statements regarding this test is true?

a. Homozygous for APOE allele is diagnostic for Alzheimer's disease.

b. This test is recommended to be done to predict the risk of dementia in asymptomatic persons.

c. The results of this test can help guide response to cholinesterase inhibitors.

d. The presence of the APOE allele is a risk factor for Alzheimer's disease.

e. The presence of APOE alleles increases the specificity of the diagnosis of Lewy body disease.

Question 23

After Alzheimer's disease, which of the following is the leading cause of dementia in elderly people?
a. Corticobasal degeneration
b. Frontal lobe dementia
c. Lewy body dementia
d. Multisystem atrophy
e. Vascular dementia

Question 24

Which of the following would be the most appropriate antidepressant to maintain a pregnant female on?
a. Amitriptyline
b. Paroxetine
c. Bupropion
d. Mirtazapine
e. Venlafaxine

Question 25

A 70-year-old man has been diagnosed to have early-onset dementia. Which of the following difficulties is the most likely to manifest earliest?
a. Apraxia
b. Comprehension of speech
c. Rapid forgetting of new information after short intervals
d. Semantic knowledge problems
e. Visuospatial problems

Question 26

Which of the following hormone levels is not decreased in patients with anorexia nervosa?
a. Corticotropin-releasing hormone (CRH)
b. Follicle-stimulating hormone (FSH)
c. Luteinizing hormone (LH)
d. Oestrogen
e. Triiodothyronine (T3)

Question 27

The cognitive impairments noted in Alzheimer's disease are most correlated with which one of the following histological abnormalities?
a. Density of neurofibrillary tangles
b. Density of senile plaques
c. Density of Lewy bodies
d. Density of Hirano bodies
e. None of the above

Question 28

A 45-year-old man with no medical or psychiatric history presents with vocal and motor tics that resemble Tourette syndrome. He is noted to have taken some

antibiotics a week ago. Which of the following antibiotics could he have taken to cause his presentation?
a. Cephalosporin
b. Clarithromycin
c. Gentamicin
d. Quinolone
e. Trimethoprim-sulfamethoxazole

Question 29
Which of the following statements is false regarding the conduction of a randomized controlled trial?
a. A multi-centred trial is preferred to assess effects of trial drug in different ethnic groups because of variation in pharmacokinetics.
b. A patient can withdraw from the randomized controlled trial at any time and a valid reason is required.
c. Placebo treatment is not recommended in chronic and severe illnesses.
d. The RCT needs to obtain ethic committee approval beforehand.
e. The RCT should be guided by the uncertainty principle, and both investigators and subjects should not know the efficacy of trial drug and gold-standard treatment.

Question 30
Which of the following statements is false regarding sample size and power?
a. Precision is increased by reducing the size of the standard error.
b. Power is increased by having a larger clinically relevant difference.
c. A power of 0.8 means that it gives an 80% chance of detecting a difference.
d. The size of the standard error is based on the size of the sample.
e. The larger the sample size, the larger the standard error.

Question 31
Which of the following statements is false?
a. Hypothalamic harmatoma is associated with epilepsy, precocious puberty and hypothalamic rage.
b. Patients with insulin-dependent diabetes mellitus (IDDM) have more cognitive impairment than patients with non-insulin-dependent diabetes mellitus (NIDDM).
c. Hyperparathyroidism can cause cognitive impairment.
d. Diabetes insipidus is associated with generalized anxiety.
e. Addison's disease is associated with hypercalcaemia, hyponatraemia and lethargy.

Question 32
Patients with AIDS can present with mania that may have a different presentation from that of primary mania. Which of the following is not a typical characteristic of AIDS mania?
a. Euphoria
b. Irritability

c. More chronic than episodic
   d. Psychomotor agitation
   e. Psychomotor slowing

Question 33
With regard to the pharmacological management of social phobia, which of the following medications has been shown to be particularly helpful?
   a. Citalopram
   b. Fluoxetine
   c. Fluvoxamine
   d. Mirtazapine
   e. Monoamine oxidase inhibitors

Question 34
The lifetime prevalence of obsessive-compulsive disorder (OCD) has been estimated to be around
   a. 2%
   b. 4%
   c. 6%
   d. 8%
   e. 10%

Question 35
The syndrome of inappropriate antidiuretic hormone (SIADH) is more likely to be associated with which of the following psychotropic medications?
   a. Carbamazepine
   b. Lithium
   c. Lamotrigine
   d. Phenytoin
   e. Valproate

Question 36
Which of the following PDs has been found to be associated with the highest rate of post-transplant non-compliance?
   a. Antisocial
   b. Borderline
   c. Dependent
   d. Histrionic
   e. Obsessive-compulsive

Question 37
Which of the following concepts regarding the stochastic damage of ageing is false?
   a. Macromolecules distort the physical and chemical properties of the human body.
   b. There is increased free-radical damage.

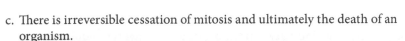

c. There is irreversible cessation of mitosis and ultimately the death of an organism.
d. The accumulation of earlier adverse events in ageing eventually leads to the end of survival.
e. There is decline in basic metabolic rate as a person gets older.

Question 38
An antidepressant was found to be more likely to reduce the score of the Hamilton Depression Scale by 50% from baseline score compared with placebo ($n = 3000$ patients, 10 centres, relative risk for remaining depressed = 0.30; 95% confidence interval (CI) 0.2–0.6; absolute risk difference = 0.42; 95% CI 0.2–0.6). What is the 95% CI number needed to treat (NNT) with this antidepressant to prevent one additional patient from remaining depressed?
a. 1.37–4.70
b. 1.47–4.80
c. 1.50–4.90
d. 1.67–5.00
e. 1.70–5.10

Question 39
Which of the following statements regarding psychosis secondary to traumatic brain injury is false?
a. Delusions are more common than hallucinations.
b. Increased severity of brain injury increases the risk of psychosis.
c. Onset of psychosis is usually gradual and occurs within 6 months after the injury.
d. Negative symptoms are less common than hallucinations.
e. Temporal lobe lesion is a risk factor for psychosis.

Question 40
Which of the following about anorexia nervosa and hormones involved is incorrect?
a. There is a decrease in CRH.
b. There is an increase in the amounts of cortisol.
c. There is an increase in growth hormone.
d. There is a decrease in both FSH and LH.
e. There is a decrease in oestrogen for females.

Question 41
Which of the following statements regarding exhibitionism is false?
a. Exhibitionism is included in both *Diagnostic and Statistical Manual of Mental Disorders* (DSM) and *International Classification of Diseases* (ICD).
b. One of the best predictors of recidivism is lack of empathy.
c. 50% of sexual offences seen by courts are related to exhibitionism.
d. Exhibitionists are more likely to be married than other sexual offenders.
e. The reconviction rate is low after a first conviction but high after second conviction.

Question 42

Which of the following findings from the National Confidential Inquiry into Suicide and Homicide (United Kingdom) is incorrect?

a. Approximately 25% of people who committed suicide had been in recent contact with mental health services before death.
b. The period of highest risk of suicide after discharge from inpatient care is the first 14 days.
c. Over one-fifth of individuals dying by suicide have not been adherent to medication in the preceding month of their death.
d. In the United Kingdom, around 50 homicides per year are committed by those in recent contact with mental health services.
e. The rate of 'stranger homicides' by those with mental illness has increased sharply.

Question 43

A 20-year-old man suffering from schizophrenia is admitted due to worsening of psychotic symptoms. The urine cannabis screen is negative (level of cannabinoids <20 ng/ml), despite the fact that his partner confirms he is a heavy user of cannabis. The core trainee wants to consult you on the underlying reason. The following are possible reasons except which one?

a. The urine screen was done on the fourth day after admission, and the active ingredient of cannabis was not detectable.
b. The person adulterated his urine sample with vinegar.
c. The person drank a lot of water and alcohol prior to the urine test.
d. The person took 10 tablets of aspirin 12 hours before the urine test.
e. The person took a lot of vitamin B prior to the test and then diluted his urine with water.

Question 44

A 22-year-old woman develops her first episode of anorexia nervosa. Her mother is very concerned and gathers some information on the outcome of her illness. Which of the following statements is correct?

a. This patient has good prognosis, as she has a relatively late onset.
b. The most common switch in pattern is from anorexia nervosa to bulimia nervosa.
c. The most common switch in pattern is from bulimia nervosa to anorexia nervosa.
d. The outpatient treatment should be 3 months, duration for those patients without hospitalization.
e. 30% will have a duration of illness longer than 12 years.

Question 45

Which one of the following deficits is unlikely to be found in a patient with caudate nucleus dysfunction (e.g. Huntington disease)?

a. Apathy
b. Body dysmorphic disorder
c. Depression
d. Disinhibition
e. Personality change

Question 46
Which of the following medications has been associated with paradoxical agitation in patients with traumatic brain injury?
  a. Carbamazepine
  b. Gabapentin
  c. Lithium
  d. Olanzapine
  e. Topiramate

Question 47
The NHS wants to decide which antidepressant is to be used to treat depression. Only cheaper antidepressants will be chosen, and outcome is not important. Which type of economic analysis is being used in this scenario?
  a. Cost minimization analysis
  b. Cost effectiveness analysis
  c. Cost–utility analysis
  d. Cost–benefit analysis
  e. None of the above

Question 48
Which of the following statements is true for disulfiram?
  a. Halitosis is an uncommon side effect.
  b. It is contraindicated in people with advanced liver disease.
  c. It decreases the level of warfarin and theophylline.
  d. It inhibits alcohol dehydrogenase leading to accumulation of acetaldehyde.
  e. The starting dose is 100 mg daily.

Question 49
Which of the following statements is false for acamprosate?
  a. It is a gamma-aminobutyric acid (GABA) antagonist and glutamate agonist.
  b. It reduces craving in people with chronic alcohol dependency.
  c. Significant benefits will continue 1–2 years after stopping.
  d. It can be combined with disulfiram.
  e. Breastfeeding is a contraindication.

Question 50
A 10-year-old boy with learning disability has fair skin and blue eyes. He also has self-mutilating and stereotyped behaviour. He suffers from epilepsy and has been eating a special diet since he was a baby, as recommended by his paediatrician. Which one of the following statements regarding his condition is false?
  a. He has to take a high-phenylalanine diet.
  b. The incidence of his condition is 1 in 4,500–15,000.
  c. This disorder involves a defect in the phenylalanine hydroxylase leading to accumulation of phenylalanine.
  d. The screening test for this disorder is the Guthrie test soon after birth.
  e. The mode of inheritance is autosomal recessive.

Question 51

A 25-year-old man who has epilepsy presents with white skin patches and gingival fibromata. Whole-body scan shows tumours in his lungs, spleen and kidneys. Several members of his family, including his father and one of his sisters, are affected. Which one of the following statements regarding his condition is true?

a. A Wood's lamp or ultraviolet light may be used to locate the hypomelanotic macules.
b. It is autosomal dominant with 70% penetrance.
c. Males are more affected than females.
d. The majority of those affected have profoundly low intelligence quotient (IQ).
e. Seizures are uncommon.

Question 52

Major depression is associated with lesion(s) in which part of the brain after a cerebrovascular accident?

a. Bilateral occipital
b. Left basal ganglia
c. Left temporal
d. Right frontal lobe
e. Right temporal

Question 53

A 12-year-old child has a happy disposition with paroxysmal laughter. He frequently flaps his hands and has jerking movements. He has a history of severe learning disability and epilepsy. Which one of the following statements about his condition is false?

a. Patients with this condition have attention-deficit syndrome and sleep disturbance.
b. The prevalence of this condition is 1 per 20,000 to 1 per 30,000.
c. Severe mental retardation is commonly seen.
d. Severe psychomotor retardation is attributed to abnormal expression of UBE3A.
e. 70% have microdeletions of chromosome 15q11–13 of paternal origin.

Question 54

Which of the following conditions is associated with severe mental retardation?

a. Cornelia De Lange syndrome
b. Klinefelter syndrome
c. Turner syndrome
d. Wilson disease
e. XYY syndrome

Question 55

Which of the following is not a strength of cohort study?

a. It is able to follow temporal relationships.
b. It measures multiple effects of a single exposure.

c. It is rapid and cheap.
d. It is useful for diseases with long latency periods.
e. It is well suited to rare exposures.

Question 56
Which of the following has the lowest incidence of mental retardation?
a. Cornelia de Lange syndrome
b. Fragile X syndrome
c. Klinefelter syndrome
d. Prader–Willi syndrome
e. Smith–Magenis syndrome

Question 57
Based on the National Institute for Health and Care Excellence (NICE) guidelines, which of the following modalities of psychological therapy has not been recommended for patients with anorexia nervosa?
a. Cognitive analytic therapy
b. Cognitive behavioural therapy
c. Dialectical behavioural therapy
d. Interpersonal therapy
e. Focal dynamic therapy

Question 58
Which of the following statements about pharmacotherapy for eating disorders is incorrect?
a. Pharmacological treatment should not be used as the sole or principle treatment for anorexia nervosa.
b. With regard to the usage of antipsychotics for anorexia nervosa, olanzapine has been the most studied antipsychotic.
c. Oestrogen administration should not be considered for use to help treat bone density problems in children and adolescents, as this might lead to problems in development.
d. Upon weight restoration, fluoxetine has demonstrated benefits for patients with anorexia nervosa.
e. Selective serotonin re-uptake inhibitors (SSRIs) are the first-line drugs of choice for the treatment of patients with bulimia nervosa.

Question 59
Which of the following statements is true for case–control studies?
a. Bias can be adjusted for at the analysis stage.
b. Confounding factors are defined as any factors that affect outcome.
c. It is often difficult to find age-matched controls.
d. In the design of case–control studies, confounding factors must be completely excluded.
e. Logistic regression can adjust for only one factor at a time.

Question 60

A 35-year-old man is brought in by the police for punching a man in the face and smashing his car window screen in his driveway. His explanation is that the other driver drove too close to his car and stared at him. This is the fourth time he has hit someone for 'pissing him off' over the last year. He admits to having difficulty controlling his temper and having a tendency to go into a rage when he gets annoyed. He usually feels guilty after the episodes. He has no psychotic symptoms, and there is no history of alcohol drinking or illicit drug use. Which of the following diagnoses is most likely?

a. Antisocial PD
b. Dissociative fugue state
c. Intermittent explosive disorder
d. Manic disorder
e. Temporal lobe epilepsy

Question 61

A university student is brought in by the school counsellor for being in a daze with purposeless overactivity after she found out that she had failed a major examination. The counsellor wants to know when her symptoms will start to disappear. Based on the ICD-10 criteria, what would the answer be?

a. 1 hour
b. 12 hours
c. 24 hours
d. 48 hours
e. 60 hours

Question 62

A 25-year-old with schizophrenia on risperidone complains of sexual dysfunction. Which of the following tests would you order?

a. Calcium and parathyroid hormone
b. Cortisol level
c. Fasting serum glucose
d. Prolactin level
e. Thyroid function test

Question 63

Which of the following statements regarding hyperthyroidism and manifestations of neuropsychiatric symptoms is true?

a. Mania or psychosis is common.
b. The prevalence of cognitive impairment in hyperthyroidism is more than in hypothyroidism.
c. The majority of patients with hyperthyroidism will exhibit some form of psychopathology.
d. In hyperthyroid patients with depressive symptoms, mood symptoms may precede physical symptoms.
e. Hypomania is the most common psychiatric manifestation.

Question 64
Which of the following is inherited in an autosomal-dominant fashion?
a. DiGeorge syndrome
b. Hunter syndrome
c. Hurler syndrome
d. Phenylketonuria
e. Mucopolysaccharidosis III

Question 65
Which of the following is a sex-linked recessive disorder?
a. Lesch–Nyhan syndrome
b. Maple syrup urine disease
c. Neurofibromatosis
d. Rett syndrome
e. Velocardiofacial syndrome

Question 66
A 7-year-old boy is brought in by his parents to see the child psychiatrist for restlessness and irritability. He has developmental delay, hypertrichosis, deafness and joint stiffness. On physical examination, he is found to have claw hand and hepatosplenomegaly. Which one of the following conditions is he most likely to have?
a. Galactosaemia
b. Martin–Bell syndrome
c. Phenylketonuria
d. Sanfilippo syndrome
e. Tay–Sachs disease

Question 67
Which of the following is relatively preserved even in the advanced stage of Huntington disease?
a. Information retrieval
b. Judgement
c. Language function
d. Mental flexibility
e. Planning

Question 68
The Family Environment Scale is a family rating scale that measures the social climate of all types of family. It has several subscales that look into different areas. Which one of the following is not an area of this rating scale?
a. Achievement
b. Bonding
c. Conflict
d. Decision making
e. Family cohesion

Question 69

Which of the following statements regarding the Conners Rating Scale–Revised is true?

a. It includes parents, teacher and youth self-report versions.
b. It includes parents and youth self-report versions only.
c. It does not assess common comorbid conditions.
d. It mostly assesses internalizing behaviour.
e. The behaviour scale does not include assessment of cognitive problems.

Question 70

Which of the following statements regarding intelligence tests is true?

a. IQ scores are weakly associated with academic achievement.
b. IQ scores are strong predictors of overall adjustment.
c. Intelligence test scores are fairly stable for children above the age of 5 years.
d. IQ scores are strongly associated with socio-emotional functioning.
e. The Kaufman Assessment Battery for Children measures socio-emotional functioning in children and adolescents.

Question 71

Which of the following is a shared commonality between the genders with regard to conduct disorder?

a. Low empathy and ability to identify interpersonal issues
b. Verbal aggression
c. Physical aggression
d. Depressive symptoms
e. Somatization disorders

Question 72

Which of the following curves is a plot of (sensitivity) versus (1 – specificity) on either axis?

a. Blobbogram
b. Forest plot
c. Funnel plot
d. Galbraith plot
e. Receiver operating characteristics curve

Question 73

Which of the following statements is false regarding screening test dimensions?

a. For a screening test, the cut-off is set towards high sensitivity.
b. If prevalence <10% or >90%, the positive and negative predictive values are not representative.
c. Sensitivity is defined as the proportion of those people who have the disease who are currently detected by the test.
d. Specificity is defined as the proportion of those people who do not have the disease who are correctly left undetected by the test.
e. The more sensitive the test, the higher the positive predictive value.

Question 74
Which of the following is a measure of external validity of a randomized control test?
a. Generalizability of study results
b. Instruments used
c. Research design
d. Reliability of study results
e. Research setting

Question 75
Which of the following is not a characteristic of the normal distribution curve?
a. 10% of the values lie beyond two standard deviations (SDs) from the median.
b. 68% of the values fall within one SD of the mean.
c. The mean, median and mode are equal.
d. The total area under the curve represents 100% of all values.
e. The spread from the mean is represented by the SD.

Question 76
Table 9.1 demonstrates important findings. Based on the table, which of the following findings is incorrect?
a. Higher levels of noradrenaline are found in patients suffering from chronic asthma, and this finding is statistically significant at the 0.1% level.
b. Patients with acute asthma have the lowest neuropeptide Y (NPY) levels among three groups.
c. The differences in number of stressful life events encountered by patients with acute asthma, chronic asthma and healthy controls are not statistically significant.
d. There are statistically significant differences in ACTH in patients with acute asthma, chronic asthma and healthy controls, and this finding is statistically significant at the 5% level.
e. There are statistically significant differences in adrenaline between patients with acute asthma, chronic asthma and healthy controls, and this finding is statistically significant at the 0.01% level.

Question 77
Based on Table 9.2, which of the following statistical tests was used to examine the independent associations?
a. Pearson's correlation analysis
b. Multivariate linear regression analysis
c. Multivariate logistic regression analysis
d. Univariate linear regression analysis
e. Univariate logistic regression analysis

Question 78
Referring to the footnotes under Table 9.2, what is the reason to control for variables such as age?
a. Age is a confounding factor, which may influence the IL-4 levels.
b. Age is an independent variable, which may influence the IL-4 levels.

Table 9.1 Measurements of interleukin (IL)-4 levels and stress-related variables in young adults aged 21–35 years (patients with acute asthma, patients with chronic asthma and healthy control subjects)

	Patients with acute asthma (n = 19)	Patients with chronic asthma (n = 51)	Healthy control subjects (n = 69)	Significance tests F value	p value
IL-4 (pg/mL)	6.96 ± 7.15‡	3.63 ± 6.79	1.57 ± 2.27	8.914	<0.001
Neuropeptide Y (NPY) (ng/ml)	0.42 ± 0.14*	0.47 ± 0.24*	0.62 ± 0.40	4.786	0.010
Cortisol (nmol/L)	387.11 ± 130.63	389.44 ± 246.32*	517.10 ± 256.58	4.876	0.009
Adrenocorticotropic hormone (ACTH; pmol/L)	6.67 ± 10.96*	4.12 ± 3.55	3.60 ± 1.75	3.172	0.045
Noradrenaline (pg/ml)	645.04 ± 329.46†	498.77 ± 413.41*	346.15 ± 179.90	8.615	<0.001
Adrenaline (pg/ml)	99.64 ± 76.79‡§	52.28 ± 43.92*	31.74 ± 18.51	20.889	<0.001
Hypothalamic–pituitary–adrenal (HPA) stress index	0.34 ± 0.51*	−0.00 ± 0.59	−0.09 ± 0.37	5.984	0.003
Stressful life events	164.14 ± 133.31	144.57 ± 101.72	139.39 ± 89.03	0.364	0.695
Perceived stress	21.43 ± 6.02*	17.53 ± 6.20	16.58 ± 6.71	3.292	0.040

Source: Lu Y, Ho R, Lim TK, Kuan WS, Goh DY, Mahadevan M, Sim TB, Van Bever HP, Larbi A, Ng TP (2014). Neuropeptide Y may mediate psychological stress and enhance T$_H$2 inflammatory response in asthma. *J Allergy Clin Immunol*, 14: 01578–4.

Notes: Data are presented as means ± SDs. Bonferroni correction was used for the *post hoc* test. The HPA stress index was created as a composite index of cortisol, noradrenaline, adrenaline and ACTH levels by the principal component analysis score (percentage of cumulative covariance, 84.467%).
*$p < 0.05$, †$p < 0.01$ and ‡$p < 0.001$ versus the healthy control group.
§$p < 0.001$ versus the chronic asthma group.

Table 9.2 Independent associations and mediation analyses of measures of perceived and HPA stress and NPY with IL-4 concentrations among asthmatic patients

	Dependent variable: IL-4 level at baseline					Dependent variable: IL-4 level at 1 year				
	R2 change	B value	SE	ß value	p value	R2 change	B value	SE	ß value	p value
Psychological stress models										
Model 1: Perceived stress	0.119	0.71	0.29	0.58	0.019	0.129	0.88	0.37	0.67	0.25
Model 2: NPY level	0.479	28.82	4.31	0.75	<0.001	0.534	32.89	4.70	0.81	<0.001
Model 3: Perceived stress controlling for NPY level	0.376	0.27	0.22	0.22	0.234*	0.416	0.28	0.28	0.21	0.324†
NPY controlling for preceived stress	0.109	26.50	4.25	0.69	<0.001	0.146	29.75	4.70	0.74	<0.001

Analyses in the psychological stress model were controlled for base model variables: age, sex, ethnicity, housing type, smoking status, body mass index, asthma severity, and asthma control score and neuroticism. R2 change is the change in the model R2 value from the base model of the candidate predictor variable.
* Sobel test: $z = 2.134$, $p = 0.033$.
† Sobel test: $z = 2.143$, $p = 0.032$.

c. Age is responsible for reverse causality, which may influence the IL-4 levels.

d. Age will cause a type I error, which may influence the IL-4 levels.

e. Age will cause a type II error, which may influence the IL-4 levels.

Question 79

Table 9.2 demonstrates important findings. Based on this table, which of the following findings is correct?

a. The NPY levels among patients with asthma was not a significant predictor of the IL-4 levels measured at baseline and 1 year later, after controlling for potential confounders.

b. Perceived stress among patients with asthma was a significant predictor of the IL-4 levels measured at baseline only but not 1 year later, after controlling for potential confounders.

c. Perceived stress among patients with asthma was a significant predictor of the IL-4 levels measured at baseline and 1 year later, after controlling for potential confounders.

d. Perceived stress among patients with asthma was a significant predictor of the IL-4 levels measured at 1 year later but not baseline after controlling for potential confounders.

e. Perceived stress among patients with asthma was not a significant predictor of the IL-4 levels measured at baseline and 1 year later, controlling for potential confounders.

Question 80

Referring to the footnotes under Table 9.2, Sobel test was performed in model 3. Which of the following statements is correct?

a. Age is a mediating factor in the association between high perceived stress levels and IL-4 overexpression in patients with asthma.

b. Asthma severity is a mediating factor in the association between high perceived stress levels and IL-4 overexpression in patients with asthma.

c. IL-4 is a mediating factor in the association between high perceived stress and NPY levels in patients with asthma.

d. NPY level is a mediating factor in the association between high perceived stress levels and IL-4 overexpression in patients with asthma.

e. Perceived stress is a mediating factor in the association between high NPY levels and IL-4 overexpression in patients with asthma.

Question 81

Which of the following factors is related to outcome in autistic patients?

a. Absence or presence of speech

b. Age of onset

c. Birth weight

d. Family history of mental illness

e. IQ of parents

Question 82

Which of the following instruments that assess autism in children does not require training?

a. Autism Diagnostic Interview (ADI)
b. Autism Diagnostic Observation Schedule (ADOS)
c. Childhood Autism Rating Scale (CARS)
d. Pervasive Developmental Disorder Behaviour Inventory (PDDBI)
e. None of the above

Question 83

One common medical comorbidity of autism is epilepsy. Which of the following statements about epilepsy in autistic children is false?

a. Approximately 5% of children with autism have epilepsy.
b. Females have greater risk of seizure than males.
c. The risk of epilepsy is highest in early childhood.
d. The most common type of seizure is grand mal seizure.
e. The use of anticonvulsants may help to reduce self-injurious behaviour.

Question 84

A 25-year-old man is arrested for trying to steal hair gel from a shop. He has a history of repeated thefts of hair gel and is suffering from OCD. Which of the following statements is incorrect regarding his condition?

a. Checking is the most common compulsion.
b. Fear of contamination is the most common obsession.
c. Obsessional image is a relatively uncommon obsession.
d. A positron emission tomography (PET) scan of this man may show hypermetabolism in the left orbital gyrus and both caudate nuclei.
e. Shoplifting is more common in OCD than in the general population.

Question 85

Which of the following substances can induce panic in an individual and provides evidence that panic disorder has a biological basis?

a. Chlorpromazine
b. Dextrose
c. Inhalation of oxygen
d. Refined sugars
e. Sodium lactate

Question 86

Which of the following statements regarding social phobia is false?

a. Alcohol abuse is not as common in social phobia as in other phobias.
b. Beta-blockers can be used to reduce autonomic arousal.
c. Taijin-kyofu-sho in Japan is a transcultural variant.
d. The first episode occurs in a public place, usually without any reason.
e. First-degree relatives of social phobics are three times more likely to be affected.

Question 87

A 50-year-old man with a history of type II diabetes, hypertension, obesity, poorly controlled asthma and osteoarthritis of the knees presents with anxiety.

He has been getting anxious easily almost every day since 6 months ago, when he was admitted to the intensive care unit for respiratory failure. His medications were then adjusted. He is currently taking an inhaled corticosteroid, regular prednisolone, metformin, naproxen, tramadol and atenolol. Which one of the following medications may be responsible for his anxiety?

a. Atenolol

b. Metformin

c. Naproxen

d. Prednisolone

e. Tramadol

Question 88

Which of the following statements regarding Fahr disease is false?

a. It is a rare autosomal-dominant disorder.

b. It is associated with hypoparathyroidism.

c. Patients present with cognitive impairment in the absence of mood or psychotic symptoms.

d. There is extensive calcification of the basal ganglia.

e. There is apathy and memory impairment but sparing of language function.

Question 89

A 22-year-old woman is brought to hospital after having fainted in class. She is found to be cachectic with a body mass index (BMI) of 16. She admits to having body image problems and restricting her diet. She has also been using laxatives and diuretics. Which abnormality would you expect to find in her case?

a. Hypochloremic acidosis

b. Hyperchloremic alkalosis

c. Hypokalaemic acidosis

d. Hypokalaemic alkalosis

e. Hyperkalaemic alkalosis

Question 90

Which of the following is not an outcome that was assessed in the multimodal treatment study?

a. Severity of attention-deficit hyperactivity disorder (ADHD)

b. Reading scores

c. Social skills

d. Extent of impairment

e. Progression to conduct disorder

Question 91

The combination of APOE e4 allele and traumatic head injury increases the risk for Alzheimer's disease by how many times?

a. Two.

b. Four.

c. Six.

d. Eight.

e. There is no increase.

Question 92

Which one of the following statements about adult sex offenders is false?

a. A majority begins their offending behaviour in middle age.

b. About 35% of sex offenders have a mental illness.

c. Lack of victim empathy predicts high risk of reoffending.

d. There is often a history of affectionless upbringing by unloving parents.

e. Treatment includes behavioural techniques on self-monitoring.

Question 93

Which one of the following statements about the Psychopathy Checklist Revised version (PCL-R) is false?

a. It is a 20-item rating scale, with each item rating from 0 (does not apply) to 2 (definitely applies).

b. It assesses interpersonal relationships of the individual.

c. It is a risk assessment tool.

d. It is able to differentiate psychopathy from antisocial PD.

e. Scores are based on both semi-structured and collateral information.

Question 94

A 14-year-old girl has been sexually assaulted by a gang of classmates around 6 months ago. Her mood has been irritable, and she is experiencing flashbacks and nightmares at the moment. Which of the following antidepressants would be most effective for her treatment?

a. Fluoxetine

b. Paroxetine

c. Sertraline

d. Venlafaxine

e. Escitalopram

Question 95

Which of the following statements regarding reading disorder is incorrect?

a. The prevalence of dyslexia in the United Kingdom is 5%.

b. The prevalence of genuine dyslexia and mild dyslexia is 10%.

c. In the United States, 17%–20% of elementary school children are estimated to suffer from reading disabilities.

d. In the United States, 17%–20% of the US population displays a reading disability.

e. A survey conducted across Japan, Taiwan and the United States concluded that, using more than one criterion, the percentage of children who were reading disabled were 8% in Japan, 8% in Taiwan and 7% in the USA.

Question 96

Which of the following statements regarding childhood disintegrative syndrome is true?

a. It is a common condition.
b. It is associated with a high prevalence of epilepsy.
c. Life expectancy is reduced.
d. Most patients suffer from mild mental retardation.
e. The age of onset is before 2 years old.

Question 97

Which of the following magnetic resonance imaging (MRI) findings is not reported in children with schizophrenia?
a. Cerebral asymmetry
b. Increase in ventricular volume
c. Decrease in temporal lobe volume
d. Decrease in midsagittal thalamic area
e. Decrease in total cerebral volume

Question 98

Children with major depression may present with atypical features. Which of the following is not a feature of childhood atypical depression?
a. Hypersomnia
b. Increased appetite
c. Mood reactivity
d. Psychomotor retardation
e. Weight loss

Question 99

You have been following up on the psychiatric care of an 11-year-old girl for major depressive disorder (MDD). Her mother recently read a newspaper article about bipolar disorder and is worried that this is the condition her daughter is suffering from, instead. What percentage of children with major depressive episodes may show signs of bipolar disorder by adolescence?
a. 20%
b. 25%
c. 33%
d. 50%
e. 75%

Question 100

Childhood mania is often misdiagnosed or under-diagnosed, as the symptoms manifested in children can be different from those in adults. Which one of the following does not usually present in children with mania?
a. Aggressive temper outbursts
b. Depression
c. Euphoria
d. Hyperactivity
e. Poor school performance

Question 101

Which of the following is not a common feature of depression in adolescents?
a. Conduct disorder
b. Increased sexual behaviour
c. Increased psychomotor retardation
d. Social withdrawal
e. Substance abuse

Question 102

Adjustment disorders are predictive of more serious mental disorders in which group of patients?
a. Adults
b. Children
c. Elderly
d. Single
e. Unemployed

Question 103

A 32-year-old man with a history of schizophrenia is brought to the emergency department by his parents. He has been prescribed with haloperidol 9 mg/day. Upon a recent relapse, with increased auditory hallucinations, his parents increased his dose to 15 mg/day. He now presents with confusion, diaphoresis, fever and hypertension. His blood investigations show a high white cell count and impaired renal function. Which one of the following is the most appropriate pharmacological treatment at this point?
a. Benztropine
b. Bromocriptine
c. Lorazepam
d. Propranolol
e. Haloperidol

Question 104

Which of the following statements regarding the immune system of depressed patients is false?
a. There is a decrease in the ratio of T-helper to T-suppressor cells in peripheral blood.
b. There is an increase in the numbers of neutrophil in peripheral blood.
c. There is an increase in the level of IL-1 in cerebrospinal fluid (CSF).
d. There is an increase in the level of IL-6 in CSF.
e. There is an increase in the levels of acute-phase proteins in peripheral blood.

Question 105

A 23-year-old university student complains of insomnia. She has never managed to sleep before 3:00 a.m. since adolescence. She always skips her morning lectures. Which one of the following is the most likely diagnosis?
a. Circadian rhythm sleep disorder
b. Delayed sleep-phase syndrome

c. Poor sleep hygiene
d. Restless leg syndrome
e. Sleep disorder related to chaotic life in studying

Question 106
What percentage of the hospitalized elderly fulfil the criteria for a major depressive episode?
  a. 5%
  b. 10%
  c. 15%
  d. 21%
  e. 31%

Question 107
Which of the following is not a common comorbid psychiatric disorder in children and adolescents with MDD?
  a. Anxiety disorder
  b. Disruptive behaviour disorder
  c. Dysthymic disorder
  d. Eating disorder
  e. Substance abuse

Question 108
Which of the following statements regarding the use of clozapine is false?
  a. The combined use of clozapine and carbamazepine is a safe practice to prevent seizures in patients on long-term clozapine.
  b. The combined use of clozapine and lithium may help to reduce neutropenia.
  c. Hyoscine may be used in the treatment of hypersalivation in clozapine users.
  d. The risk of agranulocytosis is independent of clozapine dose.
  e. The risk of seizures increases with the use of clozapine in a dose-dependent manner.

Question 109
You have diagnosed a 35-year-old Asian woman with bipolar disorder, and you want to start her on carbamazepine. Which is the most important test that you want to do for her first before starting this medication?
  a. Carbamazepine level
  b. Full blood count
  c. Human leukocyte antigen (HLA)-B 1502 allele
  d. Liver function test
  e. Renal panel

Question 110
In the use of electroconvulsive therapy (ECT) to treat schizophrenia, which particular aspect is most useful?
  a. Treating aggression
  b. Treating catatonia

c. Treating delusions
d. Treating hallucinations
e. Treating impulsivity

Question 111

You plan to start a patient with treatment-resistant schizophrenia on clozapine. In view of the potential risk of agranulocytosis, the patient's baseline white blood cell count needs to be greater than which one of the following?
a. 1,000
b. 2,000
c. 2,500
d. 3,000
e. 3,500

Question 112

Which one of the following comorbidities has been reported to occur most frequently in children diagnosed with ADHD?
a. Conduct disorder
b. Oppositional defiant disorder
c. Panic disorder
d. Speech or language impairment
e. Tics

Question 113

Which of the following statements regarding Gilles de la Tourette syndrome is false?
a. ADHD is the most frequently occurring comorbidity.
b. Coprolalia does not appear until about 6 years after onset of motor tics.
c. Habit reversal training is a form of behaviour therapy that may reduce tics.
d. It affects more males than females.
e. Obsessions and compulsions in Tourette syndrome are similar to those of pure OCD without Tourette disorder.

Question 114

Which of the following statements regarding separation anxiety is true?
a. It begins at around 15 months and peaks at 3 years.
b. It is not a normative part of development.
c. It is usually persistent and excessive.
d. The child's experiences of previous separations vary with the rate of disappearance of separation anxiety.
e. None of the above.

Question 115

Which of the following statements regarding bipolar disorder in the elderly is false?
a. Genetic factor is an important aetiology.
b. Increased cerebral vulnerabilities and insults play a more important role than life events in precipitating late-onset mania.

c. The presence of neurological abnormalities is more common, especially in elderly male patients.

d. The prognosis is the same as that for bipolar disorder in younger people.

e. More rapid recurrences tend to be more common.

Question 116

A medical social worker (MSW) is counselling a woman grieving for her husband, who died of a sudden heart attack. The social worker is concerned about the percentage of people undergoing bereavement who have MDD. Which one of the following would you advise the percentage to be?

a. 5%

b. 10%

c. 15%

d. 20%

e. 25%

Question 117

How long can cocaine metabolites remain detectable in urine?

a. 3 hours

b. 6 hours

c. 12 hours

d. 24 hours

e. 96 hours

Extended Match Items

Theme: Research Methodology

Options:

a. Level 1A

b. Level 1B

c. Level 1C

d. Level 2A

e. Level 2B

f. Level 2C

g. Level 3A

h. Level 3B

i. Level 4

j. Level 5

Lead in: Match one correct hierarchy of research evidence with each of the following study types. Each option may be used once, more than once or not at all.

Question 118

Systematic review of RCTs. (Choose one option.)

Question 119

Systematic review of cohort studies. (Choose one option.)

Question 120

Systematic review of case–control studies. (Choose one option.)

Theme: Old-Age Psychiatry

Options:
   a. Background slowing and diffuse superimposed beta activity
   b. Focal and generalized spikes, sharp waves, polyspikes and spike–wave complexes
   c. Generalized slowing of alpha rhythm, diffuse theta and delta activity with decline of low-voltage beta activity and focal delta activity in temporal areas
   d. Non-specific slow waves and irregular high-voltage delta activity
   e. Triphasic wave complexes

Lead in: Match one EEG pattern to each of the following scenarios. Each option may be used once, more than once or not at all.

Question 121

Changes seen in normal ageing. (Choose one option.)

Question 122

A 75-year-old man presents with confusion, disorientation and visual hallucinations. He has been complaining of a burning sensation on passing urine and having fever for the past few days. (Choose one option.)

Question 123

A 62-year-old woman has been going to various doctors to obtain sleeping pills. One day, she is found unconscious at home with several empty bottles of sleeping pills. (Choose one option.)

Question 124

A 65-year-old man with a background history of epilepsy is sent to the hospital after being found lying on the floor with jerking movements and urinary incontinence. He has no recollection what happened before the incident. (Choose one option.)

Theme: Research Methods and Statistics

Options:
   a. Embase
   b. Medline
   c. PsychINFO
   d. Science Direct

Lead in: A researcher wants to perform a meta-analysis. He needs to search various databases to conduct a literature review. Match the databases to each of the following descriptions.

Question 125

This database is freely accessible on the Internet via PubMed. (Choose one option.)

Question 126
This database has a greater bias towards pharmacological research. (Choose one option.)

Question 127
These two databases are operated by the publisher Elsevier. (Choose two options.)

Question 128
This database provides access to book chapters and dissertations. (Choose one option.)

Theme: Prognosis in Schizophrenia

Options:
a. Female gender
b. Male gender
c. Being married
d. Good premorbid social adjustment
e. Family history of psychosis
f. Family history of affective disorder
g. Short duration of illness prior to treatment
h. Ventricular enlargement
i. No ventricular enlargement
j. Abrupt onset of illness
k. Late onset of illness
l. Good initial response to treatment

Lead in: Match the prognostic factors with each of the following questions. Each option may be used once, more than once or not at all.

Question 129
Approximately 25% of cases of schizophrenia show good clinical and social recovery. Which of the above factors is indicative of a good prognosis? (Choose five options.)

Question 130
It has been noted that fewer than half of patients have poor long-term outcome. Which of the following factors is associated with poor prognosis? (Choose three options.)

Theme: Renal Impairment

Options:
a. Haloperidol
b. Olanzapine
c. Sulpiride
d. Amisulpride
e. Risperidone
f. Citalopram
g. Sertraline

h. Fluoxetine
i. Tricyclic antidepressants
j. Lithium
k. Valproate
l. Lamotrigine

Lead in: For patients with renal impairment, match the correct drugs to each of the following statements. Each option may be used once, more than once or not at all.

Question 131
Which antipsychotics can be used? (Choose two options.)

Question 132
Which antidepressants can be used? (Choose two options.)

Question 133
Which of the above mood stabilizers is contraindicated for usage? (Choose one option.)

Theme: Clinical Diagnosis of Learning Disabilities
Options:
a. Down syndrome
b. Fragile X syndrome
c. Turner syndrome
d. Klinefelter syndrome
e. XYY syndrome
f. Hurler syndrome
g. Lesch–Nyhan syndrome

Lead in: Match one syndrome to each of the following statements. Each option may be used once, more than once or not at all.

Question 134
A 3-year-old child presents with hepatosplenomegaly, hirustism, corneal clouding and recurrent respiratory infections. Which is the most likely diagnosis? (Choose one option.)

Question 135
A 16-year-old boy is referred to the psychiatrist because of self-harming, which includes biting of lips, inside of mouth and fingers. There is associated failure of secondary sexual development. His grandfather also suffered from the same disorder. Which is the most likely diagnosis? (Choose one option.)

Question 136
A 25-year-old married man with history of mild learning disability is referred to you. His history suggests possible fertility problems. Physical examination shows

gynaecomastia and small testes. There has not been any known family history of similar problems. Which is the most likely diagnosis? (Choose one option.)

Question 137
A 4-year-old child is referred to the psychiatrist for delayed speech and language. He was initially suspected to suffer from autism. He has gaze aversion and social avoidance. His IQ is 60. He also has attention deficit. Physical examination shows enlarged testes, large ears, long face and flat feet. Mental state examination reveals limited eye contact, perseveration of words, echolalia and stereotypical behaviour such as hand flapping. Which is the most likely diagnosis? (Choose one option.)

Theme: Learning Disabilities

Options:
a. 2
b. 3
c. 4
d. 10
e. 15
f. 20
g. 25
h. 30
i. 35
j. 40
k. 50
l. 70
m. 80
n. 85
o. 90

Lead in: Match the correct number to the following statements. Each option might be used more than once.

Question 138
What is the percentage of mild learning disability patients suffering from epilepsy? (Choose one option.)

Question 139
What is the percentage of severe learning disability patients suffering from epilepsy? (Choose one option.)

Theme: Advanced Psychology and Pharmacology

Options:
a. Multisystemic therapy
b. Duty to inform the police if not reported yet
c. Obtain informed consent from the child and his or her parents
d. Parent Management Training
e. Family therapy

f. Methylphenidate

g. Risperidone

Lead in: Match the above actions/interventions to the following situations. Each option might be used more than once.

Question 140
A 14-year-old boy has recently assaulted his classmates and is defiant with his father. His parents are finding it difficult to discipline him. He does not have ADHD. (Choose one option.)

Question 141
A 15-year-old boy is aggressive in many situations, to the point that his parents have a court injunction against him. No other symptoms have been found. The aggression is directed particularly at vulnerable people and pets at home. He does not have ADHD. He refuses psychotherapy, which his parents have also not found helpful. (Choose one option.)

Question 142
Your core trainee consults you, as she was requested by her general practitioner (GP) to perform a psychiatric assessment on a 15-year-old boy who has been involved in shoplifting over a 3-month period. (Choose two options.)

Question 143
A 15-year-old boy is referred for treatment by the children's court. He recently lit a fire that resulted in significant damage to a shop. He was previously arrested for shoplifting and fighting. Previous history shows that he does not have learning disability or attention-deficit disorder. (Choose one option.)

Question 144
An 8-year-old child has frequent loss of temper, arguments with parents and feels irritable at home but not at school. The symptoms have persisted for 8 months. The parents are asking for help. (Choose one option.)

Theme: Ethics and Psychiatry
Options:
 a. Father
 b. Mother
 c. Patient
 d. Elder brother
 e. Younger brother
 f. Male stranger

Lead in: While working in a child psychiatry department, you are dealing with an 11-year-old girl who was referred by the paediatrician. She admits that she was sexually assaulted. The gynaecologist examined her vagina, and it was partially torn. The MSW reported that the girl has been abused by her father, but he vehemently denies this.

Match the above family members to the situations below. Each option might be used more than once.

Question 145

If this is a case of incest, which family members may be involved? (Choose three options.)

Question 146

You have decided to meet the siblings of the abused child. Which family member should not be invited to the family meeting? (Choose one option.)

Question 147

The majority of abuse is committed by which family members? (Choose two options.)

Question 148

She was diagnosed as suffering from Munchausen syndrome by proxy in the past. This syndrome is associated with psychological overdependence of which person on the child? (Choose one option.)

Theme: Old-Age Psychiatry

Options:
   a. Alzheimer's disease
   b. Binswanger's disease
   c. Cerebral autosomal-dominant arteriopathy with subcortical infarcts and leukoencephalopathy (CASDIL)
   d. Frontal lobe dementia
   e. Lewy body dementia
   f. Psychogenic fugue
   g. Pseudodementia
   h. Vascular dementia
   i. Vitamin B_1 deficiency

Lead in: Match the above situations to the following diagnoses. Each diagnosis might be used more than once.

Question 149

An 80-year-old man presents with fluctuating, progressive memory loss and emotional incontinence. He has a history of falls and is being treated for hypertension by his GP. His relatives say that his personality is preserved. (Choose one option.)

Question 150

A 65-year-old woman presents with memory loss following the death of her husband 4 months ago. She also complains of poor sleep, lack of energy and weight loss. During the cognitive assessment, she is not keen to answer questions. (Choose one option.)

Question 151
A 75-year-old man presents with cognitive impairment, fluctuating levels of consciousness, particularly confusion and bizarre behaviour in the evenings. His daughter claims that he has been seeing ghosts and has not been able to turn in his bed. On physical examination, he is found to have hypertonia and hypersalivation. The Mini Mental State Examination (MMSE) score is 15/30. These above symptoms worsen following the commencement of antipsychotic medication. (Choose one option.)

Question 152
A 40-year-old woman presents with cognitive deterioration and mood changes. On physical examination, there are gait abnormalities. She has a medical history of epilepsy and migraines with aura. She also has episodes of left-sided muscular weakness. On further inquiry, you learn that her aunt also has similar problems. (Choose one option.)

Question 153
A 60-year-old woman was found wandering on the streets with some memory loss after the recent funeral of her husband. She was brought in by the police for psychiatric assessment. When you assess her, she is unable to recall her personal details. She is physically well, and all investigations are normal. (Choose one option.)

Theme: Forensic Psychiatry and Laws

Options:
  a. Adversarial system
  b. Common law
  c. Court of protection order
  d. Restriction order
  e. Hospital order
  f. Not guilty by reason of insanity (NGRI) or McNaughton rule
  g. Procedural security
  h. Relational security

Lead in: Match the above legal terminology to the following. Each option might be used more than once.

Question 154
At the time of offending, the offender does not know the act that he was doing was wrong. (Choose one option.)

Question 155
This is used by the court as an alternative to a prison sentence. (Choose one option.)

Theme: Consultation Liaison Psychiatry

Options:
  a. Anorexia nervosa
  b. Coeliac disease

c. Crohn's disease

d. Hyperthyroidism

e. Iatrogenic cause

f. Whipple's disease

Lead in: Match the above causes of weight loss to the following situations. Each option might be used more than once.

Question 156

A 68-year-old old woman with a history of type 2 diabetes mellitus was referred by the geriatrician for assessment for depression. She complains of low mood and weight loss. Physical examination reveals oedema in her lower limbs. Echocardiogram shows congestive heart failure. Her medications include fluoxetine, metformin and furosemide.

Question 157

A 40-year-old Irish woman was referred by her GP for assessment of depression. She complains of having lethargy, frequent diarrhoea with offensive stools and weight loss. She appears to be pale, and physical examination shows clubbing, abdominal distension and oral ulceration. Barium follow-through is abnormal. Her medications include iron and vitamin D supplements.

Question 158

A 16-year-old girl was referred by the paediatrician for assessment of depression. She was admitted because of fever, weight loss, diarrhoea and abdominal pain. She appears to be thin and pale. Physical examination shows clubbing, aphthous ulceration, abdominal tenderness and perianal skin tags. She is a smoker. Her medication includes paracetamol, and she is currently nil by mouth.

Question 159

A 40-year-old man was referred by the rheumatologist for assessment of depression. He complains of weight loss and migratory polyarthritis. He appears to be pale. Physical examination reveals clubbing and pigmentation. His medications include sulphamethoxazole and trimethoprim.

Theme: Schizophrenia and Psychosis

Options:

a. Paranoid schizophrenia

b. Hebephrenic schizophrenia

c. Catatonic schizophrenia

d. Simple schizophrenia

e. Residual or chronic schizophrenia

f. Undifferentiated schizophrenia

g. Post-schizophrenia depression

Lead in: Please select the correct diagnosis for each of the following.

Question 160

A 23-year-old university student has been having a gradual deterioration in his academic performance. He is currently withdrawn and does not spend time as he used to, with his peers.

Question 161

A 25-year-old university student has been recently diagnosed with schizophrenia. He has been compliant with his medications for the past year, and there are minimal residual positive symptoms. He presents to your clinic with a 4-week history of low mood associated with poor sleep and appetite.

Question 162

An 18-year-old girl has always been shy and introverted in her personality. She currently presents to the emergency services with marked affective changes, associated with fragmentary delusions.

Theme: Diagnosis

Options:
a. Acute stress disorder
b. Adjustment disorder
c. Avoidant PD
d. Asperger's syndrome
e. Bipolar disorder – manic episode
f. Catatonic schizophrenia
g. Depressive episode
h. Delirium tremens
i. Disorganized schizophrenia
j. Dysthymic disorder
k. Malignant catatonia
l. Manic stupor
m. Neuroleptic malignant syndrome
n. Obsessive-compulsive disorder
o. Obsessive-compulsive PD
p. Paranoid schizophrenia
q. Postnatal psychosis
r. Post-traumatic stress disorder
s. Psychotic depression
t. Separation anxiety disorder
u. Social phobia

Lead in: Match the above diagnoses to the following clinical scenarios. Each option might be used once, more than once or not at all.

Question 163

A 30-year-old mother gave birth to her first baby 6 months ago. She has been coping well initially. She starts feeling down, loses weight, complains of tiredness, eats poorly, wakes up before dawn and expresses guilt in her poor care to the baby. Her husband also notices that she worries constantly that an accident will happen to her baby after she read the news on a baby who died of choking after breastfeeding. She begins checking her baby every 5 minutes. (Choose one option.)

Question 164
A 40-year-old unemployed man is admitted after he was arrested by police for dangerous driving. He drove in the opposite direction at 120 km/h on the M5 southbound because he firmly believed that the paparazzi tried to harm him. He informs you that he wants to pursue a PhD degree at this moment. He has incurred £100,000 in food business although he worked as a technician before. He also sent email to the Prime Minister to advise him on how to attract investments for the United Kingdom from overseas investors. He first consulted a psychiatrist 10 years ago, and he developed psychiatric complications after taking an antidepressant. He firmly believes that he suffers from schizophrenia because he hears voices when nobody is around. (Choose one option.)

Question 165
A 50-year-old man is referred by a gastroenterologist. He firmly believes that his gut has rotted and he is already dead. The gastroenterologist is very concerned, as he has ceased to eat or drink. (Choose one option.)

Theme: Advanced Psychotherapy

Options:
  a. Isolation
  b. Intellectualization
  c. Displacement
  d. Splitting
  e. Idealization
  f. Sublimation
  g. Repression
  h. Undoing
  i. Denial
  j. Regression
  k. Projection

Lead in: Match the above defence mechanisms to the following. Each option may be used once, more than once or not at all.

Question 166
A man is passed over for promotion at work. He does not get upset while at work but loses his temper at another driver on the way home. (Choose one option.)

Question 167
It is suggested to him that perhaps some of his anger is related to his relationship with his boss. He denies this, saying that 'She's like a mother to me – always kind and supportive'. (Choose one option.)

Question 168

He suggests that his anger is due to his childhood and then begins to speak about all the books he has recently read on child-rearing across different cultures. (Choose one option.)

Theme: Old-Age Psychiatry

Options:
  a. Alzheimer's disease
  b. Fronto-temporal dementia
  c. Huntington's chorea
  d. Lewy body dementia
  e. Vascular dementia
  f. Shy–Drager syndrome

Lead in: Match the above options to the following pathological findings. Each option may be used once, more than once or not at all.

Question 169

Alpha-synuclein cytoplasmic inclusions. (Choose one option.)

Question 170

Glial cytoplasmic inclusion bodies. (Choose one option.)

Question 171

Neurofibrillary tangles. (Choose two options.)

Theme: Child Psychiatry

Options:
  a. Father
  b. Mother
  c. Patient
  d. Elder brother
  e. Younger brother
  f. Stranger

Lead in: Match the following questions with each of the following options.

Question 172

Which of the following family members is typically involved in a case of incest?

Question 173

A 10-year-old girl has admitted that she has been sexually abused and has indicated that the abuser is likely to be her father. The necessary medical examination conducted did reveal signs significant for that of an abuse. Which of the following members should not be involved if a family conference were to be conducted?

Question 174

The majority of abuse is usually committed by which of the following individuals?

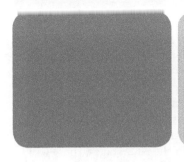

MRCPYSCH PAPER B MOCK EXAMINATION 5: ANSWERS

GET THROUGH MRCPSYCH PAPER B MOCK EXAMINATION

Question 1 Answer: d, There is per-protocol analysis
Explanation: The Consolidated Standards of Reporting Trials (CONSORT) statement, most recently updated in March 2010, is an evidence-based minimum set of recommendations, including a checklist and flow diagram for reporting randomized controlled trials (RCTs) and is intended to facilitate the complete and transparent reporting of trials and aid their critical appraisal and interpretation. In CONSORT guidelines, there is intention-to-treat analysis instead of per-protocol analysis. Another feature is that all patients assessed for the trial are accounted for, and the report is accompanied by a diagram that summarizes the outcomes of all patients involved in the trial.

Reference: Turner L, Shamseer L, Altman DG, Weeks L et al. (2012). Consolidated standards of reporting trials (CONSORT) and the completeness of reporting of randomized controlled trials (RCTs) published in medical journals. *Cochrane Database Syst Rev*, 14;11: MR000030.

Question 2 Answer: c, Quasi-randomization
Explanation: Quasi-randomization is not a proper randomization method, as it is based on subjects' characteristics, such as date of birth, and confounders can exert effects. Centralization randomization is done by a remote computer and third party to avoid selection bias. In minimization, to ensure the balance of factors between groups, the next allocation depends on the characteristics of subjects already being allocated. For stratified randomization, subjects are subdivided into strata, and individuals within each striatum are then randomized. In stepped-wedge randomization, the population is divided into groups, and then the intervention is progressively introduced, in random order, across the groups until every group is receiving it. This is used when other allocation methods would be unfeasible because of widespread belief that the intervention is beneficial.

Reference: Lewis GH, Sheringham J, Kalim K, Crayford TJB (2008). *Mastering Public Health: A Postgraduate Guide to Examination and Revalidation*. London: Royal Society of Medicine Press, pp. 48–49.

Question 3 Answer: c, Between 16% and 30%
Explanation: Early cognitive impairment occurs in 20% of patients infected with human immunodeficiency virus (HIV). It can be classified into cognitive, behavioural and motor symptoms. Cognitive symptoms include poor memory, concentration impairment and mental slowing. The patient may need a written reminder to help them to recall. Behavioural symptoms include apathy, reduced spontaneity and social withdrawal. Depression, irritability, agitation and psychotic symptoms may occur. Motor symptoms include loss of balance, poor coordination, clumsiness and leg weakness. In the later stages, there will be global deterioration of cognitive functions, and this is manifested by word-finding difficulties. Patients may exhibit psychomotor retardation and mutism. The prevalence of dementia in patients suffering from acquired immune deficiency syndrome (AIDS) is around 25%.

Reference: Puri BK, Hall AD, Ho RC (2014). *Revision Notes in Psychiatry*. Boca Raton, FL: CRC Press, p. 483.

Question 4 Answer: c, Kluver–Bucy syndrome
Explanation: Devic syndrome, also known as neuromyelitis optica, is a variant of multiple sclerosis. Churg Strauss syndrome presents with asthma, pulmonary infiltrates and vasculitic phase involving the peripheral and central nervous system (CNS), heart, lungs, kidney and gastrointestinal tract. Hallervorden–Spatz disease is a rare familial disorder with extrapyramidal symptoms, aggression and gradually developing dementia. Tolosa–Hunt syndrome presents with unilateral orbital pain with cranial nerve third, fourth and sixth nerve palsies.

Reference: Richard K (2002). *Casebook of Neurology*. Hong Kong: Lippincott William & Wilkins.

Question 5 Answer: d, Voluntary manslaughter
Explanation: The above correctly describes what is commonly referred to as voluntary manslaughter. Involuntary manslaughter refers to an unlawful and dangerous act; the actus reus (committing an act that is known to be against the law) consists of an unlawful act that is dangerous and cause death. Whereas, gross negligence refers to the actus reus, which consists of a breach of a duty of care that the accused owes to the victim, with the result that this breach leads to the victim's death.

Reference: Puri BK, Hall AD, Ho RC (2014). *Revision Notes in Psychiatry*. Boca Raton, FL: CRC Press, p. 734.

Question 6 Answer: e, Research studies have suggested that raised levels of serotonin turnover and alterations in dopamine metabolism in violent offenders
Explanation: Only 1% of offenders have depressive disorder, and the most common cause is not related to psychiatric disorder. Matricide (killing one's own mother) is more common than patricide (killing one's own father). Thirty percent of mothers who commit filicide (killing one's own children) have psychiatric illness. Physical

castration has no impact, while chemical castration shows conflicting results. Cautioning is the main disposal used for female offenders (50% in females versus 30% of males).

Reference: Chiswick D et al. (1995). *Seminars in Forensic Psychiatry*. London: Gaskell; D'Orban PT (1979). Women who kill their children. *Br J Psychiatry*, 134: 560–571.

Question 7 Answer: e, Self-injurious behaviours
Explanation: About 85% of those with Lesch–Nyhan syndrome exhibit self-injurious behaviour. The age of onset of self-injurious behaviours is usually before 3 years. Lips and fingers are often bitten. Generalized aggression with temper tantrums directed against objects and people are also seen. Other features include microcephaly, hypotonia followed by spastic choreoathetosis, dysphagia and dysarthria. The incidence of Lesch–Nyhan syndrome is 1 in 10,000 to 1 in 38,000, and it is exclusive to men. It is an X-linked recessive condition involving CAG trinucleotide repeats and is due to a defect in hypoxanthine guanine phosphoribosyltransferase resulting in accumulation of uric acid.

Reference: Puri BK, Hall AD, Ho RC (2014). *Revision Notes in Psychiatry*. Boca Raton, FL: CRC Press, p. 669.

Question 8 Answer: b, A significant increase in delta and theta frequency
Explanation: A significant increase in delta and theta frequency, together with a decrease in beta activity and slowing of dominant alpha frequencies, is a characteristic electroencephalogram (EEG) finding associated with dementia. A small decrease in alpha frequency may be seen from age 50 onwards. A small increase in beta frequency is also correlated with age. Normal age is generally associated with a non-significant increase in delta activity.

Reference: Blazer DG, Steffens DC, Busse EW (2004). *The American Psychiatric Publishing Textbook of Geriatric Psychiatry* (3rd edition). Arlington, VA: American Psychiatric Publishing, p. 66.

Question 9 Answer: c, Lewy body dementia
Explanation: The eosinophilic intracytoplasmic inclusion bodies refer to Lewy bodies that contain accumulated of alpha synuclein.

Reference: Puri BK, Treasaden I (eds) (2010). *Psychiatry: An Evidence-Based Text*. London: Hodder Arnold, pp. 1106–1107.

Question 10 Answer: a, Anxious personality disorder (PD)
Explanation: Higher levels of neuroticism, and lower scores for openness to experience and having a restricted range of interests are the personality subtype associated with suicide in the elderly.

Reference: Duberstein PR, Conwell Y, Caine ED (1994). Age differences in the personality characteristics of suicide completers: Preliminary findings from a psychological autopsy study. *Psychiatry*, 57: 213–224.

Question 11 Answer: e, 70%
Explanation: Previous epidemiological study has shown that 70% of children with autism have mental retardation. Approximately 30% have mild-to-moderate mental retardation, and around 50% have severe-to-profound mental retardation. Other comorbid disorders include academic learning problems in literacy and numeracy, attention-deficit hyperactivity disorder (ADHD), obsessive-compulsive disorder (OCD), tics or Tourette syndrome, anxiety disorders, depression, temper tantrums, oppositional defiant disorder as well as self-injurious behaviour.

Reference: Puri BK, Hall AD, Ho RC (2014). *Revision Notes in Psychiatry*. Boca Raton, FL: CRC Press, p. 627.

Question 12 Answer: b, Personality changes greatly over long periods of life
Explanation: Several longitudinal studies have shown stability of personality over long periods of life. Studies have also shown a decrease in the dimensions of neuroticism, extraversion and openness to experience and increases in agreeableness and conscientiousness across a lifetime.

Reference: Blazer DG, Steffens DC, Busse EW (2004). *The American Psychiatric Publishing Textbook of Geriatric Psychiatry* (3rd edition). Arlington, VA: American Psychiatric Publishing, pp. 127–128.

Question 13 Answer: b, The elderly have less emotional reactivity when encountering stress compared with younger adults
Explanation: Studies have shown that older people have less emotional reactivity when encountering stress and higher levels of internal control compared with younger adults. Religious involvement and having strong spiritual beliefs have been found to help alleviate the negative effects of some life experiences. Marginalized minority groups have been found to use religious coping more often when encountering problems. Retirement has not been shown to increase the risk of psychiatric disorders and poor coping skills.

Reference: Blazer DG, Steffens DC, Busse EW (2004). *The American Psychiatric Publishing Textbook of Geriatric Psychiatry* (3rd edition). Arlington, VA: American Psychiatric Publishing, pp. 128–129, 143–145.

Question 14 Answer: a, Cognitive behavioural stress management
Explanation: The most commonly effective type of psychological intervention in people with HIV/AIDS is cognitive behavioural stress management.

Reference: Levenson JL (2004). *The American Psychiatric Publishing Textbook of Psychosomatic Medicine*. Arlington, VA: American Psychiatric Publishing, p. 947.

Question 15 Answer: d, Mania
Explanation: The prevalence of chronic fatigue syndrome (CFS) in the United Kingdom ranges from 0.8% to 2.6%. The female-to-male ratio is 3:1. The age of onset is between 29 and 35 years old. People with CFS may have lower occupational

status and educational background. Aetiologies of CFS include (i) persistent viral infection, (ii) immune dysfunction, (iii) electrolyte imbalance and (iv) chronic candidiasis. Immunological changes involved include increase in expression of activation markers on the surface of T lymphocytes, increase in number of CD-8+ cytotoxic T cells and decrease in number of natural killer cell function. Endocrinological changes include abnormality in the hypothalamic–pituitary–adrenal (HPA) axis and hypocortisolism. It is most commonly associated with depression and anxiety. Individuals with CFS are at greater risk than those without for current psychiatric disorder. Patients with CFS are more likely to have received psychotropic medication or experienced psychiatric disorder in the past. There is a trend for previous psychiatric disorder to be associated with comorbid rather than non-comorbid chronic fatigue.

References: Puri BK, Hall AD, Ho RC (2014). *Revision Notes in Psychiatry.* Boca Raton, FL: CRC Press, p. 479; Wessely S, Chalder T, Hirsch S, Wallace P, Wright D (1996). Psychological symptoms, somatic symptoms, and psychiatric disorder in chronic fatigue and chronic fatigue syndrome: A prospective study in the primary care setting. *Am J Psychiatry,* 153(8): 1050–1059.

Question 16 Answer: c, Reaction formation
Explanation: In reaction formation, there is a psychological attitude that is diametrically opposed to an oppressed wish and constitutes a reaction against it. This is often seen in patients with OCD.

Reference: Puri BK, Hall AD, Ho RC (2014). *Revision Notes in Psychiatry.* Boca Raton, FL: CRC Press, p. 336.

Question 17 Answer: c, Allocation of patients by gender (subdivided into strata and individuals within each striatum undergo further randomization)
Explanation: Option C is stratified randomization, while the other options are quasi-randomization. For stratified randomization, subjects are subdivided into strata, and individuals within each striatum are then randomized. This is less likely to produce bias in RCT compared with quasi-randomization, which is not a proper randomization method, as it is based on subjects' characteristics, such as month of birth, hospitalization status and laboratory results.

Reference: Lewis GH, Sheringham J, Kalim K, Crayford TJB (2008). *Mastering Public Health: A Postgraduate Guide to Examination and Revalidation.* London: Royal Society of Medicine Press, pp. 48–49.

Question 18 Answer: d, An increase in the number of collaborating centres instead of the number of subjects
Explanation: The power of a RCT depends on sample size, total number of endpoints, difference in compliance between two groups, increased number of endpoints by selecting a high-risk population or increased duration of follow-up. Having more collaborating centres does not necessarily mean more subjects, which is important in increasing the power of an RCT.

Reference: Lewis GH, Sheringham J, Kalim K, Crayford TJB (2008). *Mastering Public Health: A Postgraduate Guide to Examination and Revalidation*. London: Royal Society of Medicine Press, p. 39.

Question 19 Answer: d, Empathetic style
Explanation: FRAMES stands for feedback about drinking, responsibility enforcement, advice to change, menu of alternatives, empathetic style and self-efficacy.

Reference: Puri BK, Hall A, Ho RC (2014). *Revision Notes in Psychiatry* (3rd edition). Boca Raton, FL: CRC Press, p. 527.

Question 20 Answer: e, The onset of symptoms occur at the age of 14 years
Explanation: Schizotypal disorder runs a chronic course (at least 2 years). People with schizotypal disorder may have odd beliefs inconsistent with cultural norms, obsessive ruminations without inner resistance, transient quasi-psychotic episodes but not as intensified as first-rank symptoms and poor rapport.

Reference: Puri BK, Treasaden I (eds) (2010). *Psychiatry: An Evidence-Based Text*. London: Hodder Arnold, pp. 593–609.

Question 21 Answer: e, Serum homocysteine level is not a good indicator of vitamin B_{12} or folate status
Explanation: Serum homocysteine level may serve as a functional indicator of vitamin B_{12} status, as it is needed to convert homocysteine to methionine in one-carbon metabolism in brain tissue. Deficiencies in vitamin B_{12} and folate can lead to neuropsychiatric disorders, including neuropathy, depression, psychosis and cognitive impairment.

Reference: Blazer DG, Steffens DC, Busse EW (2004). *The American Psychiatric Publishing Textbook of Geriatric Psychiatry* (3rd edition). Arlington, VA: American Psychiatric Publishing, pp. 128–129, 181–182.

Question 22 Answer: d, The presence of the apolipoprotein E (APOE) allele is a risk factor for Alzheimer's disease
Explanation: Several studies have shown presence of the APOE allele to be a risk factor for Alzheimer's disease. It also increases the specificity of the diagnosis of Alzheimer's disease. Homozygous for APOE allele is not diagnostic for Alzheimer's dementia. APOE testing is not currently recommended for predicting the risk of dementia in asymptomatic persons. Response to cholinesterase inhibitors in patients is also not influenced by results of APOE testing.

Reference: Blazer DG, Steffens DC, Busse EW (2004). *The American Psychiatric Publishing Textbook of Geriatric Psychiatry* (3rd edition). Arlington, VA: American Psychiatric Publishing, p. 186.

Question 23 Answer: e, Vascular dementia
Explanation: The second most common cause of dementia is vascular dementia, which accounts for 15%–30% of cases. It includes disorders arising from either large or small vessel strokes.

Reference: Blazer DG, Steffens DC, Busse EW (2004). *The American Psychiatric Publishing Textbook of Geriatric Psychiatry* (3rd edition). Arlington, VA: American Psychiatric Publishing, pp. 192–193.

Question 24 Answer: a, Amitriptyline
Explanation: Selective serotonin re-uptake inhibitors (SSRIs) can cause pulmonary hypertension (after 20 weeks) in the newborn. Neonates may experience withdrawal (agitation and irritability), especially with paroxetine and venlafaxine. Amitriptyline and imipramine have been used for many years without causing teratogenic effects. The use of tricyclic antidepressants (TCAs) in the third trimester may lead to withdrawal effects and increase the risk of preterm delivery. Fluoxetine has the most data on safety. Paroxetine is associated with foetal heart defects in the first trimester and is less safe than other SSRIs. Sertraline may also decrease Apgar scores.

Reference: Puri BK, Hall AD, Ho RC (2014). *Revision Notes in Psychiatry*. Boca Raton, FL: CRC Press, p. 561.

Question 25 Answer: c, Rapid forgetting of new information after short intervals
Explanation: Short-term memory loss is the earliest manifestation of Alzheimer's disease. Visuospatial problems and semantic knowledge problems become more prominent in the later stages of the illness. Speech comprehension, which is a fundamental element of communication, is better preserved.

Reference: Blazer DG, Steffens DC, Busse EW (2004). *The American Psychiatric Publishing Textbook of Geriatric Psychiatry* (3rd edition). Arlington, VA: American Psychiatric Publishing, p. 193.

Question 26 Answer: a, Corticotropin-releasing hormone (CRH)
Explanation: The following hormones are decreased in patients with anorexia nervosa: follicle-stimulating hormone (FSH), luteinizing hormone (LH), oestrogen and triiodothyronine (T3). In contrast, CRH, cortisol and growth hormone levels are increased. With the reduction in circulating oestrogen, there is shrunken uterus and small amorphous ovaries. As weight is gained, the uterus increases in size, and the ovaries become multifollicular. At normal weight, the ovaries become follicular: this is detected by the pelvic ultrasound and can be used to indicate correct weight. The electrolyte disturbances include hypokalaemia (leading to possible arrhythmias, cardiac arrest and renal damage), hypomagnesaemia, hypozincaemia and hypophosphataemia.

Reference: Puri BK, Hall AD, Ho RC (2014). *Revision Notes in Psychiatry*. Boca Raton, FL: CRC Press, p. 579.

Question 27 Answer: a, Density of neurofibrillary tangles

Explanation: In Alzheimer's disease, histological changes include granulovascular degeneration, Hirano bodies, neurofibrillary tangles and senile plaques. The correlation between the density of postmortem neurofibrillary tangles and cognitive impairment is more robust than with other histological abnormalities.

References: Blazer DG, Steffens DC, Busse EW (2004). *The American Psychiatric Publishing Textbook of Geriatric Psychiatry* (3rd edition). Arlington, VA: American Psychiatric Publishing, p. 213; Puri BK, Hall AD, Ho RC (2014). *Revision Notes in Psychiatry*. Boca Raton, FL: CRC Press, p. 683.

Question 28 Answer: a, Cephalosporin

Explanation: The psychiatric side effects of cephalosporins include euphoria, delusions, depersonalization and illusions. The side effects of clarithromycin include delirium and mania, whereas the side effects of gentamicin and trimethoprim-sulfamethoxazole include delirium and psychosis. The side effects of quinolones include psychosis, paranoia, mania, agitation and Tourette-like syndrome. Risk factors of neuropsychiatric side effects from antibiotics have included prior psychopathology, coexisting medical conditions, slow acetylator status, advanced age, concomitant medications and increased permeability of the blood–brain barrier, as well as high antibiotic dosage and intrathecal or intravenous administration. Psychiatric toxicity may result from various mechanisms of action, including antagonism of gamma-aminobutyric acid (GABA) or pyridoxine, adverse interactions with alcohol, or inhibition of protein synthesis.

References: Levenson JL (2004). *The American Psychiatric Publishing Textbook of Psychosomatic Medicine*. Arlington, VA: American Psychiatric Publishing, p. 592; Sternbach H, State R (1997). Antibiotics: Neuropsychiatric effects and psychotropic interactions. *Harv Rev Psychiatry*, 5(4): 214–226.

Question 29 Answer: b, A patient can withdraw from the RCT at any time, and a valid reason is required

Explanation: This option is contrary to the Declaration of Helsinki that states that research subjects can withdraw from study without giving any reason. Steps involved in the conduction of RCT include identify and engage investigational sites, develop trial governance procedures, develop trial procedures according to good clinical practice, apply and obtain funding, develop recruitment strategies and methods to identify and overcome recruitment problems, develop data capture methods, engage in oversight of trial progress, develop procedures for adverse event reporting and complete trial termination procedures.

References: Lewis GH, Sheringham J, Kalim K, Crayford TJB (2008). *Mastering Public Health: A Postgraduate Guide to Examination and Revalidation*. London: Royal Society of Medicine Press, pp. 48–49; Smith A, Palmer S, Johnson DW, Navaneethan S et al. (2010). How to conduct a randomized trial. *Nephrology (Carlton)*, 15(8): 740–746.

Question 30 Answer: e, The larger the sample size, the larger the standard error
Explanation: The larger the sample size, the smaller the standard error. Increased statistical power is associated with larger sample size, larger meaningful difference and smaller standard deviation.

Reference: Lewis GH, Sheringham J, Kalim K, Crayford TJB (2008). *Mastering Public Health: A Postgraduate Guide to Examination and Revalidation*. London: Royal Society of Medicine Press, p. 97.

Question 31 Answer: b, Patients with insulin-dependent diabetes mellitus (IDDM) have more cognitive impairment than patients with non-insulin-dependent diabetes mellitus (NIDDM)
Explanation: Patients with IDDM tend to have less cognitive impairment than patients with NIDDM.

Reference: Puri BK, Treasaden I (eds) (2010). *Psychiatry: An Evidence-Based Text*. London: Hodder Arnold, pp. 621–622.

Question 32 Answer: d, Psychomotor agitation
Explanation: AIDS mania has a clinical picture that is rather different from primary mania. There is irritable mood, which can be prominent, although euphoria may still be observed. There can be psychomotor slowing that accompanies the cognitive slowing of the AIDS dementia, replacing the expected hyperactivity of mania. This form of mania is also more chronic than episodic, with infrequent spontaneous remissions.

Reference: Levenson JL (2004). *The American Psychiatric Publishing Textbook of Psychosomatic Medicine*. Arlington, VA: American Psychiatric Publishing, pp. 587–588.

Question 33 Answer: e, Monoamine oxidase inhibitors
Explanation: Monoamine oxidase inhibitors are effective in agoraphobics and social phobics, with at least 80%–90% of pure social phobia individuals being asymptomatic with 16 weeks of treatment. However, patients who are withdrawn from treatment suffer from relapse. Selective serotonin reuptake inhibitors such as citalopram, fluvoxamine, paroxetine and sertraline are usually used as first-line treatment. Benzodiazepines can also help to prevent the reinforcement of fear through avoidance. Beta blockers can be particularly useful for individuals to help them with performance anxiety.

Reference: Puri BK, Hall AD, Ho RC (2014). *Revision Notes in Psychiatry*. Boca Raton, FL: CRC Press, pp. 407–408.

Question 34 Answer: a, 2%
Explanation: Based on the Epidemiologic Catchment Area (ECA) study, it was found that OCD is very rare in children. Rutter found no cases among the 2,000 10- and 11-year-olds in the Isle of Wight. Other findings were that the 6-month prevalence of OCD has been estimated to be around 1.3%–2.0%; the lifetime prevalence has been estimated to be around 1.9%–3.0%; there is an equal sex ratio, and there has been noted to be a bimodal peak of onset, with peaks occurring at

12–14 and also around 20–22 years of age. There is a noted decline in onset after the age of 55 years. The ECA study prevalence findings were consistently higher than earlier accepted estimates.

Reference: Puri BK, Hall AD, Ho RC (2014). *Revision Notes in Psychiatry*. Boca Raton, FL: CRC Press, p. 416.

Question 35 Answer: a, Carbamazepine
Explanation: Carbamazepine may cause syndrome of inappropriate antidiuretic hormone (SIADH). The mechanism for this is uncertain but may involve increased release of antidiuretic hormone (ADH) (vasopressin) and/or potentiation of the action of this hormone.

Reference: Puri BK, Treasaden I (eds) (2010). *Psychiatry: An Evidence-Based Text*. London: Hodder Arnold, p. 431.

Question 36 Answer: b, Borderline
Explanation: Perioperative psychosocial characteristics are strong and significant predictors of noncompliance. Pretransplantation screening for background and demographic variables may have limited utility for compliance outcomes. Strategies to improve compliance should focus on psychosocial risk factors pertaining to early psychologic reactions to transplantation, the quality of family relationships and patient styles of coping. These risk factors are each potentially modifiable through appropriate educational and supportive interventions.

References: Levenson JL (2004). *The American Psychiatric Publishing Textbook of Psychosomatic Medicine*. Arlington, VA: American Psychiatric Publishing, pp. 686–687; Dew MA, Roth LH, Thompson ME, Kormos RL, Griffith BP (1996). Medical compliance and its predictors in the first year after heart transplantation. *J Heart Lung Transplant*, 15(6): 631–645.

Question 37 Answer: c, There is irreversible cessation of mitosis and ultimately the death of an organism
Explanation: The essential concept of stochastic damage talks about wear and tear as a result of ageing. Macromolecules distorting the physical and chemical properties of the human body, free-radical damage, accumulation of earlier adverse events and a decline in the basic metabolic rate are concepts related to this theory. Irreversible cessation of mitosis and ultimately the death of an organism are related to the Hayflick limit theory, which involves genetically programmed ageing.

Reference: Puri BK, Hall AD, Ho RC (2014). *Revision Notes in Psychiatry*. Boca Raton, FL: CRC Press, p. 682.

Question 38 Answer: d, 1.67–5.00
Explanation: The number needed to treat (NNT) is a useful statistic that indicates how many patients would need to be treated with a particular intervention to

reduce by one the expected number of a defined outcome. It is the reciprocal of the absolute risk difference. It is particularly useful since it takes into account the frequency of the outcome and thus reflects the public health impact of the intervention. For this scenario, the confidence interval (CI) is obtained by 1/0.6 to 1/0.2 while NNT = 2 (1/0.42).

Reference: Lewis GH, Sheringham J, Kalim K, Crayford TJB (2008). *Mastering Public Health: A Postgraduate Guide to Examination and Revalidation*. London: Royal Society of Medicine Press, pp. 42–43.

Question 39 Answer: c, Onset of psychosis is usually gradual and occurs within 6 months after the injury

Explanation: The onset of psychotic symptoms is usually gradual and delayed, often occurring more than 1 year after the injury. Risk factors for psychosis include temporal lobe and left-hemisphere lesions, closed head injury and increasing severity of brain injury. Delusions are more common than hallucinations. Negative symptoms (deficits of normal emotional responses or of other thought processes such as flat expressions or little emotion, poverty of speech, inability to experience pleasure, lack of desire to form relationships and lack of motivation) are not as common as hallucinations and delusions.

Reference: Levenson JL (2004). *The American Psychiatric Publishing Textbook of Psychosomatic Medicine*. Arlington, VA: American Psychiatric Publishing, pp. 794–795.

Question 40 Answer: a, There is a decrease in CRH

Explanation: There are multiple hormonal changes in anorexia nervosa. The typical changes increased a decrease in T3, an increase in CRH, an increase in cortisol, an increase in growth hormone and a decrease in FSH and LH. The 24 hours pattern of secretion of LH would resemble that normally seen in the pre-pubertal individual. There is a decrease in oestrogen in women.

Reference: Puri BK, Hall AD, Ho RC (2014). *Revision Notes in Psychiatry*. Boca Raton, FL: CRC Press, p. 579.

Question 41 Answer: c, 50% of sexual offences seen by courts are related to exhibitionism

Explanation: The true answer is only 25%. Less than 20% of indecent exposers will re-offend.

References: Stone JH, Roberts M, O'Grady J, Taylor AV, O'Shea K (2000). *Faulk's Basic Forensic Psychiatry* (3rd edition). Oxford, UK: Blackwell Science; Gelder M, Mayou R, Cowen P (2001). *Shorter Oxford Textbook of Psychiatry*. Oxford, UK: Oxford University Press; Gunn J, Taylor PJ (1993). *Forensic Psychiatry: Clinical, Legal and Ethical Issues*. Oxford, UKJ: Butterworth-Heinemann.

Question 42 Answer: e, The rate of 'stranger homicides' by those with mental illness has increased sharply
Explanation: There is no increase in 'stranger homicide' committed by psychiatric patients. In the United Kingdom, 35% of homicide is committed by offenders with psychiatric illnesses. Among those with psychiatric illnesses, schizophrenia is the most common psychiatric disorder associated with homicide (55%), followed by PD (26%) and affective disorder (19%). Less than 50% of psychotic offenders describe psychotic motivation; 160–200 psychiatric inpatients die by suicide annually, and the most common method is hanging.

References: Gelder M, Mayou R, Cowen P (2001). *Shorter Oxford Textbook of Psychiatry*. Oxford, UK: Oxford University Press; Swinson N (2007). National confidential inquiry into suicide and homicide by people with mental illness: New directions. *Psychiatric Bulletin*, 31: 161–163.

Question 43 Answer: a, The urine screen was done on the fourth day after admission, and the active ingredient of cannabis was not detectable
Explanation: This usually applies to a first-time user but not a heavy user. The active ingredient is detectable in the urine after 48–72 hours in the first-time or occasional user but up to 6 weeks in heavy users, as it is stored in the body fat. B is possible, and other possible agents include toilet-cleaning agent. D is possible, as aspirin may interfere with the enzyme immunoassays. E is possible, and the excessive consumption of vitamin B has darkened his urine. This would make the laboratory staff less suspicious that his urine was diluted.

Reference: Puri B, Treasaden I (eds) (2010). *Psychiatry: An Evidence-Based Text*. London: Hodder Arnold, pp. 412, 1031.

Question 44 Answer: b, The most common switch in pattern is from anorexia nervosa to bulimia nervosa
Explanation: The course and the outcome are variable. Some patients recover fully after a single episode. Some exhibit fluctuating patterns of weight gain followed by a relapse. For adolescents, around 80% recover in 5 years, and 20% may develop chronic anorexia nervosa. For adults, 50% recover, 25% have intermediate outcome and 25% have poor outcomes. Fifty percent of restrictive anorexia nervosa patients may develop bulimia after 5 years. This is a serious disorder with substantial mortality (5%–20%). The aggregate mortality rate is 5.6% per decade. This is 12 times the annual death rate for all causes for females aged 15 to 24. The aggregate mortality rate is substantially greater than that reported for psychiatric inpatients and the general population.

Reference: Puri BK, Hall AD, Ho RC (2014). *Revision Notes in Psychiatry*. Boca Raton, FL: CRC Press, p. 577.

Question 45 Answer: e, Personality disorder
Explanation: Huntington disease is a genetic disorder resulting in a condition characterized by continuous involuntary movements and a slowly progressive dementia. There are five cases per 100,000 in the United Kingdom. The onset of

symptoms is usually between ages of 35 and 45, but childhood onset accounts for 10%–20% of cases. The onset is insidious with fidgety movements or non-specific psychiatric symptoms in the early stages. The more commonly reported deficits seen in caudate nucleus dysfunction include apathy, depression, disinhibition, change in personality, aphasia, psychosis and predisposition for delirium.

References: Yudofsky SC, Hales RE (2002). *The American Psychiatric Publishing Textbook of Neuropsychiatry and Clinical Neurosciences* (4th edition). Arlington, VA: American Psychiatric Publishing, p. 269; Puri BK, Hall AD, Ho RC (2014). *Revision Notes in Psychiatry*. Boca Raton, FL: CRC Press, pp. 706–707.

Question 46 Answer: b, Gabapentin

Explanation: Gabapentin is an anticonvulsant structurally related to GABA. It has been reported to cause paradoxical agitation in some patients with traumatic brain injury. This is not reported in other medications. Physicians treating brain-injured patients and prescribing gabapentin for neuropathic pain may wish to closely monitor patients for similar signs of restlessness or anxiety.

Reference: Childers MK, Holland D (1997). Psychomotor agitation following gabapentin use in brain injury. *Brain Inj*, 11: 537–540.

Question 47 Answer: a, Cost minimization analysis

Explanation: Cost minimization analysis study is used to find the least expensive method of achieving a single outcome. The advantage of this analysis study is that it is simple to conduct. However, the disadvantage is that it assumes that interventions have an equivalent effect and compares programmes solely on the criterion of cost. Cost effectiveness analysis compares alternative treatments where both the costs and the benefits vary. Benefits are measured in natural units. For cost utility analysis, it measures the effect of an intervention on both morbidity and mortality. Cost–benefit analysis involves measuring both costs and benefits in monetary terms.

Reference: Lewis GH, Sheringham J, Kalim K, Crayford TJB (2008). *Mastering Public Health: A Postgraduate Guide to Examination and Revalidation*. London: Royal Society of Medicine Press, pp. 437–440.

Question 48 Answer: b, It is contraindicated in people with advanced liver disease

Explanation: The mechanism of action of disulfiram is to inhibit aldehyde dehydrogenase and lead to aldehyde accumulation after drinking alcohol, resulting in unpleasant effects (flushing, tachycardia and hypotension). The starting dose is 800 mg, reducing to 100–200 mg daily. It increases the blood levels of warfarin, theophylline and diazepam via drug–drug interactions. It is contraindicated in people with advanced liver disease, cardiac failure, coronary artery disease, cerebrovascular disease and in pregnancy and breastfeeding.

Reference: Taylor D, Paton C, Kapur (2012). *The Maudsley Prescribing Guidelines in Psychiatry* (11th edition). Oxford, UK: Wiley-Blackwell, p. 371.

Question 49 Answer: c, Significant benefits will continue 1–2 years after stopping
Explanation: Acamprosate is a GABA agonist and glutamate antagonist. It inactivates N-methyl-D-aspartate (NMDA) receptors and prevents calcium ion influx. This reverses the GABA and glutamate imbalance when abstaining from alcohol and reduces the long-lasting neuronal hyperexcitability. The treatment effect is most pronounced at 6 months, although it remains significant for up to 12 months. It can be used in combination with disulfiram. Contraindications to its use include severe renal or hepatic impairment, pregnancy and breastfeeding.

Reference: Taylor D, Paton C, Kapur S (2012). *The Maudsley Prescribing Guidelines in Psychiatry* (11th edition). Oxford, UK: Wiley-Blackwell, p. 370.

Question 50 Answer: a, He has to take a high-phenylalanine diet
Explanation: The boy is suffering from phenylketonuria. It is caused by a defect in the phenylalanine hydroxylase, leading to accumulation of phenylalanine. Thus, this group of patients needs to take a low phenylalanine diet before 6 months of age. Initiation of such a diet before 3 months of age may preserve normal intelligence. However, the side effects of this diet include anaemia, hypoglycaemia and oedema.

Reference: Puri BK, Hall AD, Ho RC (2014). *Revision Notes in Psychiatry*. Boca Raton, FL: CRC Press, p. 668.

Question 51 Answer: a, A Wood's lamp or ultraviolet light may be used to locate the hypomelanotic macules
Explanation: The mode of inheritance of tuberous sclerosis is autosomal dominant with 100% penetration. Males and females are equally affected. The majority have normal intelligence quotient (IQ) but, if there is learning disability, it is usually profound. Seizures are common, and initial presentation is often infantile spasms.

Reference: Puri BK, Hall AD, Ho RC (2014). *Revision Notes in Psychiatry*. Boca Raton, FL: CRC Press, pp. 671–672.

Question 52 Answer: b, Left basal ganglia
Explanation: The prevalence of major depression is 30% amongst patients suffering from cerebrovascular accident. The incidence of depression is lower amongst patients suffering from an occlusion of the posterior cerebral arteries in comparison with occlusions in anterior and middle cerebral arteries. Major depression is associated with left frontal lobe and left basal ganglia lesions, with the strongest correlation of risk during the acute period after stroke. Patients who develop depression after right-sided stroke are associated with family history of depression. The volume of the lesion is directly proportional to the severity of depression.

Reference: Yudofsky SC, Hales RE (2002). *The American Psychiatric Publishing Textbook of Neuropsychiatry and Clinical Neurosciences* (4th edition). Arlington, VA: American Psychiatric Publishing, p. 729.

Question 53 Answer: e, 70% have microdeletions of chromosome 15q11–13 of paternal origin
Explanation: This child is suffering from Angelman syndrome. It is autosomal dominant with deletion on chromosome 15q11–13 of the maternal origin. Clinical features include paroxysms of laughter, cheerful disposition, ataxia, axial hypotonia, jerky movements, epilepsy, gastrointestinal problems and severe or profound learning disability.

Reference: Puri BK, Hall AD, Ho RC (2014). *Revision Notes in Psychiatry*. Boca Raton, FL: CRC Press, pp. 675–676.

Question 54 Answer: a, Cornelia De Lange syndrome
Explanation: Cornelia De Lange syndrome is associated with severe-to-profound learning disability, while Klinefelter syndrome, Turner syndrome, Wilson disease and XYY syndrome are associated with milder forms of mental retardation.

Reference: Puri BK, Hall AD, Ho RC (2014). *Revision Notes in Psychiatry*. Boca Raton, FL: CRC Press, p. 679.

Question 55 Answer: c, It is rapid and cheap
Explanation: In a cohort study, a group of individuals is selected who do not initially have the outcome of interest. A range of exposures is quantified for cohort members, and at the end of the study, those people who have developed the outcome of interest are compared (according to the exposure of interest) with those who have not. Strengths of cohort studies include able to follow temporal relationships, well suited to rare exposures, multiple effects of a single exposure, minimize selection bias and useful for diseases with long latency periods. Weaknesses of cohort studies include expensive and time consuming, risk of loss to follow-up and inefficient for rare disease.

Reference: Lewis GH, Sheringham J, Kalim K, Crayford TJB (2008). *Mastering Public Health: A Postgraduate Guide to Examination and Revalidation*. London: Royal Society of Medicine Press, p. 38.

Question 56 Answer: c, Klinefelter syndrome
Explanation: Only about 30% of Klinefelter syndrome patients have a learning disability, which, when it does occur, is usually mild with some difficulty in acquiring verbal skills. This condition is usually diagnosed only when patients undergo evaluation for infertility. 48XXXY and 49XXXXY are associated with severe learning disability and marked hypogonadism.

Reference: Puri BK, Hall AD, Ho RC (2014). *Revision Notes in Psychiatry*. Boca Raton, FL: CRC Press, pp. 667–668.

Question 57 Answer: c, Dialectical behavioural therapy
Explanation: For patients with anorexia nervosa, cognitive analytical therapy, cognitive-behavioural therapy, interpersonal therapy, focal dynamic therapy and

family interventions focusing on eating disorders are the recommended modalities of treatment. The main aim of psychotherapy is to reduce the risk, enhance their motivation, help encourage healthy eating and also reduce the other symptoms related to anorexia nervosa. It has been suggested that the minimum duration for outpatient psychological treatment should be at least 6 months.

Reference: Puri BK, Hall AD, Ho RC (2014). *Revision Notes in Psychiatry*. Boca Raton, FL: CRC Press, p. 580.

Question 58 Answer: d, Upon weight restoration, fluoxetine has demonstrated benefits for patients with anorexia nervosa

Explanation: Fluoxetine has failed to demonstrate any benefits in the treatment of patients with anorexia nervosa following weight restoration. Olanzapine has been studied extensively, and it has been associated with greater weight gain, reduction in obsessive symptoms, reduction in anxiety and increase in compliance. Case report has highlighted that risperidone is associated with weight gain and reduction in anxiety when combined with an antidepressant. Oestrogen administration should not be used to treat bone density problems in children and adolescents, as it might lead to premature fusion of the epiphyses. SSRIs are usually the drugs of first choice for the treatment of bulimia nervosa. The effective dose of fluoxetine is 60 mg per day. Other psychotropic medications are not usually recommended for the treatment of bulimia nervosa.

Reference: Puri BK, Hall AD, Ho RC (2014). *Revision Notes in Psychiatry*. Boca Raton, FL: CRC Press, p. 587.

Question 59 Answer: c, It is often difficult to find age-matched controls

Explanation: For case–control studies, individuals with the outcome of interest (cases) are matched with individuals who do not have the outcome of interest (controls). It is often difficult to find age-matched controls. Bias cannot be adjusted for, confounding factors cannot be completely excluded and regression is able to adjust for several factors simultaneously.

Reference: Lewis GH, Sheringham J, Kalim K, Crayford TJB (2008). *Mastering Public Health: A Postgraduate Guide to Examination and Revalidation*. London: Royal Society of Medicine Press, p. 37.

Question 60 Answer: c, Intermittent explosive disorder

Explanation: Intermittent explosive disorder is a behavioural disorder characterized by extreme expressions of anger, often to the point of uncontrollable rage, which are disproportionate to the situation at hand. Impulsive aggression is unpremeditated and is defined by a disproportionate reaction to any provocation, real or perceived. Some individuals have reported affective changes prior to an outburst (e.g. tension, mood changes, energy changes). It is diagnosed by the presence of the following: several episodes of uninhibited aggression leading to assault or vandalism; aggression out of proportion to the precipitating situation and aggression not accounted for by another diagnosis such as mania, psychosis, anti-social personality or medical conditions.

Reference: McElroy SL (1999). Recognition and treatment of DSM-IV intermittent explosive disorder. *J Clin Psychiatry*, 60(Suppl 15): 12–16.

Question 61 Answer: d, 48 hours
Explanation: The student is suffering from acute stress reaction. This is a transient disorder developing in an individual without other mental disorders in response to exceptional stress. Exposure to the stressor is followed by an immediate onset of symptoms within 1 hour, which begin to diminish after not more than 48 hours. The risk is increased if physical exhaustion or organic factors are present. There is a mixed and changing picture – initial state of daze, depression, anxiety, anger, despair, overactivity and withdrawal may all be seen, with no one symptom predominating for long. Pharmacological treatment includes beta blockers (e.g. propranolol) and alpha-2 receptor antagonist (e.g. clonidine), which reduces nightmares and emotional reactivity.

Reference: Puri BK, Hall AD, Ho RC (2014). *Revision Notes in Psychiatry*. Boca Raton, FL: CRC Press, pp. 426–427.

Question 62 Answer: d, Prolactin level
Explanation: Risperidone leads to an increase in prolactin level and sexual dysfunction.

Reference: Puri BK, Treasaden I (eds) (2010). *Psychiatry: An Evidence-Based Text*. London: Hodder Arnold, p. 632.

Question 63 Answer: d, In hyperthyroid patients with depressive symptoms, mood symptoms may precede physical symptoms
Explanation: Serious psychopathology is present only in a minority of patients. Major depression is the most common psychiatric manifestation, and mania, hypomania or psychoses are uncommon. The prevalence of cognitive impairment in hyperthyroidism is less than that in hypothyroidism. Mood symptoms may precede development of physical signs and symptoms of hyperthyroidism.

Reference: Yudofsky SC, Hales RE (2002). *The American Psychiatric Publishing Textbook of Neuropsychiatry and Clinical Neurosciences* (4th edition). Arlington, VA: American Psychiatric Publishing, pp. 858–860.

Question 64 Answer: a, DiGeorge syndrome
Explanation: The incidence of the disorder is 1 in 4000 live births. It is caused by a micro-deletion in chromosome 22q11.12. More than 50% of the patients have mild-to-moderate learning disability. It is inherited in an autosomal dominant fashion. The clinical features include cardiac abnormalities, hypocalcaemia, seizures and short stature.

Reference: Puri BK, Hall AD, Ho RC (2014). *Revision Notes in Psychiatry*. Boca Raton, FL: CRC Press, p. 673.

Question 65 Answer: a, Lesch–Nyhan syndrome
Explanation: Lesch–Nyhan syndrome is a sex-linked recessive disorder involving CAG trinucleotide repeats.

- Maple syrup urine disease – autosomal recessive
- Neurofibromatosis – autosomal dominant
- Rett syndrome – X-linked dominant
- Velocardiofacial syndrome – either sporadic or autosomal dominant

Reference: Moore DP, Puri BK (2012). *Textbook of Clinical Neuropsychiatry and Behavioral Neuroscience* (3rd edition). London: Hodder Arnold, p. 463.

Question 66 Answer: d, Sanfilippo syndrome
Explanation: Sanfilippo syndrome or mucopolysaccharidosis is a rare autosomal-recessive lysosomal storage disease. It is caused by deficiency in one of the enzymes needed to break down heparin sulphate. It causes severe learning disability, and the cause of death is usually respiratory tract infections between the age of 10 and 20 years.

Reference: Puri BK, Hall AD, Ho RC (2014). *Revision Notes in Psychiatry*. Boca Raton, FL: CRC Press, p. 670.

Question 67 Answer: c, Language function
Explanation: Huntington disease is a genetic disorder resulting in a condition characterized by continuous involuntary movements and a slowly progressive dementia. There are 5 cases per 100,000 in the United Kingdom. The onset of symptoms is usually between the ages of 35 and 45 years, but childhood onset accounts for 10%–20% of cases. The onset is insidious with fidgety movements or nonspecific psychiatric symptoms in the early stages. Planning, organizing and mental flexibility are affected early in Huntington disease. Judgement is also poor, although there may be awareness of deficits. Language functions are relatively preserved in the advanced cases.

References: Yudofsky SC, Hales RE (2002). *The American Psychiatric Publishing Textbook of Neuropsychiatry and Clinical Neurosciences* (4th edition). Arlington, VA: American Psychiatric Publishing, pp. 928–929; Puri BK, Hall AD, Ho RC (2014). *Revision Notes in Psychiatry*. Boca Raton, FL: CRC Press, pp. 706–707.

Question 68 Answer: b, Bonding
Explanation: The Family Environment Scale was developed to measure social and environmental characteristics of all families. It can be used in several ways, including family counselling and psychotherapy, teaching program evaluators about family systems and in program evaluation. This scale has also been widely used in many research projects. The other area that this rating scale looks at is independence.

Reference: Boyd CP, Gullone E, Needleman GL, Burt T (1997). The family environment scale: Reliability and normative data for an adolescent sample. *Fam Process*, 36(4): 369–373.

Question 69 Answer: a, It includes parents, teacher and youth self-report versions
Explanation: The Conners Rating Scale-Revised is a diagnostic scale for ADHD using *Diagnostic and Statistical Manual of Mental Disorders, Fourth Edition (DSM-IV)* criteria. It includes parents, teacher and youth self-report versions. The behaviour scale includes ADHD symptoms, anxiety, cognitive problems, oppositional behaviour, perfectionism and social problems.

Reference: Puri BK, Hall AD, Ho RC (2014). *Revision Notes in Psychiatry*. Boca Raton, FL: CRC Press, p. 632.

Question 70 Answer: c, Intelligence test scores are fairly stable for children above the age of 5 years
Explanation: Intelligence test scores are generally considered to be unstable for normal developing preschool children. However, the scores are fairly stable above the age of 5 years. IQ scores are strongly associated with academic achievement but only modestly predictive of overall adjustment. The Kaufman Assessment Battery for Children measures the cognitive and intellectual functioning in children and adolescents.

Reference: Wiener JM, Dulcan MK (2004). *The American Psychiatric Publishing Textbook of Child and Adolescent Psychiatry* (3rd edition). Arlington, VA: American Psychiatric Press, pp. 169, 171.

Question 71 Answer: a, Low empathy and ability to identify interpersonal issues
Explanation: Both boys and girls with conduct disorder demonstrate low empathy and ability to identify interpersonal issues. Girls with conduct disorders are more likely to engage in covert behaviours and prostitution. Boys tend to be more concrete and egocentric. Girls with conduct disorder are more verbal and use indirect and relational aggression. Boys use physical aggression. Girls with conduct disorders are more likely to develop depression, anxiety and somatization.

Reference: Puri BK, Hall AD, Ho RC (2014). *Revision Notes in Psychiatry*. Boca Raton, FL: CRC Press, p. 638.

Question 72 Answer: e, Receiver operating characteristic (ROC) curve
Explanation: A ROC curve is a plot of the sensitivity of a diagnostic test against one minus its specificity as the cut-off criterion for indicating a positive test is varied. It is often used in choosing between competing tests, although the procedure takes no account of the prevalence of the disease being tested for.

Reference: Lewis GH, Sheringham J, Kalim K, Crayford TJB (2008). *Mastering Public Health: A Postgraduate Guide to Examination and Revalidation*. London: Royal Society of Medicine Press, p. 170.

Question 73 Answer: e, The more sensitive the test, the higher the positive predictive value

Explanation: The more sensitive the test, the less likely it is that a negative result will be a true positive and hence the higher the negative predictive value. Conversely, the more specific the test, the less likely it is that a positive result will be true negative, and hence the higher the positive predictive value.

Reference: Lewis GH, Sheringham J, Kalim K, Crayford TJB (2008). *Mastering Public Health: A Postgraduate Guide to Examination and Revalidation*. London: Royal Society of Medicine Press, p. 171.

Question 74 Answer: a, Generalizability of study results

Explanation: External validity refers to the extent to which causal relationships can be generalized to different measures, persons, settings and times. Factors affecting external validity include subject characteristics, the effect of the research environment, researcher or experimenter effects and data collection methodology. Internal validity refers to the degree to which the results are attributable to the independent variables and no other rival explanations. Factors affecting internal validity include subject variability, size of subject population, time given for the data collection or experimental treatment and instrument/task sensitivity. Options B–E are measures of internal validity of RCT.

Reference: Steckler A, McLeroy KR (2008). The importance of external validity. *Am J Public Health*, 98(1): 9–10.

Question 75 Answer: a, 10% of the values lie beyond two standard deviations from the median

Explanation: Normal distribution is a probability distribution assumed by many statistical procedures. The distribution is bell-shaped and depends on two parameters: the population mean and the population variance. The standard normal distribution has a mean of 0 and variance of 1. In the standard normal distribution, 68% of the area under the curve is within 1 standard deviation of the mean, 95% of the area is within 1.96 standard deviations and 99% of the area is within 2.58 standard deviations.

Reference: Lewis GH, Sheringham J, Kalim K, Crayford TJB (2008). *Mastering Public Health: A Postgraduate Guide to Examination and Revalidation*. London: Royal Society of Medicine Press, p. 77.

Question 76 Answer: a, Higher levels of noradrenaline are found in patients suffering from chronic asthma, and this finding is statistically significant at the 0.1% level

Explanation: Higher levels of noradrenaline are found in patients suffering from acute asthma (mean = 645.04) but not in patients suffering from chronic asthma (mean = 498.77). This finding is statistically significant at the 0.1% level. In Table 9.1, the authors first evaluated differences in the levels of psychological stress, HPA-related biological stress indices and NPY levels among patients with acute asthma, patients with chronic asthma and healthy control subjects. Although the number of life events did not differ among groups, asthmatic patients, especially those with acute asthma, experienced higher levels of perceived stress than their healthy counterparts, as corroborated by increased levels of ACTH, noradrenaline and adrenaline and HPA stress index scores and decreased levels of cortisol and NPY.

Question 77 Answer: b, Multivariate linear regression analysis
Explanation: In this study, there is more than one independent continuous variable (i.e. perceived stress, NPY level). As a result, multivariate linear regression analysis was used to examine the relationship between dependent continuous variable (interleukin (IL)-4 levels) and several independent variables together. Logistic regression analysis is used when dependent and independent variables are categorical (e.g. disease status) rather than continuous. Univariate analysis examines the relationship between the dependent variable and one independent variable at a time. Pearson's correlation analysis generates correlation coefficient but not slope (i.e. *B* value).

Question 78 Answer: a, Age is a confounding factor, which may influence the IL-4 levels
Explanation: Age is a confounding factor, which is an extraneous variable that may correlate with both the dependent variable (IL-4 levels) and the independent variables (e.g. perceived stress, NPY levels). Age is not an independent variable based on analysis performed in Table 9.2, The variable age does not cause type I and type II errors. Type I error refers to a statistically significant association may have occurred by chance. Type II error occurs when null hypothesis is false, and the researchers fail to reject the false null hypothesis. Age is not responsible for reverse causality because it is not a dependent variable.

Question 79 Answer: c, Perceived stress among asthmatic patients was a significant predictor of the IL-4 levels measured at baseline and 1 year later, after controlling for potential confounders
Explanation: Perceived stress among asthmatic patients was a significant predictor of IL-4 levels measured at baseline ($p = 0.19$, $p < 0.05$) and 1 year later ($p = 0.025$, $p < 0.05$), after controlling for potential confounders. Similarly, NPY levels among asthmatic patients was a significant predictor of IL-4 levels measured at baseline ($p < 0.001$) and 1 year later ($p < 0.001$), after controlling for potential confounders.

Question 80 Answer: d, NPY level is a mediating factor in the association between high perceived stress levels and IL-4 overexpression in asthmatic patients
Explanation: The Sobel test is a method of testing the significance of a mediation effect. In the above study, the relationship between the independent variable (i.e. perceived stress) and the dependent variable (i.e. the IL-4 levels) is hypothesized to be an indirect effect that exists due to the influence of the mediator (i.e. the NPY levels). As a result when the NPY levels are included in a regression analysis model with perceived stress, the effect of the perceived stress is reduced (p value for IL-4 at baseline is 0.234 ($p > 0.05$) and p value at 1 year is 0.324 ($p > 0.05$), and the effect of

the NPY remains significant (Sobel test at baseline $p = 0.033$ [$p < 0.05$] and at 1 year $p = 0.032$ [$p < 0.05$]).

Reference: Sobel ME (1982). Asymptotic confidence intervals for indirect effects in structural equation models. *Sociological Methodology,* 13: 290–312.

Question 81 Answer: a, Absence or presence of speech
Explanation: Factors that have been shown to consistently relate to outcome in autistic patients include absence or presence of speech by 5 years old, the IQ of the patient and the severity of the disorder. Nonverbal IQ <60 is associated with severe social impairment and lack of independent living. Childhood autism often causes lifelong disability. Ten percent of people with autism will ultimately lose language skills with intellectual deterioration. Age of onset, birth weight, family history of mental illness and the IQ of parents are not related to outcome in autistic patients.

References: Wiener JM, Dulcan MK (2003). *The American Psychiatric Publishing Textbook of Child and Adolescent Psychiatry* (3rd edition). Arlington, VA: American Psychiatric Press, p. 296; Puri BK, Hall AD, Ho RC (2014). *Revision Notes in Psychiatry*. Boca Raton, FL: CRC Press, p. 628.

Question 82 Answer: d, Pervasive Developmental Disorder Behaviour Inventory (PDDBI)
Explanation: The PDDBI is an instrument that does not require training. It is used to evaluate children with age range 6 months to 12 years who have been diagnosed with a pervasive developmental disorder as defined by the DSM-IV. Rating forms completed by parents and teachers yield age-standardized scores, which are helpful in planning treatment, monitoring progress, assessing outcome and making placement decisions. In contrast, Autism Diagnostic Interview (ADI), Autism Diagnostic Observation Schedule (ADOS) and Childhood Autism Rating Scale (CARS) all require training before use.

Reference: Puri BK, Hall AD, Ho RC (2014). *Revision Notes in Psychiatry*. Boca Raton, FL: CRC Press, p. 626.

Question 83 Answer: d, The most common type of seizure is grand mal seizure
Explanation: Independent associations have been found between epilepsy and older age and lower cognitive ability. Other risk factors, such as poor language and developmental regression, are not associated with epilepsy after controlling for IQ. The most common type of seizure is partial seizure, and females have greater risk of seizures than males. A prospective study of epilepsy in children with autistic spectrum disorder found that about 5% of those with autistic condition had epilepsy (Wong 1993).

References: Wiener JM, Dulcan MK (2003). *The American Psychiatric Publishing Textbook of Child and Adolescent Psychiatry* (3rd edition). Arlington, VA: American Psychiatric Press, p. 267; Wong V (1993). Epilepsy in children with autistic spectrum disorder. *J Child Neurol*, 8: 316–322; Viscidi EW, Triche EW, Pescosolido MF, McLean RL, Joseph RM et al. (2013). Clinical characteristics of children with autism spectrum disorder and co-occurring epilepsy. *PLoS One*, 8(7):e67797.

Question 84 Answer: e, Shoplifting is more common in OCD than in the general population

Explanation: Shoplifting is not common among OCD patients. The most common obsessions are fear of contamination (45%), doubting (42%), fear of illness, germs or bodily fear (36%), symmetry (31%) and sexual or aggressive thoughts (28%). The most common compulsions are checking (63%), washing (50%) and counting (36%). In neuroimaging of OCD, diffuse-tensor imaging shows decreased cortico-striato-thalamo-striato-cortical circuitry, while functional magnetic resonance imaging (MRI) shows increased orbitofrontal cortex, anterior cingulate cortex and striatum. Favourable prognostic factors include mild symptoms, predominance of phobic ruminative ideas and absence of compulsions, short duration of symptoms and no childhood symptoms or abnormal personality traits. Poor prognostic factors include males with early onset, symptoms involving the need for symmetry and exactness, presence of hopelessness, hallucinations or delusions, family history of OCD and a continuous episodic or deteriorating course.

Reference: Puri BK, Hall AD, Ho RC (2014). *Revision Notes in Psychiatry*. Boca Raton, FL: CRC Press, pp. 417–418.

Question 85 Answer: e, Sodium lactate

Explanation: Hypersensitivity of presynaptic alpha 2-receptor and increase in adrenergic activity, subsensitivity of 5-hydroxytryptamine 1A (5-HT1A) receptors and exaggerated postsynaptic receptor response and reduction in GABA receptor sensitivity have been implicated in the aetiology of panic disorder. Yohimbine, d-fenfluramine, flumazenil, cholecystokinin, sodium lactate, 1-(3-chlorophenyl) piperazine (mCPP) (MCCP) (5-HT receptor agonist) and the inhalation of carbon dioxide have been found to induce panic in individuals. In terms of neuroimaging, structural MRI shows decreased medial temporal lobe volume, while functional MRI shows increased haemodynamic responses in the amygdala, hippocampus and insula.

References: Argyropoulos S, Campbell A, Stein G (2007). Anxiety disorders, in Stein G, Wilkinson G (eds). *Seminars in General Adult Psychiatry*. London: Gaskell, pp. 332–334; Puri BK, Hall AD, Ho RC (2014). *Revision Notes in Psychiatry*. Boca Raton, FL: CRC Press, pp. 413–414.

Question 86 Answer: a, Alcohol abuse is not as common in social phobia as in other phobias

Explanation: Social phobias are characterized by a fear of scrutiny by others in small groups. This may progress to panic attacks. Avoidance is often marked. Beta-blockers can be used to reduce autonomic arousal, which can be particularly helpful for performance anxiety. The relatives of socially phobic probands have a threefold-elevated risk of social phobia. The course is continuous, but it may improve gradually. Alcohol and drug abuse are common, with alcohol abuse being more common in social phobia than in other phobias.

Reference: Puri BK, Hall AD, Ho RC (2014). *Revision Notes in Psychiatry*. Boca Raton, FL: CRC Press, pp. 408–409.

Question 87 Answer: d, Prednisolone
Explanation: Steroids are known to cause anxiety symptoms. Other drugs that can cause anxiety include amphetamines and other stimulants, appetite suppressants, caffeine, cocaine, decongestants, thyroxine, antihypertensives, antiarrhytmics, anticholingerics, anticonvulsants and nonsteroidal anti-inflammatory drugs. About 70% of patients have mild or no impairment, and 9% have severe impairment. Poor prognostic factors include severe anxiety symptoms, syncope, agitation, derealization and suicide.

Reference: Puri BK, Hall AD, Ho RC (2014). *Revision Notes in Psychiatry*. Boca Raton, FL: CRC Press, pp. 410–411.

Question 88 Answer: c, Patients present with cognitive impairment in the absence of mood or psychotic symptoms
Explanation: Fahr disease is a rare autosomal dominant neuropsychiatric disorder. It commonly affects young to middle-aged adults. Aetiology of this syndrome does not identify a specific agent, but associations with a number of conditions have been noted, the most common of which are endocrine disorders, mitochondrial myopathies, dermatological abnormalities and infectious diseases. Patients may present with a schizophrenia-like psychosis or mood disorder in early adulthood. Apathy, memory impairment and poor judgement are prominent with language function being spared. It is associated with hypoparathyroidism.

Reference: Yudofsky SC, Hales RE (2002). *The American Psychiatric Publishing Textbook of Neuropsychiatry and Clinical Neurosciences* (4th edition). Arlington, VA: American Psychiatric Publishing, p. 942.

Question 89 Answer: d, Hypokalaemic alkalosis
Explanation: The patient is likely to have hypokalaemic alkalosis because of the use of laxatives, diuretic and self-induced vomiting. The electrolyte disturbances seen in patients with anorexia nervosa include hypokalaemia, hypomagnesaemia, hypozincaemia and hypophosphataemia. A multivitamin/multimineral supplement in oral form is recommended in people with anorexia nervosa during both inpatient and outpatient weight restoration. Total parenteral nutrition should not be used unless there is significant gastrointestinal dysfunction.

Reference: Puri BK, Hall AD, Ho RC (2014). *Revision Notes in Psychiatry*. Boca Raton, FL: CRC Press, pp. 579–580.

Question 90 Answer: e, Progression to conduct disorder
Explanation: In the study, a total of 485 children took part in a 3-year follow-up study. Their mean age was that of 12 years. The primary outcome measures were

the severity of ADHD and oppositional defiant disorder, reading scores, social skills, level of impairment and diagnosis. The four treatment groups demonstrated reduction in their ADHD symptoms over time.

Reference: Puri BK, Hall AD, Ho RC (2014). *Revision Notes in Psychiatry*. Boca Raton, FL: CRC Press, p. 635.

Question 91 Answer: d, Eight

Explanation: Traumatic brain injury reduces the time to onset of Alzheimer's disease among persons at risk of developing the disease. The presence of APOE E4 allele combined with traumatic head injury increases the risk for Alzheimer's disease by eight times. Among traumatic brain injury cases who developed Alzheimer's disease, the observed time to onset was shorter than the expected time to onset, and the effect of traumatic brain injury on time to onset was greatest when the injury occurred before age 65 years.

Reference: Nemetz PN, Leibeson C, Naessens JM et al. (1999). Traumatic brain injury and time to onset of Alzheimer's disease: A population-based study. *Am J Epidemiol*, 149: 32–40.

Question 92 Answer: a, A majority begin their offending behaviour in middle age

Explanation: The majority of adult sex offenders begin their offending behaviour in adolescence.

References: Chiswick D, Cope R (1995). *Seminars in Forensic Psychiatry*. London: Gaskell; Murrey GJ, Briggs D, Davis C (1992). Psychopathic disordered, mentally ill, and mentally handicapped sex offenders: A comparative study. *Med Sci Law*, 32: 331–336.

Question 93 Answer: c, It is a risk assessment tool

Explanation: It is a tool to identify psychopathy at multiple aspects, including (i) personality, (ii) behavioural, (iii) cognitive, (iv) interpersonal relationships and (v) forensic. It is not a risk assessment tool.

Reference: Hare RD (2003). *Hare Psychopathy Checklist–Revised* (2nd edition). Toronto, Ontario: Multi-Health Systems.

Question 94 Answer: c, Sertraline

Explanation: Based on National Institute for Health and Care Excellence (NICE) guidelines, fluoxetine, paroxetine, sertraline, venlafaxine and escitalopram have been found to be beneficial for post-traumatic stress disorder (PTSD). These drugs usually require at least 8 weeks of duration before the effects are evident. The Food and Drug Administration (FDA), however, has approved sertraline for OCD in children more than 6 years and PTSD in adults. Hence, for adolescents, sertraline has the best evidence compared with other antidepressants.

References: Puri BK, Hall AD, Ho RC (2014). *Revision Notes in Psychiatry*. Boca Raton, FL: CRC Press, p. 424; Cohen JA et al. (2007). A pilot randomized controlled trial of combined trauma-focused CBT and sertraline for childhood PTSD symptoms. *J Am Acade Chil Adolesc Psychiatry*, 46(7): 811–819.

Question 95 Answer: c, In the United States, 17%–20% of elementary school children are estimated to suffer from reading disabilities

Explanation: There has been a recent study that showed that the epidemiology of reading disorder is similar in the United States, Taiwan and Japan. In the United Kingdom, the prevalence is approximately 45 among 9- to 10-year-olds. The male-to-female ratio is 3:1. A score on reading and/or under comprehension that is 2 SE below the level expected on the basis of the children's chronological age, and intelligence is the defined criteria.

References: Stevenson HW et al. (1982). Reading disabilities: The case of Chinese, Japanese and English. *Child Development*, 53: 1164–1181; Puri BK, Hall AD, Ho RC (2014). *Revision Notes in Psychiatry*. Boca Raton, FL: CRC Press, p. 646.

Question 96 Answer: b, It is associated with a high prevalence of epilepsy

Explanation: In a study of 13 patients with childhood disintegrative disorder, Mouridsen et al. (1999) found that 77% of the patients had epilepsy. It is a rare condition with prevalence of 1.7 per 10,000. Life expectancy is normal. Most patients suffer from moderate mental retardation. People with this condition have normal or near-normal development until the age of 3 or 4 years.

References: Mouridsen SE, Rich B, Isager T (1999). Epilepsy in disintegrative psychosis and infantile autism: A long-term validation study. *Dev Med Child Neurol*, 41: 110–114; Puri BK, Hall AD, Ho RC (2014). *Revision Notes in Psychiatry*. Boca Raton, FL: CRC Press, p. 631.

Question 97 Answer: c, Decrease in temporal lobe volume

Explanations: In children with schizophrenia, there is uneven development with delay in language and social behaviour. There is also cognitive impairment and behavioural abnormalities. Other common features include visual hallucinations, ideas of reference and negative symptoms. MRI studies in children have reported larger volumes of the superior temporal lobe gyrus (Jacobsen et al. 1996), increased ventricular volume, a decrease in total cerebral volume (Rapoport et al. 1997, 1999) and a smaller midsagittal thalamic area (Frazier et al. 1996).

References: Frazier JA, Giedd JA, Hamburger SD et al. (1996). Brain anatomic magnetic resonance imaging in childhood onset schizophrenia. *Arch Gen Psychiatry*, 53: 617–624; Jacobsen LK, Giedd JN, Vaituzis AC et al. (1996). Temporal lobe morphology in childhood-onset schizophrenia. *Am J Psychiatry*, 153: 355–361; Rapoport JL, Giedd J, Kumra S et al. (1997). Childhood onset schizophrenia: Progressive ventricular change during adolescence. *Arch Gen Psychiatry*, 54: 897–903; Rapoport JL, Giedd JN, Blumenthal J (1999). Progressive cortical change during adolescence in childhood onset schizophrenia: A longitudinal magnetic resonance imaging study. *Arch Gen Psychiatry*, 56: 649–654.

Question 98 Answer: e, Weight loss
Explanation: Atypical depression is more common in younger individuals and women. Childhood atypical depression is more likely to present with weight gain rather than weight loss. Patients may have hypersomnia, increased appetite, mood reactivity and psychomotor retardation. It is more likely to have chronic course with poor inter-episode recovery. It responds better to monoamine oxidase inhibitors (MAOI). Patients with atypical depression are more likely to suffer from PDs and anxiety disorders such as borderline PD, avoidant PD, generalized anxiety disorder and OCD.

Reference: Wiener JM, Dulcan MK (2003). *The American Psychiatric Publishing Textbook of Child and Adolescent Psychiatry* (3rd edition). Arlington: American Psychiatric Press, pp. 413–414.

Question 99 Answer: c, 33%
Explanations: Studies have shown that as many as one-third of children with major depressive episodes may show signs of bipolar disorder by adolescence. Childhood bipolar disorder is ranked as having the second worst prognosis among all psychiatric disorders in childhood. Reduction of sleep is often the first indicator for childhood bipolar disorder and is associated with ADHD. The first line of treatment is olanzapine.

Reference: Geller B, Fox LW, Clark KA (1995). Rate and predictors of prepubertal bipolarity during follow-up of 6- to 12-year-old depressed children. *J Am Acad Child Adolesc Psychiatry*, 33: 461–468.

Question 100 Answer: c, Euphoria
Explanation: Compared with adults, children with mania seldom present with euphoric mood. Children with mania present with irritability, hyperactivity, aggressive temper outbursts, moodiness, insomnia, impulsivity, poor concentration, depression and poor school performance. Reduction of sleep is often the first indicator for childhood bipolar disorder. It is ranked as having the second worst prognosis among all psychiatric disorders in childhood. The first line of treatment is olanzapine.

Reference: Wiener JM, Dulcan MK (2003). *The American Psychiatric Publishing Textbook of Child and Adolescent Psychiatry* (3rd edition). Arlington, VA: American Psychiatric Press, p. 415.

Question 101 Answer: c, Increased psychomotor retardation
Explanation: Studies have shown that conduct disorder, promiscuous sexual behaviour, social withdrawal, substance abuse and poor school performance are common among depressed adolescents. Mood symptoms are generally similar to adults, and severe cases may present with mood-congruent psychotic features. Adolescents are less likely to have psychomotor retardation in comparison with

adults. Aetiology includes adverse life events, arguments with parents, multiple family disadvantages and positive family history of depression.

Reference: Wiener JM, Dulcan MK (2003). *The American Psychiatric Publishing Textbook of Child and Adolescent Psychiatry* (3rd edition). Arlington, VA: American Psychiatric Press, p. 439.

Question 102 Answer: b, Children
Explanation: The onset of adjustment disorder is within 1 month of the stressor. The duration is usually less than 6 months, expect for prolonged depressive reaction. The manifestations vary, including depressed mood, anxiety, worry, an inability to cope and some inability to manage daily routine. Conduct disorders may be associated, especially in adolescents. Regressive phenomena in children are frequently seen. In children, adjustment disorders are predictive of more serious mental illnesses for late adolescence and adulthood. In the younger age groups, unlike adults, adjustment disorder carries with it significant morbidity and a poor outcome, frequently developing into major psychiatric illness.

References: Puri BK, Hall AD, Ho RC (2014). *Revision Notes in Psychiatry.* Boca Raton, FL: CRC Press, p. 432; Casey P, Bailey S (2011). Adjustment disorders: The state of the art. *World Psychiatry*, 10(1): 11–18.

Question 103 Answer: b, Bromocriptine
Explanation: The patient is suffering from neuroleptic malignant syndrome, which is a serious adverse effect of antipsychotics, mostly seen in young males. It is an idiosyncratic reaction towards antipsychotics and caused by a sudden hypodopaminergic state that affects the hypothalamus. Treatment is supportive with use of dantrolene (direct muscle relaxant) followed by bromocriptine (dopamine receptor agonist). Sometimes, amantadine, levodopa, carbidopa, or electroconvulsive therapy (ECT) is used.

References: Ahuja N, Cole AJ (2009). Hyperthermia syndromes in psychiatry. *Adv Psychiatric Treat*, 15: 181–191; Caroff SN, Mann SC (1993). Neuroleptic malignant syndrome. *Med Clin N Am*, 77: 185–202.

Question 104 Answer: d, There is an increase in the level of IL-6 in cerebrospinal fluid (CSF)
Explanation: As a product of monocytes and macrophages, IL-6 is one of the most frequently investigated immune parameters in patients with major depression. IL-6 is involved in modulation of the HPA axis. Activation of the HPA axis is one of the best-documented changes in major depression. CSF studies of depressed patients have shown decreased levels of IL-6 and soluble IL-6 receptor. Studies have also shown that lower levels of CSF IL-6 are associated with current depression, with future depression during a follow-up of almost two decades and that lower levels of CSF IL-6 may be related to depression vulnerability in later life.

References: Mössner R, Mikova O, Koutsilieri E, Saoud M et al. (2007). Consensus paper of the WFSBP Task Force on Biological Markers: Biological markers in depression. *World J Biol Psychiatry*, 8(3): 141–174; Kern S, Skoog I, Börjesson-Hanson A, Blennow K et al. (2013). Lower CSF interleukin-6 predicts future depression in a population-based sample of older women followed for 17 years. *Brain Behav Immun*, 32: 153–158.

Question 105 Answer: b, Delayed sleep-phase syndrome (DSPD)
Explanation: DSPD is a circadian rhythm sleep disorder affecting the timing of sleep, peak period of alertness, the core body temperature rhythm, hormonal and other daily rhythms, compared with the general population and relative to societal requirements. The prevalence of DSPD is 3 in 2000. There is no known cause. Sleep architecture and total time of sleep are normal. People with DSPD generally fall asleep some hours after midnight and have difficulty waking up in the morning. Treatment involves adaptation to late night sleep, sleep schedule and good sleep hygiene, light therapy and melatonin.

Reference: Stuart CY, Robert EH (2010). *Essentials of Neuropsychiatry and Behavioral Neurosciences* (2nd edition). Arlington, VA: American Psychiatric Publishing, pp. 5–324.

Question 106 Answer: d, 21%
Explanation: It is estimated that up to 21% of the hospitalized elderly fulfil the criteria for a major depressive episode, and an additional 20%–25% have a minor depression.

Reference: Koenig HG, George LK, Peterson BL, Pieper CF (1997). Depression in medically ill hospitalized older adults: Prevalence, characteristics, and course of symptoms based on six diagnostic schemes. *Am J Psychiatry*, 154: 1376–1383.

Question 107 Answer: d, Eating disorder
Explanation: Approximately 40%–70% of children and adolescents with major depressive disorder (MDD) have a comorbid psychiatric disorder. The most frequent comorbid psychiatric disorders include anxiety disorder (30%–80%), dysthymic disorder (30%–80%), substance abuse (20%–30%) and disruptive disorder (10%–80%). Eating disorder is not common in children and adolescents with MDD. For adolescent-onset depressive disorder, there is a high conversion rate to bipolar disorder at 40% by 2 years. Furthermore, depression and conduct disorder are associated with increased risk of suicide, alcoholism, substance misuse and antisocial PD.

References: Wiener JM, Dulcan MK (2003). *The American Psychiatric Publishing Textbook of Child and Adolescent Psychiatry* (3rd edition). Arlington, VA: American Psychiatric Press, pp. 444–445; Puri BK, Hall AD, Ho RC (2014). *Revision Notes in Psychiatry*. Boca Raton, FL: CRC Press, p. 649.

Question 108 Answer: a, The combined use of clozapine and carbamazepine is a safe practice to prevent seizures in patients on long-term clozapine
Explanation: Clozapine may cause neutropenia and potentially fatal agranulocytosis. It can also cause seizure at high doses. The incidence of clozapine-induced seizures appears to be highest in patients treated with doses of ≥600 mg per day.

Other factors that increase the risk of seizures in patients treated with clozapine include rapid titration of clozapine dose, patients with histories of previous seizures, head trauma with loss of consciousness, recent electroconvulsive therapy, and/or concomitant therapy with other drugs that lower the seizure threshold. Anticonvulsants can be used to prevent seizures in those aforementioned high-risk patients or as treatment for clozapine-induced seizures. When choosing an anticonvulsant, it is important to consider the risk of potentiation of adverse effects such as agranulocytosis. Combining carbamazepine with clozapine greatly increases the risk of agranulocytosis. Carbamazepine is a potent inducer of CYP1A2, known to decrease serum clozapine concentrations. In addition, carbamazepine by itself has been associated with leukopenia and agranulocytosis.

Reference: Taylor D, Paton C, Kapur S (2012). *The Maudsley Prescribing Guidelines in Psychiatry* (11th edition). Oxford, UK: Wiley-Blackwell, pp. 62–63, 68.

Question 109 Answer: c, human leukocyte antigen (HLA)-B 1502 allele
Explanation: Administration of carbamazepine to patients with Asian ancestry who carry the HLA-B 1502 allele is especially likely to cause Stevens–Johnson syndrome. Before prescribing carbamazepine to Asian patients, doctors should first test them for this allele; however, if they have been taking carbamazepine for longer than several months without the adverse reaction of Stevens–Johnson syndrome, their risk of subsequently developing it is low. Stevens–Johnson syndrome begins as a rash, consists of blisters on the mucous membranes around the mouth, eyes and other areas of the skin. The blisters often weep and reach a confluent appearance. Disrupted skin and mucous membranes leak serum, fluid and electrolytes. In severe cases, bacteria can invade the bloodstream.

Reference: Kaufman DM, Milstein MJ (2013). *Kaufman's Clinical Neurology for Psychiatrists* (7th edition). Philadelphia, PA: Saunders, p. 215.

Question 110 Answer: b, Treating catatonia
Explanation: ECT has been shown to be especially helpful in treatment of catatonia. The physical seriousness of catatonia – which can present as psychomotor disturbances leading to extreme behaviour such as hyperkinesis, stupor, catalepsy, negativism and anomalies of voluntary movement, which in turn are associated with dehydration, malnutrition, hyperpyrexia and outbursts of violence – merits urgent physical treatment. In such circumstances, ECT has long been considered the treatment of choice. The American Psychiatric Association (1990) endorsed ECT as an effective treatment for the catatonic subtype of schizophrenia.

Reference: Lock T (1994). Advances in the practice of electroconvulsive therapy. *Adv Psychiatric Treat*, 11: 150–156.

Question 111 Answer: e, 3500
Explanation: Clozapine treatment can potentially cause agranulocytosis, defined as an absolute neutrophil count (ANC) less than 500/mm^3. Agranulocytosis can

lead to serious infection and death. Before initiating treatment with clozapine, there is a need to obtain a baseline white blood cell (WBC) count and ANC. The ANC must be greater than or equal to 2000/mm³, and the WBC must be greater than or equal to 3,500/mm³ before a patient can begin treatment with clozapine. During treatment, patients must have regular monitoring of ANC and WBC.

Reference: Clozapine Important Safety Information, from Clozapine Registry. http://www.clozapineregistry.com/Clozapine_Fair_Balance_Professional.pdf.ashx

Question 112 Answer: d, Speech or language impairment
Explanation: The frequency of speech and language impairment in children with ADHD is about 50%. For oppositional defiant disorder, the frequency is 40%; for conduct disorder, it is 30%–50%; for anxiety disorder, it is 25% and for tic, it is 11%. Compared with children with ADHD alone, those with language problems had poorer word reading, math computation and academic competence. Language problems were not associated with poorer social functioning in those with ADHD.

References: Puri BK, Hall AD, Ho RC (2014). *Revision Notes in Psychiatry*. Boca Raton, FL: CRC Press, p. 632; Sciberras E, Mueller KL, Efron D, Bisset M, Anderson V et al. (2014). Language problems in children with ADHD: A community-based study. *Pediatrics*, 133(5):793–800.

Question 113 Answer: e, Obsessions and compulsions in Tourette syndrome are similar to those of pure OCD without Tourette disorder
Explanation: The obsessions and compulsions in Tourette syndrome differ somewhat from those of pure OCD. For example, obsessions in Tourette syndrome relate to sex, violence and aggression; whereas, in pure OCD, they relate to dirt, germs and illness. Compulsions in Tourette syndrome typically involve checking and ordering while those in pure OCD consist of more elaborate activities such as handwashing or housecleaning.

Reference: Kaufman DM, Milstein MJ (2013). *Kaufman's Clinical Neurology for Psychiatrists* (7th edition). Philadelphia, PA: Saunders, pp. 425–427.

Question 114 Answer: d, The child's experiences of previous separations vary with the rate of disappearance of separation anxiety
Explanation: Separation anxiety is the fear of an infant being separated from his or her caregiver. It is a normal part of development, usually beginning at around 6–7 months, peaking at around 18 months and decreasing after 30 months. When separation anxiety becomes persistent and excessive, a diagnosis of separation anxiety disorder needs to be considered. The rate of disappearance of separation anxiety varies with the child's experience of previous separations (real or threatened), handling by mother, perception of whether mother will die or not and temperament.

References: Puri BK, Hall AD, Ho RC (2014). *Revision Notes in Psychiatry*. Boca Raton, FL: CRC Press, p. 64; Wiener JM, Dulcan MK (2003). *The American Psychiatric Publishing Textbook of Child and Adolescent Psychiatry* (3rd edition). Arlington, VA: American Psychiatric Press, p. 557.

Question 115 Answer: a, Genetic factor is an important aetiology
Explanation: Late-onset cases appear to have less genetic loading than younger-onset cases, with fewer of the former giving a family history of affective disorder. There is a tendency towards more rapid recurrence late in the illness, with decreasing periods of normality. Increased cerebral vulnerabilities and insults play a more important role than life events in precipitating late-onset mania.

References: Blazer DG, Steffens DC, Busse EW (2004). *The American Psychiatric Publishing Textbook of Geriatric Psychiatry* (3rd edition). Arlington, VA: American Psychiatric Publishing, pp. 245–246; Puri BK, Hall AD, Ho RC (2014). *Revision Notes in Psychiatry*. Boca Raton, FL: CRC Press, pp. 711–712.

Question 116 Answer: d, 20%
Explanation: Bereavement is a term that can apply to any loss event, from the loss of a relative by death to unemployment, divorce or loss of a pet; it refers to being in a state of mourning. Parks described the five stages of bereavement: alarm, numbness, pining for the deceased (illusions or hallucinations of the deceased may occur), depression and recovery and reorganization. About 20% of bereaved people meet the criteria for MDD. The diagnosis of MDD can only be made 2 months following the bereavement. Symptoms that point towards MDD rather than mere bereavement include guilt about things other than actions taken or not taken by the survivor at the time of death, thoughts of death, morbid preoccupation with worthlessness, marked psychomotor retardation, prolonged and marked psychomotor retardation and hallucinatory experiences other than thinking he or she hears the voice of, or transiently sees the image of, the deceased person.

References: American Psychiatric Association (2010). *American Psychiatric Association Practice Guidelines. Practice Guideline for the Treatment of Patients with Major Depressive Disorder* (3rd edition). Arlington, VA: American Psychiatric Publishing; Puri BK, Hall AD, Ho RC (2014). *Revision Notes in Psychiatry*. Boca Raton, FL: CRC Press, pp. 76–77.

Question 117 Answer: e, 96 hours
Explanation: Cocaine can be detected in urine for 6–8 hours, but its metabolites can be detected for up to 2–4 days. However, the behavioural effects of cocaine last for only a relatively short time (30–60 minutes); thus, users require repeated doses of the drug to maintain the feeling of intoxication.

Reference: Sadock BJ, Sadock VA (2003). *Kaplan and Sadock's Synopsis of Psychiatry* (9th edition). Philadelphia, PA: Lippincott Williams & Wilkins, p. 430.

Extended Match Items

Theme: Research Methodology

Question 118 Answer: a, Level 1A

Question 119 Answer: d, Level 2A

Question 120 Answer: g, Level 3A
Explanation: The Centre for Evidence Basic Medicine (CEBM) has ranked the different types of research evidence based on how likely they are to be true. The strongest evidence comes from a systematic review that demonstrates consistent findings from several high-quality RCTs. This is termed as level 1 evidence, and recommendations based on level 1 results are called grade A. Further down the hierarchy come more heterogeneous findings and evidence from less robust sources.

Reference: Lewis GH, Sheringham J, Kalim K, Crayford TJ (2008). *Mastering Public Health*. London: Royal Society of Medicine Press Ltd, p. 62.

Theme: Old-Age Psychiatry

Question 121 Answer: c, Generalized slowing of alpha rhythm, diffuse theta and delta activity with decline of low-voltage beta activity and focal delta activity in temporal areas
Explanation: In normal ageing (after the age of 60 years), there is generalized slowing of alpha rhythm, diffuse theta and delta activity with decline of low-voltage beta activity and focal delta activity in temporal areas.

Question 122 Answer: d, Non-specific slow waves and irregular high-voltage delta activity
Explanation: This man is suffering from delirium, and the EEG is most likely to show diffuse non-specific slowing. Delta activity, asymmetry in delta waves and localized spike and sharp waves complexes occur more frequently in those with intracranial pathology. Alpha activity correlates with cognitive functioning, and delta activity correlates with length of illness.

Question 123 Answer: a, Background slowing and diffuse superimposed beta activity
Explanation: This is most suggestive of benzodiazepine intoxication. In general, benzodiazepines cause background slowing and increase in beta activity and sometimes decreased alpha activity.

Question 124 Answer: b, Focal and generalized spikes, sharp waves, polyspikes and spike–wave complexes
Explanation: This is most suggestive of epilepsy. Focal and generalized spikes, sharp waves, polyspikes and spike–wave complexes are typical features of an EEG seen in epilepsy.

Reference: Puri BK, Hall AD. Ho RC (2014). *Revision Notes in Psychiatry*. Boca Raton, FL: CRC Press, pp. 217, 690, 691.

Theme: Research Methods and Statistics

Question 125 Answer: b, Medline

Question 126 Answer: a, Embase

Question 127 Answer: a, Embase, d, Science Direct

Question 128 Answer: c, PsychINFO

Explanation: Medline contains over 21 million records and approximately 7000 publications. It contains records relating to medicine and biological research in humans and animals. It is compiled by the United States National Library of Medicine and is freely accessible on the Internet via the PubMed.

Embase was first created by a group of Dutch physicians who promoted the flow of medical knowledge shortly after the World War II in 1946. In 1972, the publisher, Elsevier, acquired the Embase. Since its establishment, Embase has a greater bias towards pharmacological research and provides valuable information on drugs and adverse effects.

PsychINFO is a database that contains journal articles, book chapters and dissertations related to the field of psychology and created by the American Psychological Association.

Science Direct is a database created by Elsevier and contains articles in physical sciences, biological sciences and social sciences.

References: Kleijnen J, Knipschild P (1992). The comprehensiveness of medline and embase computer searches. *Pharmaceutisch Weekblad Scientific Edition*, 14(5): 316–320; De Petro TG (n.d.). ScienceDirect – Elsevier Science's MegaSource. *Econtent*, 23(6): 56–61.

Theme: Prognosis in Schizophrenia

Question 129 Answer: a, Female gender, c, Being married, d, Good premorbid social adjustment, f, Family history of affective disorder, i, No ventricular enlargement

Question 130 Answer: b, Being male, e,Family history of psychosis, h, Ventricular enlargement

Explanation: Schizophrenia is considered to be a heterogeneous disorder, and there are no reliable predictors of outcome. Approximately 25% of cases of schizophrenia show good clinical and social recovery, while most studies show that fewer than a half of patients have poor long-term outcome. Factors associated with a good prognosis include being female, being married, good premorbid social adjustment, family history of affective disorder, short duration of illness prior to treatment, no ventricular enlargement, abrupt onset of the illness, later onset of the illness, having an affective component to the illness, paranoid ideations, lack of negative symptoms, lack of cognitive impairment and good initial response to treatment.

Reference: Puri BK, Hall AD, Ho RC (2014). *Revision Notes in Psychiatry*. Boca Raton, FL: CRC Press, p. 370.

Theme: Renal Impairment

Question 131 Answer: a, Haloperidol, b, Olanzapine
Explanation: Haloperidol of dosage between 2 and 6 mg per day can be used. Olanzapine at 5 mg per day can also be used.

Question 132 Answer: f, Citalopram, g, Sertraline
Explanation: Citalopram and sertraline are indicated for usage in patients with renal impairment and depressive disorder. Tricyclic antidepressants are not indicated, largely due to their anticholinergic side effects.

Question 133 Answer: j, Lithium
Explanation: Valproate, carbamazepine and lamotrigine can be used for patients with renal impairments. Lithium is contraindicated.

Reference: Puri BK, Hall AD, Ho RC (2014). *Revision Notes in Psychiatry*. Boca Raton, FL: CRC Press, p. 474.

Theme: Clinical Diagnosis of Learning Disabilities

Question 134 Answer: f, Hurler syndrome
Explanation: This is the classical presentation of this disorder. In addition, children may have short stature. The associated psychiatric features include anxiety and fearful feelings. There may be moderate-to-severe learning disabilities. There may be recurrent respiratory infections and death before the age of 10 years.

Question 135 Answer: g, Lesch–Nyhan syndrome
Explanation: This is the classical presentation of the disorder. In addition, there will associated errors in metabolism, thus resulting in the accumulation of uric acid. During infancy, orange uricosuric acid sand is found in the nappy. The child then develops hypotonia followed by spastic choreoathetosis, dysphagia and dysarthria. The age of onset of self-injurious behaviours is usually before the age of 3 years. Lips and fingers are often bitten.

Question 136 Answer: d, Klinefelter syndrome (XXY)
Explanation: The classical clinical features are that newborn boys are usually normal. Sexual orientation is usually normal and results in heterosexual marriage. The child tends to be passive and compliant in childhood but more aggressive and antisocial past puberty.

Question 137 Answer: b, Fragile X syndrome
Explanation: Fragile X syndrome is the most common inherited cause of learning disability. It accounts for 10%–12% of mental retardation in men. It is an X-linked dominant genetic disorder with low penetrance.

Reference: Puri BK, Hall AD, Ho RC (2014). *Revision Notes in Psychiatry*. Boca Raton, FL: CRC Press, pp. 663–673.

Theme: Learning Disabilities

Question 138 Answer: e, 15
Explanation: For individuals diagnosed with mild learning disability, the estimated prevalence of epilepsy is that of 12%–18%.

Question 139 Answer: h, 30
Explanation: Approximately 30%–37% of individuals diagnosed with severe mental retardation or learning disability do suffer from comorbid condition such as epilepsy.

Further Reading: Puri BK, Treasaden I (eds) (2010). *Psychiatry: An Evidence-Based Text*. London: Hodder Arnold, pp. 538, 1080, 1086.

Theme: Advanced Psychology and Pharmacology

Question 140 Answer: d, Parent Management Training
Explanation: The Parent Management Programme draws on operant-behavioural and cognitive-behavioural approaches involving consistent strategies that reward desired behaviours but ignore undesired behaviours.

Further Reading: Puri BK, Treasaden I (eds) (2010). *Psychiatry: An Evidence-Based Text*. London: Hodder Arnold, p. 1059.

Question 141 Answer: g, Risperidone
Explanation: Short-term risperidone (at a dose of 0.25–2 mg) can be used in adolescents with conduct disorder with aggressive behaviour who refuse psychological treatment.

Further Reading: Puri BK, Treasaden I (eds) (2010). *Psychiatry: An Evidence-Based Text*. London: Hodder Arnold, pp. 1058–1059.

Question 142 Answer: b, Duty to inform the police if not reported yet, c, Obtain informed consent from the child and his or her parents
Explanation: This may be a case of juvenile delinquency with ethical, legal and clinical problems. Aetiological factors may include living in an inner city area, lack of caring supervision and lower socio-economic class. The male-to-female ratio is 3–10:1. In the United Kingdom, the African-Caribbean rates are around double the rates in Caucasians. The trainee needs to be aware that there are differences between potential forensic and therapeutic assessments. The trainee needs to obtain consent from the adolescent and his parents. She also needs to inform them that there are circumstances in which the clinical information gathered could be used in court proceedings. From the forensic aspect, she needs to assess the mode of shoplifting and the nature of the items stolen. Risk assessment is important. She also needs to assess the adolescent's awareness of the implications

of conviction and the impact on himself and his family. The forensic history may shed light on how previous offences may affect the current situation. Clinical issues involve assessment of the developmental stage, school situation, family reaction to the shoplifting, the adolescent's reaction to and explanation for the shoplifting, evidence of psychiatric illness, substance abuse and social history. One quarter of juvenile offenders will be repeat offenders.

Reference: Goodman R, Scott S (2005). *Child Psychiatry* (2nd edition). Oxford, UK: Blackwell Publishing.

Question 143 Answer: a, Multisystemic therapy
Explanation: This is a case of juvenile delinquency after excluding common causes for fire-setting in young people. Multisystemic therapy is the treatment of choice in juvenile delinquency. It involves family therapy focusing on effective communication, systematic reward and punishment systems and taking a problem-solving approach to day-to day conflicts. It also encourages the adolescent to spend more time with his or her peers without delinquency and to avoid those with delinquency. Individual therapy involves assertiveness training against negative peer influences. The therapist also needs to liaise with the education authority (to improve learning and academic performance), the correctional services (regular monitoring of antisocial behaviour) and social worker (to help the family to cope).

Further Reading: Puri BK, Treasaden I (eds) (2010). *Psychiatry: An Evidence-Based Text*. London: Hodder Arnold, pp. 1156–1157.

Question 144 Answer: d, Parent Management Training, e, Family therapy
Explanation: Family therapy and parent management training are both possible treatments for oppositional defiant disorder.

Theme: Ethics and Psychiatry
Question 145 Answer: a, Father, d, Elder brother, e, Younger brother
Explanation: Incest is generally forbidden across cultures. In law, it is an offence for a man to have sexual intercourse with a woman he knows to be his daughter, granddaughter, mother, sister or half-sister and for a women over 16 years to allow a man whom she knows to be her son, father, grandfather, brother, or half-brother to have sexual intercourse with her.

Sibling incest relationships are the most common, but father–daughter relationships are most commonly seen in court. They often reflect some breakdown in the martial relationship.

Further Reading: Puri BK, Treasaden I (eds) (2010). *Psychiatry: An Evidence-Based Text*. London: Hodder Arnold, p. 773.

Question 146 Answer: a, Father

Question 147 Answer: a, Father, b, Mother

Question 148 Answer: b, Mother

Explanation: In childhood sexual abuse, the abuse is usually inside the family, and disclosure is less likely if incest occurs. In the United Kingdom, sexual intercourse under 13 years is regarded in law as statutory rape. Father–daughter incest usually takes place when the girl is aged about 10 or 11 years. The father who has an incestuous relationship with his daughter usually does not suffer from a psychiatric abnormality. Mother–son incest is often associated with neurotic states, personality difficulties and occasionally psychosis. Victims of sexual abuse are more likely to develop inability to control sexual impulses, precocious sexual play, weakened gender identity, increased incidence of homosexuality, increased incidence of child molestation and eating disorders.

In the United Kingdom, incest is legally defined as occurring when a man has sexual intercourse with a female whom he knows to be his daughter, granddaughter, sister, half-sister or mother, or when a woman aged over 16 years permits a man whom she knows to be of such consanguinity to have sexual intercourse with her. Family relationships that do not involve consanguinity (e.g. stepfather–daughter) generally do not fall within the legal definition of incest.

Munchausen syndrome (or factitious illness) by proxy was first described by Meadow in 1977. The main psychiatric associations with the mother are personality, somatization, affective and eating disorders. The perpetrator often appears to be an exemplary mother with nursing experience, and the father is either emotionally or physically absent.

Reference: Chiswick D, Cope R (1995). *Seminars in Forensic Psychiatry*. London: Gaskell.

Theme: Old-Age Psychiatry

Question 149 Answer: h, Vascular dementia

Explanation: Vascular dementia is characterized by a stepwise deteriorating course with a patchy distribution of neurological and neuropsychological deficits. There is evidence of vascular diseases on physical examination (hypertensive changes on fundoscopy, carotid bruits, enlarged heart and focal neurological signs suggestive of cerebrovascular accidents).

Further Reading: Puri BK, Treasaden I (eds) (2010). *Psychiatry: An Evidence-Based Text*. London: Hodder Arnold, p. 1105.

Question 150 Answer: g, Pseudodementia

Explanation: In psuedodementia, the onset is usually acute in nature. There is a lack of motivation, and the individual does not attempt to answer any of the questions. They tend to answer don't know for most of the questions. Memory deficits are usually reported by the patients and not by caregivers.

Further Reading: Puri BK, Treasaden I (eds) (2010). *Psychiatry: An Evidence-Based Text*. London: Hodder Arnold, p. 93.

Question 151 Answer: e, Lewy body dementia
Explanation: In this particular form of dementia, there is enduring and progressive cognitive impairment with impairments in consciousness, alertness and attention. Cognition is fluctuating, and short-term memory is not affected in early stages. Patients suffering from this form of dementia tend to have less episodic amnesia, more executive dysfunction and more apraxagnosia compared with patients suffering from Alzhemier's.

Further Reading: Puri BK, Treasaden I (eds) (2010). *Psychiatry: An Evidence-Based Text*. London: Hodder Arnold, p. 1106.

Question 152 Answer: c, Cerebral autosomal-dominant arteriopathy with subcortical infarcts and leukoencephalopathy (CASDIL)
Explanation: Cerebral autosomal-dominant arteriopathy with subcortical infarcts and leukoencephalopathy is a genetic disease with Notch 3 mutations in chromosome 19 and results in subcortical CVAs (80%), cognitive deterioration (50%), mood changes (30%), epilepsy (10%) and gait abnormalities.

Question 153 Answer: f, Psychogenic fugue
Explanation: Fugue is present with loss of semantic memory (details of events or facts), but procedural memory is usually retained.

Reference: Kay R (2002). *Casebook of Neurology*. Hong Kong: Lippincott Williams & Wilkins Asia; Butler R, Pit B (1998). *Seminars in Old Age Psychiatry*. London: Gaskell.

Theme: Forensic Psychiatry and Laws
Question 154 Answer: f, Not guilty by reason of insanity (NGRI) or McNaughton rule
Explanation: The offender meets the requirements of the rule if he or she fulfils the following criteria: That by reason of such defect from disease of the mind, the person did not know the nature of the quality of his or her act; that person did not know that what he or she was doing was wrong (forbidden by law); if the person was suffering from a delusion – his or her actions would be judged by the relationship to the delusion, that is, if he or she believed his or her life to be immediately threatened, he or she would not be justified in striking out, but not otherwise.

Further Reading: Puri BK, Treasaden I (eds) (2010). *Psychiatry: An Evidence-Based Text*. London: Hodder Arnold, pp. 1162–1163, 1168.

Question 155 Answer: e, Hospital order
Explanation: Approximately 15% of hospital orders are created with restriction on discharge.

Further Reading: Puri BK, Treasaden I (eds) (2010). *Psychiatry: An Evidence-Based Text*. London: Hodder Arnold, p. 1168.

Theme: Consultation Liaison Psychiatry

Question 156 Answer: e, Iatrogenic cause
Explanation: The three medications mentioned can cause unintentional weight loss in the elderly. Fluoxetine is stronger than other SSRIs in causing an anorectic effect.

Question 157 Answer: b, Coeliac disease
Explanation: This patient suffers from coeliac disease. Investigations include full blood count (FBC) (↓haemoglobin) and detection of antigliaden antibody. Treatment involves a gluten-free diet, iron supplementation and immunosuppression.

Question 158 Answer: c, Crohn's disease
Explanation: This patient suffers from Crohn's disease. Investigations include FBC (↓haemoglobin), ↑C reactive protein (CRP), ↑erythrocyte sedimentation rate (ESR), ↓B$_{12}$ and folate. Sigmoidoscopy and colonoscopy show patch inflammation, and biopsy may show granuloma. Small bowel follow-through may show fistulae. Corticosteroids and azathioprine may be prescribed in the short-term and long-term, respectively.

Question 159 Answer: f, Whipple's disease
Explanation: This patient suffers from Whipple's disease, which is caused by *Tropheryma whipplei* (formerly *whippelii*). Jejunal biopsy characteristically shows large foamy macrophages in the lamina propria, which contain positive periodic acid-Schiff staining material. The treatment is to continue sulphamethoxazole and trimethoprim for 1 year. Other causes of malabsorption include chronic pancreatitis, tropical sprue (rare in the United Kingdom), giardiasis (often with a history of travelling to infected areas), small bowel syndrome and following gastric surgery.

Reference: Firth JD, Collier JD (2001). *Medical Masterclass: Gastroenterology and Hepatology*. London: Royal College of Physicians.

Theme: Schizophrenia and Psychosis

Question 160 Answer: d, Simple schizophrenia
Explanation: In this condition, there is an insidious onset of decline in functioning. Negative symptoms develop without any preceding positive symptoms. Diagnosis would require changes in behaviour over at least 1 year, with marked loss of interest, idleness and social withdrawal.

Question 161 Answer: g, Post-schizophrenia depression
Explanation: In this condition, schizophrenic illness must have occurred within the last 12 months, some symptoms still being present. Depressive symptoms must fulfil at least the criteria for a depressive episode and are present for at least 2 weeks. There is an increased risk of suicide.

Question 162 Answer: b, Hebephrenic schizophrenia
Explanation: The age of onset is usually between 15 and 25 years. There is a poor prognosis. Affective changes are prominent. Fleeting and fragmentary delu-

sions and hallucinations, irresponsible behaviour, fatuous, disorganized thought, rambling speech and mannerisms are common. Negative symptoms, particularly flattening of affect and loss of volition, are prominent. Drive and determination are lost, goals abandoned and behaviour becomes aimless and empty.

Reference: Puri BK, Hall AD, Ho RC (2014). *Revision Notes in Psychiatry*. Boca Raton, FL: CRC Press, p. 354.

Theme: Diagnosis

Question 163 Answer: g, Depressive episode

Explanation: This woman suffers from moderate-to-severe depressive episode. The childbirth is a distractor because this patient does not meet the diagnostic criteria for post-natal depression, as the onset of depression is too late. Her checking behaviour is secondary to low mood and pessimism.

Reference And Further Reading: Puri BK, Treasaden I (eds) (2010). *Psychiatry: An Evidence-Based Text*. London: Hodder Arnold, pp. 614–624.

Question 164 Answer: e, Bipolar disorder – manic episode

Explanation: This man is in the manic phase as evidenced by grandiosity (pursuing a PhD degree, advising the Prime Minister), delusion of persecution as a result of grandiosity (probably he thought that he was a celebrity and chased by paparazzi), dangerous driving and foolhardy investment in the food business. The patient firmly believes that he suffers from schizophrenia, but this is a distractor, as he may hear mood-congruent auditory hallucination. The antidepressant was stopped as a result of antidepressant-induced mania.

Reference And Further Reading: Puri BK, Treasaden I (eds) (2010). *Psychiatry: An Evidence-Based Text*. London: Hodder Arnold, pp. 624–634.

Question 165 Answer: s, Psychotic depression

Explanation: This 50-year-old man exhibits nihilistic delusion, and it is considered to be a mood congruent delusion in patients with severe depressive episode.

Theme: Advanced Psychotherapy

Question 166 Answer: c, Displacement

Explanation: This is displacement. Negative emotions are transferred from their original object to a less threatening substitute.

Question 167 Answer: i, Denial

Explanation: This is denial. The external reality of an unwanted or unpleasant piece of information is denied.

Question 168 Answer: b, Intellectualization

Explanation: He avoids disturbing feelings by engaging in excessive abstract thinking. This is intellectualization.

Reference And Further Reading: Puri BK, Hall AD (2002). *Revision Notes in Psychiatry*. London: Hodder Arnold, pp. 168–169.

Theme: Old-Age Psychiatry

Question 169 Answer: d, Lewy body dementia
Explanation: Alpha-synuclein cytoplasmic inclusions are found in patients with Lewy body dementia.

Question 170 Answer: f, Shy–Drager syndrome
Explanation: Glial cytoplasmic inclusion bodies are found in patients with Shy–Drager syndrome (also known as multiple system atrophy). Shy–Drager syndrome is characterized by autonomic dysfunction, parkinsonism and ataxia.

Question 171 Answer: a, Alzheimer's dementia, d, Lewy body dementia
Explanation: Neurofibrillary tangles are found in patients with Alzheimer's disease and Lewy body dementia.

Reference: Puri BK, Hall AD, Ho RC (2014). *Revision Notes in Psychiatry*. Boca Raton, FL: CRC Press, pp. 681–695.

Theme: Child Psychiatry

Question 172 Answer: a, Father, d, Elder brother, f, Male stranger
Explanation: Ten percent of children have been victims of sexual abuse including exhibitionism, lascivious talk, and being sexually active at the age of 15 years. The male-to-female ratio has been estimated to be 1:2.5.

Question 173 Answer: a, Father

Question 174 Answer: a, Father and b, Mother
Explanation: In childhood sexual abuse, the abuse is usually inside the family, and disclosure is less likely if incest occurs. In the United Kingdom, sexual intercourse under 13 years is regarded in law as statutory rape. Father–daughter incest usually takes place when the girl is aged about 10 or 11 years. The father who has an incestuous relationship with his daughter usually does not suffer from a psychiatric abnormality. Mother–son incest is often associated with neurotic states, personality difficulties and occasionally psychosis. Victims of sexual abuse are more likely to develop inability to control sexual impulses, precocious sexual play, weakened gender identity, increased incidence of homosexuality, increased incidence of child molestation and eating disorders.

In the United Kingdom, incest is legally defined when a man has sexual intercourse with a female whom he knows to be his daughter, granddaughter, sister, half-sister or mother or when a woman aged over 16 years permits a man whom she knows to be of such *consanguinity* to have sexual intercourse with her. Family relationships that do not involve consanguinity (e.g. stepfather–daughter) generally do not fall within the legal definition of incest.

Reference: Puri BK, Hall AD, Ho RC (2014). *Revision Notes in Psychiatry*. Boca Raton, FL: CRC Press, p. 653.

Additional Reference: Johnstone EC, Cunningham ODG, Lawrie SM, Sharpe M, Freeman CPL (2004). *Companion to Psychiatric Studies* (7th edition). London: Churchill Livingstone; Chiswick D, Cope R (1995). *Seminars in Forensic Psychiatry*. London: Gaskell.

INDEX